Clinical Manual of Small Animal Endosurgery

Clinical Manual of Small Animal Endosurgery

Edited by

Alasdair Hotston Moore
and
Rosa Angela Ragni

WILEY-BLACKWELL

A John Wiley & Sons, Ltd., Publication

This edition first published 2012
© 2012 by Blackwell Publishing Ltd

Wiley-Blackwell is an imprint of John Wiley & Sons, formed by the merger of Wiley's global Scientific, Technical and Medical business with Blackwell Publishing.

Registered office: John Wiley & Sons, Ltd, The Atrium, Southern Gate, Chichester, West Sussex, PO19 8SQ, UK

Editorial offices: 9600 Garsington Road, Oxford, OX4 2DQ, UK
The Atrium, Southern Gate, Chichester, West Sussex, PO19 8SQ, UK
2121 State Avenue, Ames, Iowa 50014-8300, USA

For details of our global editorial offices, for customer services and for information about how to apply for permission to reuse the copyright material in this book please see our website at www.wiley.com/wiley-blackwell.

Library of Congress Cataloging-in-Publication Data
Clinical manual of small animal endosurgery / edited by Alasdair Hotston Moore and Rosa Angela Ragni.
p. cm.
Includes bibliographical references and index.
    ISBN 978-1-4051-9001-5 (hardcover :alk. paper)   1. Veterinary endoscopy.
I. Moore, Alasdair Hotston.   II. Ragni, Rosa Angela.
    [DNLM: 1. Endoscopy–veterinary.   2. Animal Diseases–diagnosis.   3. Endoscopes.
4. Endoscopy–methods. SF 772.55]
    SF772.55.C55 2012
    636.089'705–dc23
                                        2012002559

A catalogue record for this book is available from the British Library.

Wiley also publishes its books in a variety of electronic formats. Some content that appears in print may not be available in electronic books.

Cover image: iStockphoto.com
Cover design by Meaden Creative

Set in 10/12 pt Sabon by Toppan Best-set Premedia Limited, Hong Kong
Printed and bound in Singapore by Markono Print Media Pte Ltd

1   2012

Contents

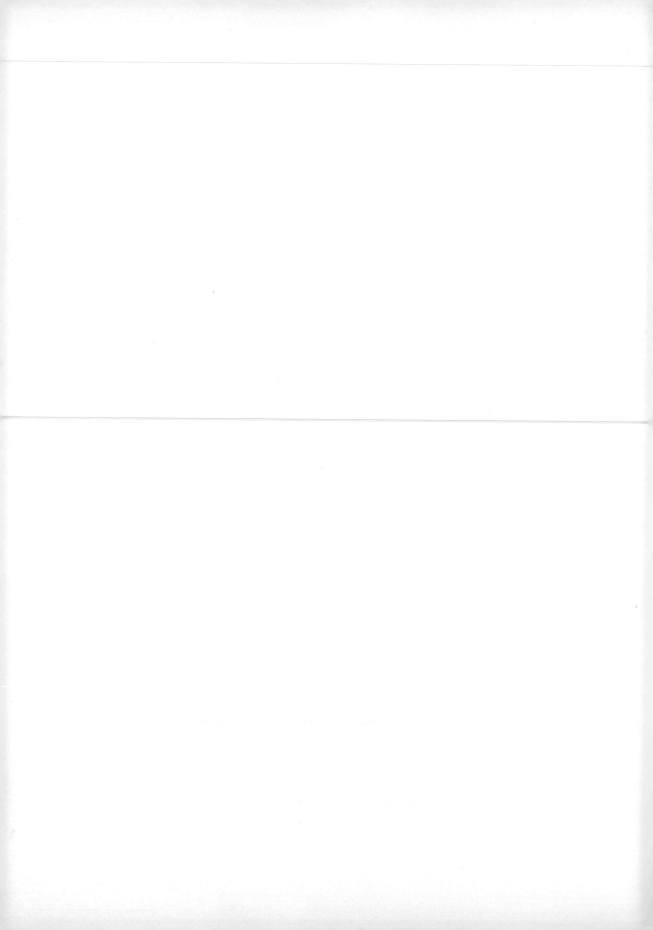

Contributors

Lynetta J. Freeman, DVM, MS, MBA, Diplomate ACVS
Associate Professor of Small Animal Surgery and Biomedical Engineering, Purdue University, West Lafayette, IN, USA

Alasdair Hotston Moore, MA, VetMB, CertSAC, CertVR, CertSAS, CertMedEd, MRCVS
Head of Surgical Referrals, Bath Veterinary Referrals, Rosemary Lodge Veterinary Hospital, Wellsway, Bath, UK

Philip J. Lhermette, BSc (Hons), CBiol, MSB, BVetMed, MRCVS
Special Lecturer in Veterinary Endoscopy and Endosurgery, The University of Nottingham, School of Veterinary Medicine and Science; Head of Referral Services, Elands Veterinary Clinic, Sevenoaks, Kent, UK

Martin R. Owen, BSc, BVSc, PhD, DSAS (Orth), DipECVS, MRCVS, RCVS
Specialist in Small Animal Surgery (Orthopaedics), European Specialist in Small Animal Surgery; Honorary Associate Professor, University of Nottingham and Head of Orthopaedic Referrals, Dick White Referrals, Six Mile Bottom, Suffolk, UK

Romain Pizzi, BVSc, MSc, DZooMed, FRES, MACVSc (Surg), MRCVS
Royal College of Veterinary Surgeons, recognised Specialist in Zoo and Wildlife Medicine; Special Lecturer in Zoo and Wildlife Medicine, the University of Nottingham, School of Veterinary Medicine and Science; Veterinary Surgeon, Edinburgh Zoo, Royal Zoological Society of Scotland, Edinburgh Zoo; Veterinary Cardiorespiratory Centre, Kenilworth; Director, Zoological Medicine Ltd; Borders Veterinary Cardiology, Biggar; Scottish SPCA Wildlife Rescue Centre

Rosa Angela Ragni, DVM, DSPCA, MRCVS
Veterinary Surgeon, The Blue Cross Animal Hospital, Merton, London, UK

David S. Sobel, BA, DVM, MRCVS
Director of Medicine, Metropolitan Veterinary Consultants, Hanover, NH, USA; Consultant, Elands Veterinary Clinic, Sevenoaks, Kent, UK; Staff Consultant, Minimally Invasive Surgery, Valley CARES, Hanover, NH, USA; Small Animal Veterinary Emergency Services, Lebanon, NH, USA; Capital Area Veterinary Emergency Services, Concord, NH, USA

Foreword

Endoscopic surgery has been on the forefront of human medicine for the last 25 years and slowly is penetrating the veterinary market. The obvious reason for this delay is that the surgeon needs extra skills and investment to be able to perform endoscopic surgery. Routine visible and tactile stimuli are missing and one often feels inadequate in the beginning, delaying the practical use of endoscopic procedures. Additionally, endoscopy was often regarded as a skill set that only internal medicine specialists possessed, not necessarily surgeons or practitioners. Lately, a surge of interest in the veterinary field has lead to endoscopic surgery being embraced by specialist surgeons and private practitioners alike.

The advantages of endoscopic surgery are obvious: why perform major surgery through a big incision if three small puncture wounds can result in the same success rate? Procedures such as laparoscopic ovariectomy and thoracoscopic pericardectomy have quickly become the gold standard in veterinary medicine, leaving the conservative therapies trailing far behind.

Thus, the question is, why has this excellent new technique not skyrocketed (as in human medicine) and changed veterinary medicine forever? The answer is simple: you need to have experience to be able to do it safely and a solid base of knowledge so as not to do harm to the animal. Halstedt's major principle – above all, do not harm –should still resonate in every surgeon's mind. Experience comes by doing a lot of procedures and practising as much as one can. Knowledge comes from books such as the one in front of you. Why read it? Because it is written by veterinary clinicians with a wealth of experience in veterinary endoscopic surgery, and it is presented in a way that it will appeal to both practitioners and specialists. It is practical and explains the procedures clearly. It answers the questions that most clinicians have and poses problems with a view to solving them. I personally enjoyed reading this book, edited by Dr Hotston Moore and Dr Ragni. With its clinical view it is a welcome addition to the number of books now available, and it will not disappoint you.

Jolle Kirpensteijn, DVM, PhD
Professor in Surgery
Department of Clinical Sciences of Companion Animals
Faculty of Veterinary Medicine
Utrecht University
Utrecht, The Netherlands

Preface

In producing this book, we have been fortunate in finding contributors who are leaders in their field, enthusiastic practitioners of endosurgery and friends. We have ourselves been active in rigid endoscopy since the 1990s and during this time have observed a growth in the use of the technique for both diagnosis and intervention. Rigid endoscopy makes a contribution to the welfare of our patients by improving diagnosis and increasingly by allowing interventions with reduced morbidity compared to traditional open surgery. Diagnoses that would otherwise not have been possible can now be made and techniques that would not be possible in other ways can be used. To the veterinarian, rigid endoscopy also provides new way of looking at our patients (literally) and enhances our understanding of diseases and their management. We confidently expect the applications of this equipment and technique to continue to expand over the next decade and one of our intentions with this book was to allow practitioners to see how broadly useful the equipment is, and to encourage them to acquire it and use it as widely as possible. This is one reason for focusing on rigid endoscopy: much of the equipment can be used for a variety of organ systems and species.

Bringing together any book requires the support and forbearance of friends, colleagues and family. We gratefully acknowledge the help of our families during the 'gestation' of this book, together with the assistance of colleagues and the team at Wiley Blackwell. We owe a particular thank you to the friends who agreed to become contributors and who have delivered the excellent material that makes this book all that it is.

Alasdair Hotston Moore
Rosa Angela Ragni
April 2012

Chapter 1
Rigid Endoscopy
Alasdair Hotston Moore and Rosa Angela Ragni

Introduction

Endoscopy is a minimally invasive technique that uses a flexible or rigid viewing instrument (endoscope) to look inside a body cavity or organ for diagnostic or therapeutic purposes. Over the last three decades, the importance of endoscopy has greatly increased in veterinary medicine and practitioners are now more often requested to be proficient in it. This chapter gives an overview of the equipment necessary to perform rigid endoscopy, to allow the novice endoscopist to choose and maintain the proper equipment, thus containing costs and enhancing professional satisfaction.

Although rigid endoscopes cannot be manoeuvred around corners in the way that a flexible endoscope can, they generally offer better optics (particularly compared to traditional fibre-optic flexible scopes), are more difficult to damage and are cheaper. Their rigidity permits better manoeuvrability inside non-tubular structures, and consequently they are preferred for many applications in small animal practice. Rhinoscopy, otoscopy, cystoscopy and vaginoscopy using rigid scopes offer unparalleled views of different body cavities and allow the possibility of minimally invasive therapeutic interventions; more advanced techniques, such as arthroscopy, laparoscopy and thoracoscopy, allow 'keyhole' surgery, thus minimising patient discomfort and recovery times. Some surgeons also prefer rigid endoscopes for tracheobronchoscopy, oesophagoscopy and colonoscopy.

Rigid endoscopy is extremely versatile, and a few core pieces of equipment (a multipurpose telescope, a video system and some ancillary

Clinical Manual of Small Animal Endosurgery, First Edition. Edited by Alasdair Hotston Moore and Rosa Angela Ragni.
© 2012 Blackwell Publishing Ltd. Published 2012 by Blackwell Publishing Ltd.

instruments) are used for many different diagnostic and therapeutic procedures.

The rigid endoscope

Rigid endoscopes (also referred to as telescopes) are hollow tubes able to direct light into a body area or cavity by way of a fibre-optic bundle and to return the image via a series of lenses. In conventional telescopes, a central glass lens chain is embedded in an air medium, whereas most recent telescopes use the Hopkins rod lens technology (Fig. 1.1), in which the glass lenses have been replaced with glass rods, and air acts as a negative lens. This system transmits more light, produces better magnification and allows a better field of view in terms of both depth of focus and the width of the angle of view.

Telescopes are available in a wide range of diameters, ranging from 1.2 to 10 mm. Larger scopes provide more light transmission, superior image resolution and a larger field of view. Smaller scopes need to be positioned close to the target area to transmit a clear view, but as they are used for procedures in smaller areas such as joints or nasal cavities this is rarely a problem. Larger-diameter endoscopes are preferred for procedures involving a larger animal, and to obtain panoramic views of large body cavities.

As no single size of telescope is suitable for all procedures in all patients, endoscopes are purchased according to the procedures most commonly performed. A 5 mm telescope is usually adequate for laparoscopy and thoracoscopy in most small animal patients, whereas for other purposes such as arthroscopy, cystoscopy and rhinoscopy a 2.7 mm telescope (or smaller) is preferable. Smaller telescopes (4 mm or less) are very fragile, and consequently a protective sheath is recommended to avoid damage. The outer sheath (Fig. 1.2) usually has also attachments for influx and efflux of fluids, and sometimes an instrument channel for a small flexible biopsy instrument. This determines an increase in the overall diameter of approximately 1–1.5 mm (for instance a 2.7 mm telescope with its associated sheath approaches 4–4.5 mm in width), which has to be considered in scope choice.

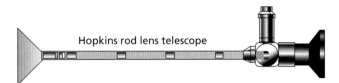

Hopkins rod lens telescope

Fig. 1.1 Line drawing of the internal structure of a Hopkins (rod lens) telescope. The arrangement of rod lenses improves light transmission and offers a wider field of view compared to a conventional telescope.

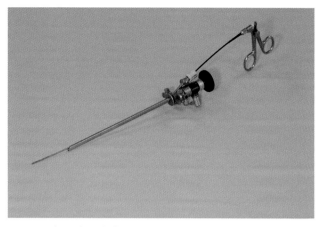

Fig. 1.2   An operating sheath for a 2.7 mm cystoscope. It is equipped with two Luer lock stopcocks for fluid infusion and drainage, and a working channel. A pair of biopsy forceps are located in the channel.

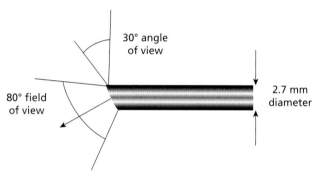

Fig. 1.3   Line drawing illustrating the effect of rotation on the field of view of an angled scope.

Other important considerations in choosing a telescope are length and angle of view. Wider endoscopes are usually longer than narrow ones, with the 5 and 10 mm-diameter scopes typically having a working length of 30 or 35 cm, whereas a 1.9 mm scope is only about 10 cm in length. The most common length of the 2.7 mm scope is 18 cm. Due to the increased length of the lever arm, longer telescopes can be difficult to manoeuvre in limited spaces. If a sheath is required (e.g. for cystoscopy), the length of the sheath must be matched to the scope.

The viewing angle of the telescope affects its orientation and visualisation of the operative field. The 0° or forward-viewing scope provides the simplest orientation, as the visual field is in line with the true field. However, this field of view is the most limited. An angled scope enables the surgeon to widen the field of view simply by rotation of the longitudinal axis, which allows better examination of relatively inaccessible areas (Fig. 1.3). However, angled-view scopes are less intuitive to use,

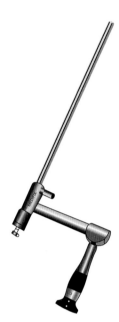

Fig. 1.4   Line drawing of an operating telescope. The offset eyepiece allows straight rigid instruments to be passed in parallel with the scope.

and have a slightly steeper learning curve. As the angled view is opposite the insertion of the light guide cable, when the operator holds the endoscope with the light cable up, the surgeon has a more 'anatomical' spatial orientation. Telescopes are available with viewing angles up to 70°, and even 120°; the forward-oblique 30° ones are a good compromise between increase in the field of view and ease of orientation, and are particularly indicated for more advanced procedures such as thoracoscopy. Scopes with viewing angles over 30° are used for particular purposes in human surgery but are rarely used in animals.

Some telescopes (operating or single-portal scopes) have a working channel (Fig. 1.4), which can be up to 5–6 mm in diameter, and allows the introduction of instruments for biopsy or surgical procedures. These scopes are usually wider and longer than conventional ones, and their eyepiece is offset. These telescopes are used in human surgery and are designed for specialised applications; they are rarely used in animals.

In small animal practice, two scopes are useful for performing the majority of endoscopic procedures: a 2.7 mm, 18 cm-long scope and a 5 mm, 30 cm-long scope. The 2.7 mm scope is used for rhinoscopy, otoscopy, cystoscopy in female dogs, and arthroscopy, and can be used for endoscopy in birds and exotic species. It should have a 30° angle of view. The 5 mm scope is ideal for laparoscopy and thoracoscopy of any size dog or cat. If only one 5 mm scope is chosen, a 0° scope is most suitable. An outer sheath with channels for fluid influx/efflux and instruments is useful for cystoscopy and otoscopy and is used with the 2.7 mm scope.

When only one telescope is being purchased, a long (30 cm) 2.7 mm scope is preferred. This long endoscope, often called the universal or multipurpose telescope, can be used for numerous endoscopic techniques. When choosing a scope, it is also important to check its compatibility with ancillary equipment purchased from another manufacturer.

Older rigid endoscopes are not suitable for sterilising other than by soaking in a proprietary cold sterilising solution or by exposure to ethylene oxide gas. Newer scopes have been manufactured to allow them to be sterilised in an autoclave. However, care must be taken to use the correct cycle (typically 121° rather than 134°). Additionally, bench-top autoclaves used in veterinary practices heat up and cool down very rapidly, which may damage even those scopes designed to be autoclavable. For this reason, many clinics choose to use cold sterilisation. Variously using sterilising solutions and autoclaving is not recommended because this may damage the seals on the equipment.

Video system

Although endoscopic images can be observed directly through the eyepiece (oculus), video systems are preferable for most applications of rigid endoscopy, as they allow the operator to work more comfortably, to see a magnified image and to benefit from the help of assistants. Furthermore, with a video system there is the possibility of documenting the procedure and using it for educational purposes.

An endoscopic video camera system consists of camera head with integrated video cable (Fig. 1.5), camera control unit (CCU; Fig. 1.6) and monitor.

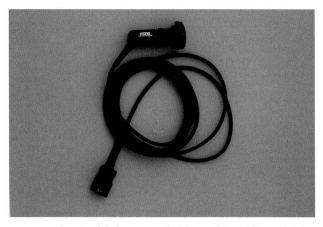

Fig. 1.5 Camera head with integrated video cable. This model is suitable for sterilising by soaking but not by autoclaving.

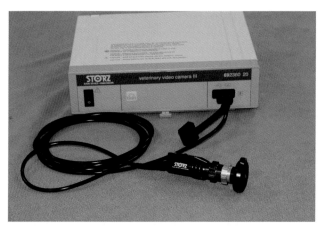

Fig. 1.6   CCU with camera head plugged in. Photograph courtesy of Mr P.J. Lhermette.

The camera head is connected to the endoscope via an adaptor, which focuses and magnifies the image between five and 15 times. Different adaptors have different focal lengths, and zoom lenses are also available.

The camera head can use one or three chips (or camera-coupling devices, or CCD) to convert the optical (analogue) image into an electronic (digital) signal, which is then transmitted to the CCU. Although single-chip cameras have lower horizontal resolution and less accurate colour reproduction than three-chip cameras, they produce images that are adequate for many procedures, and are more widely used. Three-chip cameras use a prism to separate light into the three primary colours (red, green and blue), and use a separate camera-coupling device to transmit each of them. In this way colours are more accurate, and images obtained are of higher quality, as all the signal available for resolution is used only for that purpose. However the cost of these cameras is higher and they are less commonly used.

Recently, high-definition cameras have become available, providing five times the resolution of standard cameras. Some of these high-definition cameras also provide images in widescreen format, which more resemble three-dimensional images on the video monitor.

The CCU decodes the information and distributes it to the monitor and other video devices, and also houses other features such as white balancing and automatic exposure control. The former allows the camera to compensate for variations in the colour of light, thus reproducing colours accurately. With the latter, an automatic iris measures the available light and selects the shutter speed that will provide the best exposure. In fact, bright reflections from white and/or shiny surfaces may otherwise create the white-out phenomenon, causing light-coloured objects to appear white as well and to lack detail.

Video signals are then sent to a monitor, which can vary in size and resolution. Although a high-resolution monitor cannot improve a poor image, it is important for it to match or surpass the video camera's resolution (500 lines for single-chip cameras and 750 lines for three-chip ones). It is also important that the video input format quality equals the video camera quality. In particular, Y/C (also called S) video format is recommended for single-chip cameras, and RGB video input should be used for a three-chip camera. These signal formats are capable of high resolution (the latter more than the former), as they separate different aspects of signal information (such as brightness, colour and synchronisation) into more than one signal (two in S format and four in RGB format), thus minimising artefacts. Flat widescreen LCD high-resolution monitors are required for use with high-definition cameras, in order to benefit from the perceived three-dimensional effect.

Cameras are not generally autoclavable. They can be sterilised by cold soaking in most instances, but during surgery it is more common to use a disposable camera sheath to provide asepsis (Fig. 1.7).

Finally, a series of different video accessories completes the video system. Until some years ago the most widespread devices were video printers and VHS recorders. With the advances in digital technology, digital recording devices have become readily available and affordable. Still images and/or video clips can be captured and stored for editing, printing and reproduction. The main advantages of digital devices are the lack of degradation in photo quality over time and in successive passages, and the saving of storage space.

More recent devices combine all video system components (CCU, light source and image recording) into one unit, apart from the camera head (Fig. 1.8). Their compactness makes them easy to use in clinic or field settings but the set-up cost may be greater than using modular

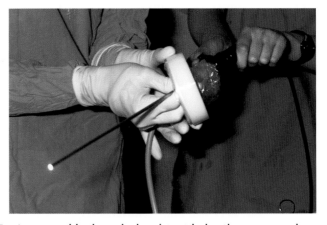

Fig. 1.7 An unscrubbed surgical assistant helps the surgeon place a sterile disposable camera sleeve over the camera head.

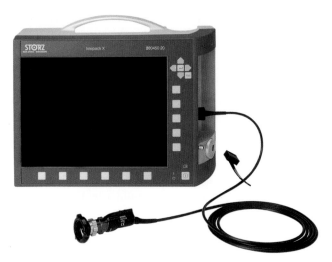

Fig. 1.8 Combined CCU, light source and monitor. This unit combines the light source, CCU, monitor and image capture in a single package.
Photograph courtesy of Karl Storz GmbH & Co. KG, Tuttlingen, Germany.

components. Additionally, the light intensity from these units is lower than is obtained with a separate light source. Although adequate for most applications, the image may be poor in large cavities (e.g. in laparoscopy of giant-breed dogs).

All the components of the video system are arranged in a video cart (called a tower) to minimise space and set-up times. The cart should have a large-wheeled base with lockable wheels in order for it to be moved around the surgical suite easily. The cart usually also accommodates the insufflator and the light source, and should have drawers for cables and equipment not in use, and the capability to secure a carbon dioxide canister for insufflation. Some carts are also equipped with a power strip with electrical surge protection, which allows the various devices to be plugged in and enables use of a single mains cable. The video monitor is usually located on the top shelf of the cart, at the surgeon's eye level; to allow more versatility in its position, some surgeons prefer to have it on a mechanical arm.

Light source

Since the development of fibre-optic cables in 1960, light has been transmitted to the endoscope from a remote source. Two main different types of high-intensity light source are in use: xenon and halogen. The intensity of light from different technology types cannot be compared accurately using wattage, as this measures how much power the bulb consumes, rather how much light it produces. Light output is measured in *lumens*:

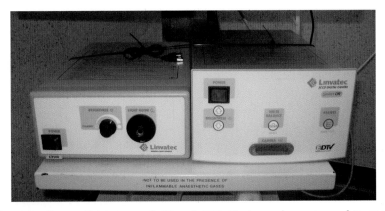

Fig. 1.9 Xenon light source (left) and CCU. Photograph courtesy of Dr M.R. Owen.

xenon light sources produce 50% more lumens per watt than halogen light sources.

Sources using xenon bulbs (Fig. 1.9) provide excellent colour reproduction, and, although more expensive, are recommended when light intensity and colour reproduction are essential. The life span of xenon lamps is approximately 400–1000 h. Halogen lamps emit a red-yellow light, and are unable to provide a very high intensity of light, especially after some length of time (about 100 h, only a fraction of their estimated life span). However, they are relatively inexpensive.

The intensity of light needed depends on the specific application: a bright source (e.g. a 300 W xenon light) is necessary when illuminating a large cavity, as in laparo- or thoracoscopy, whereas in smaller spaces, such as in otoscopy or arthroscopy, a lower-intensity source (e.g. 150 W halogen light) is usually adequate. This is because the brightness of the image depends on the distance between the endoscope and the object being examined, and on the reflective quality of its surface: pigmented tissues and blood absorb light. Dark images cause loss of detail and depth perception. Similarly, fine detail is lost when a highly reflective tissue is illuminated: the image is too bright, and the visual field appears white.

Other factors contributing to image brightness are diameter of the endoscope, light sensitivity of the camera, light-carrying capacity and condition of light cables and cleanliness of all the lenses and interfaces.

Most modern systems have an automatic iris-adjustment feature, with no need for the operator to manually adjust the light intensity. Another available feature of modern light sources is the ability to measure bulb life, thus minimising the risk of loss of illumination during a procedure (and the consequent necessity of converting to an open procedure in the case of endoscopic surgery). A spare bulb should in any case always be available (and a staff member be taught how to change it), and – in case no bulb-life meter is present – the dates of bulb changes should be recorded.

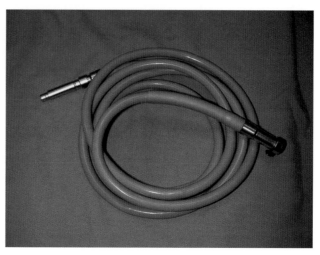

Fig. 1.10   Typical fibre-optic light guide.

Light guide cable

Light guide cables (Fig. 1.10) transmit the light to the endoscope, and generally consist of thousands of small fibres (from 30 μm to hundreds of micrometres in diameter) surrounded by a protective jacket. For rigid endoscopy (rather than flexible endoscopy), the light guide is a separate unit, equipped with metal ends, which are inserted into the endoscope at one end, and introduced into the light source at the other. They can be fitted with adapters for endoscopes from different manufacturers, and are available in various diameters for use with the different-diameter endoscopes available. Smaller endoscopes require smaller cables, thus preventing overheating. In fact, although fibre-optic light is defined as 'cold' light, significant heat is generated. This can pose a hazard to the patient, especially when the cable is laid on the skin or the end of the scope or light guide is allowed to rest on the tissues. Incidents of drapes igniting have also been reported.

When an insufficient amount of light transmission is noticed, the cable and connections need to be checked for cleanliness and/or damage. Light guide cables are delicate, and need to be handled with care. If any fibres are broken the ability of the cable to transmit light is reduced; single broken fibres appear as black dots when the light is projected on a white surface. When more than 20% of the fibres are damaged the cable needs replacing. Another type of degradation is discoloration, when changes in the colour of the light transmitted will be noticed.

Less commonly, liquid-filled light guides are used, which are less prone to damage by mechanical means but are more expensive and less tolerant of heat. Light guides are commonly sterilised in the autoclave.

Specialised instrumentation

Basic rigid-endoscopy sets can be used for different applications, such as rhinoscopy, cystoscopy and video-otoscopy. More specialised procedures (arthroscopy, laparoscopy and thoracoscopy) are also possible, but require larger investments in equipment and time (due to the steep learning curve).

Instrumentation typically used for video-otoscopy – besides the standard video system – are small-diameter rigid endoscopes (18 cm long, 1.9 or 2.7 mm diameter) with a 0 or 30° viewing angle. These are inserted into specialised video-otoscopic cones, or into cystoscope or arthroscope sheaths, which provide an irrigation channel. In anaesthetised animals, fluids are used to provide an optical space and ensure complete cleansing and examination.

Cystoscope sheaths have a rounded tip, and have the advantage of also having an outflow and an operating channel, which is useful for the insertion of forceps (for biopsies and removal of foreign bodies), and of curettes and ear loops. These instruments, as well as suction and catheters for flushing, can otherwise be inserted along the scope.

The endoscope most useful in rhinoscopy is one with a 30° viewing angle, 2.7 mm diameter and 18 cm in length (1.9 mm diameter/10 cm length for cats and very small dogs), and can be used 'naked' or with a cystoscopy or arthroscopy sheath, depending on the surgeon's preference. The advantage of using a sheath is the presence of irrigation and – in cystoscopy sheaths – biopsy channels; however, the sheath increases considerably the outer diameter of the endoscope, thus limiting its use in smaller patients. Furthermore, the samples retrieved through the biopsy channel are very small, and therefore this technique may produce less reliable biopsy results. Biopsy samples are preferably to be collected with 3 mm oval biopsy forceps, which allow collection of larger diagnostic samples (Fig. 1.11). The forceps are inserted alongside the endoscope

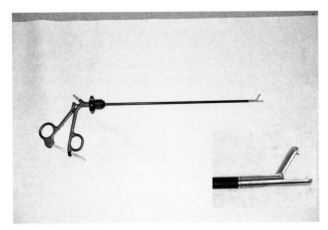

Fig. 1.11 Cup biopsy forceps: these 3 mm oval biopsy forceps allow collection of large diagnostic samples.

shaft, and their tip is not always visible; consequently sample collection using this technique requires considerable practice.

High fluid rates are required to flush the nasal cavities, to obtain increased optical space and to flush away haemorrhage and discharge from the visual field. Vigorous flushing can also be exploited to obtain biopsy samples.

Another diagnostic and therapeutic application achievable with the basic rigid-endoscopy kit is transurethral cystoscopy in female dogs and cats. The preferred endoscope again has a diameter of the 2.7 mm (or 1.9 mm for cats and dogs less than 5 kg), is 18 cm long with a 30° viewing angle, and is used with a cystoscopy sheath. Although the sheath increases the outer diameter (the most used sheath is the 14 French), its use is preferred for the presence of fluid-inflow and -outflow channels, which allow fluid infusion to increase the optical space and avoid clouding of the operating field.

An instrument channel is also present, useful for insertion of biopsy forceps and various operating instruments. Grasping forceps and basket catheters are commonly used for removal of small uroliths and foreign bodies such as sutures protruding in the bladder lumen, whereas energy-assisted devices allow removal of intraluminal inflammatory polyps and masses, and correction of mucosal defects such as ectopic ureters and strictures.

This cystoscope permits examination of the urethra and the bladder of bitches from 5 to 20 kg. For larger bitches, due to urethral length, a cystoscope with a longer shaft (30 cm, with a diameter of 3.5–4 mm) is necessary for bladder examination.

A 1.9 mm rigid endoscope allows examination of the bladder and urethra in bitches smaller than 5 kg, queens, and male cats after perineal urethrostomy. A flexible endoscope is necessary for male dogs and cats. Laparoscopic-assisted cystoscopy is also useful for diagnostic purposes and treatment, for example when the presence of large uroliths does not allow transurethral removal.

A more specialised procedure feasible with rigid endoscopes is tran-scervical catheterisation in the bitch, useful for collection of uterine samples and for insemination (Wilson, 1993, 2001). Due to vaginal length in bitches, a specialised 29 cm-long telescope is necessary. A cystoscope with a 30° oblique viewing angle and an outer-diameter 3.5 mm sheath is typically used.

Finally, in the last 20 years rigid endoscopes have been used more and more often to minimise the extent of the surgical approach to the abdomen, thorax and joints. These techniques (laparoscopy, thoracoscopy and arthroscopy, respectively) allow evaluation, biopsy and more advanced surgical procedures via the insertion of a telescope through a small incision in the surgical site.

As for all the other procedures examined so far, the core pieces of equipment required are the same (camera system and light source).

Accessories

Numerous accessories can be added to the basic endoscopic kit to increase diagnostic and therapeutic capabilities, and to perform more specialised techniques, such as laparoscopy and thoracoscopy. They include sheaths, devices for insufflation, irrigation and suction (Fig. 1.12), tools to control haemorrhage and a variety of grasping (Fig. 1.13) and biopsy (Fig. 1.11) instruments and trocars. Sheaths are tubes that lock on to the endoscope to protect it and to provide a channel for the passage of gas, fluids or instruments used in the specific procedure. They are commonly used for cystoscopy, otoscopy, arthroscopy and, sometimes, rhinoscopy.

With a minimally invasive approach, the presence of working space is essential to obtain adequate access to the structures examined. Often a potential space has to be created with specific techniques, according to the area in question; for instance, a liquid medium is used to create an optical cavity in arthroscopy and cystoscopy, whereas gas insufflation is exploited in laparoscopy and in flexible endoscopy.

Irrigation and suction units are also used to keep the operating field clean, by removing blood, accumulated fluid and debris, thus allowing better visualisation and minimising postoperative inflammation.

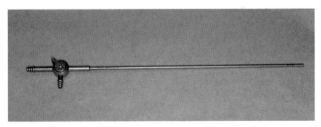

Fig. 1.12 Irrigation/suction device: multipurpose tool with irrigation and suction capabilities.

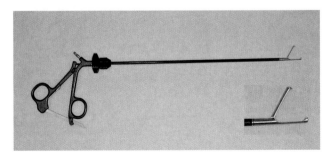

Fig. 1.13 Babcock grasping forceps.

Irrigation can be provided by devices that apply pressure on a fluid bag, but electronically controlled irrigators guarantee precise flux and irrigation pressure. Suction tips can be reusable or disposable: the latter are preferable, especially in laparoscopy, as they allow fine regulation of the intensity and duration of suction. This avoids loss of pneumoperitoneum, which otherwise can occur with excessive removal of gas by suction.

Insufflator

In flexible endoscopy an air pump is adequate for displacing the mucosa from the distal end of the endoscope, thus allowing visualisation. In thoracoscopy, a working space is created by creation of a controlled partial pneumothorax and/or selective lung ventilation, and thoracic insufflation is needed only rarely. In laparoscopy, introduction of gas is instead required to induce pneumoperitoneum. Air, nitrous oxide and carbon dioxide have all been used for this purpose; carbon dioxide is the gas of choice because it is more readily absorbed in blood, thus minimising the risk of gas embolism, and spark ignition is prevented when diathermy is used. The carbon dioxide is delivered from a cylinder of compressed gas (or via piped gas supply) by an insufflator (Fig. 1.14).

Carbon dioxide can be delivered initially either with a Veress needle or using a semi-open technique (Hasson or paediatric technique), in which the gas is insufflated directly through a cannula. After cannula

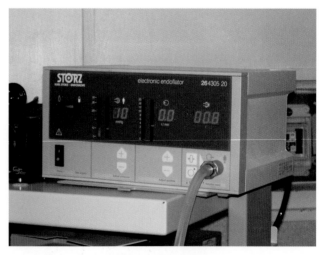

Fig. 1.14 An electronic insufflator. The operator sets the pressure level at which insufflation is maintained as well as the maximum instantaneous flow rate.

introduction, the gas insufflation tubing is attached to the cannula via a Luer-lock extension to maintain pneumoperitoneum during the procedure. The carbon dioxide should be infused via an automatic regulating device (insufflator), which controls abdominal pressure, gas flow rate and total volume of gas delivered. Automatic insufflation is another feature of insufflators: the intra-abdominal pressure is set at a predetermined value, and the device insufflates gas if the pressure within the abdominal cavity falls below it. The intra-abdominal pressure should not exceed 12–13 mmHg in cats and 13–15 mmHg in dogs: higher abdominal pressures decrease venous return and reduce ventilating ability. The carbon dioxide flow rate can usually be regulated to between 1 and 20 L/min in 0.1 L increments.

A filter is placed at the outlet of the insufflator to provide microbiological filtration of the insufflating gas and to prevent retrograde contamination of the machine. Such filters are disposable and intended for single use, although they are commonly used repeatedly in veterinary surgery, unless soiled. An insufflation hose connects the insufflator to the patient (via trocar or Veress needle).

Veress needles

Veress needles are the most common type of insufflation needle and can be disposable or reusable (Fig. 1.15). Although disposable needles are always sharp, their cost usually precludes their use in veterinary medicine; as with other disposable items they could be re-sterilised a number of times. However, this would cause loss of sharpness and therefore defeat the purpose of their use. Veress needles have a spring-loaded obturator that retracts when the needle is in contact with tissues. When the needle enters the abdomen, the pressure on the tip is released, and

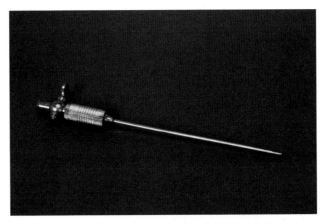

Fig. 1.15   A reusable Veress needle suitable for establishing pneumoperitoneum by the closed technique.

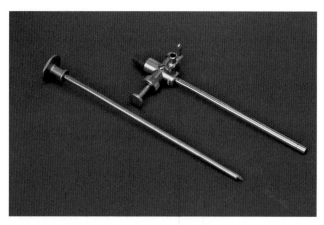

Fig. 1.16   A reusable 10 mm trocar-cannula unit. This example has a pyramidal tip, insufflation port and trumpet valve.

the obturator advances beyond the tip, thus protecting abdominal organs from injury. Insufflation tubing attaches to the hub of the needle.

Cannulae

During laparoscopy, the telescope and working instruments are introduced into the abdomen via trocar-cannula units (Fig. 1.16). Trocars are sharp-pointed stylets enclosed in a sleeve (cannula) used to penetrate fascia and muscles. Once the abdominal cavity has been entered, the trocar is removed, and the cannula is used to introduce the scope and instruments. These are freely movable within the cannula, as there is no locking mechanism.

The presence of a one-way valve prevents gas escape and loss of pneumoperitoneum during instrument passage; a rubber washer seals the space between the cannula and the endoscope or instrument when in place. Most cannulae have also a Luer-lock stopcock for gas insufflation. Trocar-cannula assemblies can be made of stainless steel (reusable) or hard plastic. The latter are intended for single use, but can be re-sterilised a limited number of times. Three trocar-cannula assemblies are typically required to perform laparoscopic interventions. This number can increase to four for more advanced procedures. The size of the cannula depends on the size of the scope and instruments used: the cannula is usually chosen to be 0.5–1 mm larger than the item inserted through it (commonly 6–11.5 mm); reducers are available to permit insertion of smaller instruments without loss of pneumoperitoneum. Larger cannulae (18–33 mm) are used to insert particular instruments such as large staplers and specimen bags. Cannulae can have straight or threaded shafts; the latter, although more difficult to insert, are more secure, and minimise the risk of dislodgement during introduction and removal of instruments.

Laparoscopic instruments

Virtually all surgical instruments are available in a laparoscopic version (grasping forceps, scissors, retractors and needle holders, for example). An additional instrument is the palpation probe. This is a blunt metal calibrated probe used as a finger to 'palpate' or move organs. The probe is marked at 1 cm intervals, allowing for accurate measurement of organs or lesions, which is otherwise difficult in the presence of magnification.

Energy sources

Haemostasis is a critical step in minimally invasive surgery, as even minor haemorrhages have a detrimental effect on surgical performance. During video-assisted surgery the presence of blood in the surgical field not only obscures the organs but absorbs light, resulting in loss of image quality. It can also be difficult to remove from the site. For this reason, as well as minimising blood loss, haemostasis is critical for these surgeries. Although numerous modalities are available to achieve haemostasis, energy-assisted devices such as electrosurgical units, lasers and ultrasonic cutting/coagulating appliances are usually preferred. All these devices have been shown to significantly decrease surgical time (Mayhew and Brown, 2007).

Energy sources are also used for tissue debridement and capsule shrinkage in arthroscopy, and for lithotripsy in cystoscopy.

Electrosurgery

Electrosurgical modalities are the most commonly used energy sources, since they are the most economical. These entail the use of an alternating current passing through the patient to complete the circuit. In monopolar electrosurgery, the current flows from the active electrode (in the handpiece) through the patient towards the passive electrode (grounding pad), whereas in bipolar devices both the active and return electrodes are housed in the handpiece.

Monopolar applications are less safe during rigid endoscopy than bipolar ones, because as current flow follows the path of least resistance, coupling can occur when the electrosurgical tip comes into contact with the scope or other instruments outside the field of view. Similarly, insulation defects and sparking can cause damage to adjacent tissues. These injuries are usually outside the surgical field of view, increasing the hazard. Monopolar electrosurgery also causes the generation of more aerosolised particles (smoke or plume) than bipolar surgery; this plume is a potential hazard to operating-room personnel and also obscures the surgical field. Monopolar electrosurgery can only be used in a non-conducting medium. Therefore it can be used during laparoscopy and thoracoscopy but cannot be used during fluid instillation (e.g.

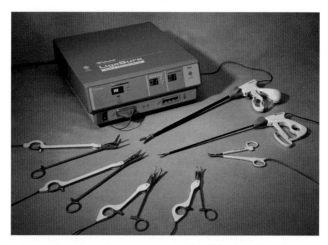

Fig. 1.17 Vessel-sealing electrosurgery unit with variety of handpieces for endosurgery and open surgery This sophisticated bipolar electrosurgery generator produces vessel sealing through a combination of a closely monitored electrical current and pressure applied by the handpieces. Copyright © 2011 Covidien. All rights reserved. Reprinted with the permission of the Energy-based Devices Division of Covidien.

urethrocystoscopy) unless a non-conducting irrigating medium (e.g. lysine solution) is used, rather than saline.

In bipolar electrosurgery devices, the electrodes are similar in size, and the current passes only through the tissue confined between them, thus limiting the amount of heat generated and minimising the risk of damage to surrounding tissues. Recent advances in bipolar technology have introduced electrothermal bipolar vessel-sealing devices (e.g. Ligasure, Valleylab, Boulder, CO, USA; Fig. 1.17), able to seal vessels up to 7mm in diameter, and lymphatics and tissue bundles, by denaturing collagen and elastin within the vessel wall and connective tissue. These seals have bursting strengths comparable to those of clips and ligatures; furthermore, since they are intrinsic to the vessel wall structure there is no risk of dislodgement. The vessel-sealing devices have dedicated handpieces for laparoscopy and thoracoscopy that allow both tissue sealing and tissue division. The handpieces are relatively expensive (compared to monopolar electrosurgery) and generally designed as disposable devices: this is a limitation to their use in veterinary surgery.

Lasers in rigid endoscopy

Laser is an acronym which stands for light amplification by stimulated emission of radiation: a laser beam is formed by light photons having all the same wavelength and travelling all in the same direction. This is achieved by passing light (or electrons) through a lasing medium,

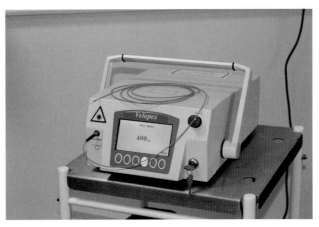

Fig. 1.18 Diode laser with flexible insertion tube suitable for endosurgery. Photograph courtesy of Mr P.J. Lhermette.

such as gases (carbon dioxide, helium, argon), crystals (usually neodymium:yttrium-aluminium-garnet or Nd:YAG), liquid dyes or diode semiconductors. The energy absorbed by atoms of the lasing medium at the passage of light is emitted as photons of a wavelength characteristic of that medium, which in turn strike other atoms, and so on. The result is a laser beam of a characteristic wavelength, which is focused in a set direction by the use of partially reflective mirrors: the light is thus concentrated and released in a coherent and powerful manner.

In the animal tissues, substances (called chromophores) absorb laser light, thus generating heat; these include water, haemoglobin and other pigments, each absorbing light in a specific portion of the electromagnetic spectrum. For instance, lasers emitting light at the wavelength absorbed by water will heat and vaporise tissues with high water content.

Carbon dioxide, diode (Fig. 1.18) and Nd:YAG lasers are the most commonly used surgical lasers. Carbon dioxide lasers emit light that does not penetrate fluids well, and is therefore used for cutting and vaporisation of surface lesions. Diode and Nd:YAG lasers instead penetrate fluids very well, and can be used for precise cutting and coagulation of deeper tissues. Consequently, they are preferred for veterinary endoscopy. Additionally, diode lasers can be directed to the surgical site through flexible fibre-optic shafts, which makes them more practical for endoscopic application. Diode lasers are particularly useful for resection of soft tissues during rhinoscopy and urethrocystoscopy.

Ultrasonic haemostasis and tissue division

Ultrasonic waves are created by applying electromagnetic energy to a piezoelectric transducer, usually located in the handpiece. These ultrasonic waves travel from the handpiece to the blade, producing mechanical vibrations. Ultrasonic (harmonic) devices (e.g. Harmonic Scalpel, Ethicon) have different tissue effects depending on pressure exerted, activation time, blade speed, blade configuration and power level. Four different actions (cutting, coagulation, coaptation and cavitation) can be achieved singularly or in combination with one another. In surgical procedures, all of these effects are typically applied consecutively. Before activating the blade, a combination of tension and pressure is used to rapidly stretch tissue. When the tissue reaches its elastic limit, the blade or device tip is able to cut smoothly through it. The blade usually vibrates 55 500 times per second, and the mechanical energy produced when it comes into contact with the tissue breaks hydrogen bonds, defragmenting the protein in the cells (coaptation). This mechanical energy propagates in the direction in which force is applied, with minimal collateral thermal damage. When ultrasound energy is applied to tissues a few seconds longer than it takes to achieve coaptation, a rise in temperature leads to the release of water vapour and then denaturation of protein. The denatured protein forms a coagulum, which seals the compressed blood vessels.

Cavitation occurs when the rapid vibration of a harmonic device is transmitted to the surrounding tissue, causing cell disruption and vaporisation of intracellular water at body temperature. This leads to separation of the tissue planes in advance of the blade, which enhances visibility and allows careful dissection. As with electrosurgical vessel-sealing technology, the capital cost of the generator and the high cost of the disposable handpieces limit the application of this technology in animals.

Powered instrumentation

Power-operated instruments for arthroscopy consist of motorised blades (shavers) and burrs, available in multiple sizes and shapes. These power instruments are used to remove cartilage, bone and soft tissues. Disposable blades are available, which can be reused six to eight times in veterinary patients (until no longer sharp). All the powered instruments are cannulated to allow suction of the debris produced by the cutting action of the instrument out of the joint. The most useful sizes in veterinary medicine are 2.0–4.0 mm.

Operating-room requirements

Whereas some procedures involving rigid endoscopy (notably rhinoscopy, otoscopy, tracheoscopy and urethrocystoscopy) can be performed in a non-sterile setting, surgical procedures such as arthroscopy, laparoscopy or thoracoscopy should only be performed with proper aseptic technique, and in an operating room. In fact, the operating team must be ready to convert the minimally invasive approach to an open procedure for any reason. In any case, a dedicated operating room is preferred whenever possible.

Operating-room layout

The video tower should be close to the table and in full view of the surgeon; when an assistant is present, the monitor must be easily viewable by both operators. To allow easier orientation during the procedure, the surgeon(s), patient and monitor should be positioned in a straight line (Fig. 1.19). The surgical telescope should be pointed towards the video monitor for most of the time; thus, for example in laparoscopic procedures caudal to the umbilicus, the monitor is positioned at the foot of the patient, whereas procedures in the cranial abdomen require the monitor to be positioned at the head of the table (Fig. 1.20). Ideally this should be considered during operating-room design and certainly each time surgery is planned, and the positioning and access to anaesthetic equipment, and gas and electrical outlets, must also be considered. The

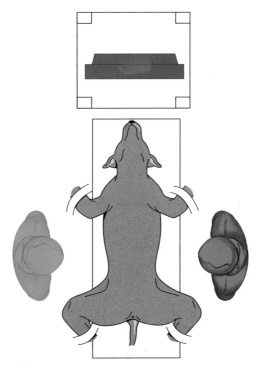

Fig. 1.19 Layout of the operating theatre with two surgeons and a single monitor. The theatre must be arranged so that the surgeon is looking along the endoscope, across the surgical site and towards the monitor. This makes directing the scope and instruments easier and more comfortable for the surgeon.

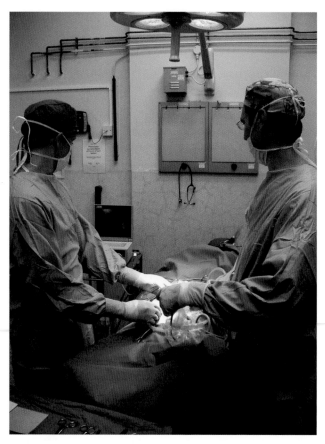

Fig. 1.20   Combined monitor/CCU in use during laparoscopic liver biopsy. The lead surgeon is to the left and is looking cranially over the patient to the monitor.

surgeon may have to move around the table to operate with the dominant hand and to examine the entire body cavity, and look at the monitor without straining. This may need the tower or monitor to be moved. Having the image on more than one monitor considerably reduces the need for repositioning of equipment and hanging the monitors on adjustable mounts (on the wall or from the light pendants) is also helpful. When the procedure is in progress the lights will need to be dimmed and thus avoiding cable cluttering is important to prevent tripping hazards. Electrical interference when the electrosurgical unit is in use can be minimised by using separate electrical outlets for the video cart and the electrosurgical unit.

For laparoscopy, the insufflator should be positioned at eye level, close to the video monitor; this allows easy monitoring of the intra-abdominal pressure. Both the surgeon and anaesthetist should be able to see the insufflator settings.

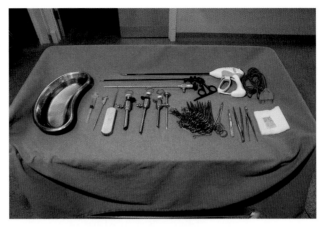

Fig. 1.21   Sterile trolley laid out in an orderly fashion for endosurgery (e.g. laparoscopic ovariectomy). Photograph courtesy of Mr P.J. Lhermette.

Operating-room equipment

The variety and length of instruments used in this type of surgery (especially laparoscopy and thoracoscopy) requires the provision of one or more large instrument trolleys to allow the instruments to be laid out in an orderly and secure fashion (Fig. 1.21). During laparoscopy and thoracoscopy the use of gravitational forces to displace other organs is a very effective means of retraction to increase visualisation of the operative site. A surgical table that allows the patient to be positioned with the head down or up (the Trendelenburg and reverse Trendelenburg positions respectively), as well as to be rotated from side to side, is therefore of great help in improving exposure of the area of interest. The height of the table should also be adjustable. Table height is generally lower during endoscopic procedures than conventional procedures. This is because of the greater length of the instruments and because the surgeons are looking across the table to the monitor rather than down onto the patient.

Nearly all rigid endoscopic procedures require the patient to be under general anaesthesia. To improve a patient's safety this requires a dedicated member of the team and appropriate monitoring should be available. Furthermore, some endoscopic procedures such as laparoscopy and thoracoscopy require special anaesthetic considerations. The cardiovascular status of the animal must be closely evaluated in laparoscopy because of the induction of pneumoperitoneum. Carbon dioxide diffuses across the peritoneum, causing a significant increase in arterial blood carbon dioxide levels (Duke et al., 1996). There is often a corresponding decrease in oxygenation, even in patients receiving mechanical ventilation. Insufflation of the abdomen also increases intra-abdominal pressure, compressing the vena cava, depressing venous return, and cranially displacing the diaphragm, inhibiting spontaneous ventilation. Access to mechanical ventilation is therefore recommended in animals undergoing laparoscopy and is an absolute requirement for thoracoscopy. Monitoring should include electrocardiography, blood pressure monitoring, capnography and pulse oximetry. A simple oesophageal stethoscope is also of help in such cases, as development of heart murmurs is a feature of gas embolism. If an arterial catheter is placed, blood-gas analysis will be facilitated and this form of monitoring is especially helpful in prolonged procedures.

Adverse effects can also be induced by changes in body position in an anaesthetised, dorsally recumbent patient. Inhalant anaesthetics depress the baroreflex, thus diminishing reflex control of circulation following changes in body posture (Joris et al., 1993; Bailey and Pablo, 1999).

The head-down tilt (Trendelenburg position) tends to decrease ventilation and cardiac output, whereas the head-up tilt (reverse Trendelenburg position) leads to reflex vasoconstriction, with increased heart rate and blood pressure (Abel et al., 1963). Limiting the increase in abdominal pressure to no more than 15 mmHg and the Trendelenburg angle to no more than 15° ('the rule of 15') is used as a general guideline to minimise these effects (Bailey and Pablo, 1999).

Instrument care and sterilisation

Proper care of endoscopy equipment maximises its longevity, and includes careful cleaning, lubricating, sterilising and storing in accordance with the manufacturer's guidelines. It is highly recommended to train all people using and responsible for processing the equipment in its handling and care. All instrumentation should be cleaned immediately after use, removing organic material from all surfaces. For example, if body fluids are allowed to dry onto the lens of the endoscope it is difficult to clean later without risking physical damage. Disassembly is often required for proper cleaning of hand instruments; similarly, seals and protective caps must be removed. Surfaces, inner cavities and jaws have to be mechanically cleaned with soft brushes or sponges specifically designed for the respective instruments. Not all the components of the kit are submersible for cleaning, especially the less-modern telescopes and camera heads. Pieces of equipment that are not submersible can usually be cleaned by wiping with medical disinfectant wipes (e.g. camera lenses, light cables and optical surfaces of telescopes). Use always a detergent approved by the manufacturer. All the items containing optics should be handled with particular care to prevent damage to the delicate glass fibres or lenses. Bending and sudden impacts (e.g. dropping on to hard surfaces) are particular hazards.

For the initial phase of cleaning commercial enzymatic cleaning solutions are commonly used to clean both the scope and instruments. Cleaning solutions specifically designed for endoscopes are preferred whenever possible. Although equipment with glass fibres or lenses is not suitable for ultrasonic cleaning, this technique can be extremely useful for hand instruments, facilitating cleaning of hard to reach areas.

After cleaning, the equipment should be rinsed thoroughly. Working channels, stopcocks on cannulae and all ports are flushed until clear water runs through. Distilled or demineralised water must be used to avoid mineral deposits that can prevent smooth operation of moving parts; it is also important to remember not to leave instruments in saline solution as this may cause corrosion and pitting. After cleaning, instruments are thoroughly dried, especially optical surfaces of telescopes, before sterilisation, using soft cloths for external surfaces and compressed air or alcohol flushes for inaccessible areas. All moving parts are lubricated according to the manufacturer's instructions using proprietary instrument lubricant. After lubricant has been applied, the working parts are opened and closed and then any excess lubricant wiped away.

Before sterilising, the equipment is inspected for damaged areas, and telescopes and light cables are checked for light transmission. Plastic components are inspected for discoloration, porosity and flexibility, and instrument channels are checked for patency. Alignment of jaws of scissors and grasping forceps is checked.

Instruments and telescopes may be sterilised by steam, ethylene oxide or soaking in a chemical solution, depending on manufacturer's recommendations. Stopcocks and valves on cannulae should be left disassembled for sterilisation, and ratcheting closures should be left in the open position. This ensures that all components are exposed to the sterilising agent or process. Instruments can be autoclaved similarly to other surgical equipment, and specialised trays are available for their sterilisation. Telescopes, camera heads, light cables and other delicate instruments require careful storage in padded, rigid boxes. They can be stored after steam or ethylene oxide sterilisation, ready for the next use, or stored non-sterile, then immersed in sterilising solutions shortly before use.

Only certain telescopes and cameras are autoclavable, and specific cycles and temperatures may be required. However, autoclaving reduces the life expectancy of optical devices due to heat damage, and therefore cold sterilisation is often preferred for endoscopes. Rather than being sterilised, the camera head is usually covered with a disposable sterile sleeve during use. Plastic items are usually sterilised with ethylene oxide, and some camera heads are suitable for this type of sterilisation too. The manufacturer's recommendations for cycle and aeration times should be consulted. More commonly, high-level disinfection is achieved by soaking instruments and telescopes in a proprietary disinfectant solution. The equipment should be thoroughly cleaned after soaking by rinsing with sterile lavage solution, as disinfectant solutions can cause significant tissue reaction. Sterile soft cloths are then used to dry it completely; alcohol wipes are used for lenses and glass surfaces.

Disposable, reposable and reusable instruments

Many endoscopic instruments and accessories (e.g. cannulae, instruments, needles) are available as pre-sterilised plastic items (disposable), or as items intended for limited reuse (reposable) or in-clinic re-sterilisation (reusable). Disposable items are typically manufactured from plastic (with non-replaceable blades if necessary) and have a lower capital cost. They are intended to be single-use items but in veterinary practice are sometimes cleaned and reused. If this approach is chosen, certain limitations must be recognised. Notably, such items are often complicated in structure and cannot be disassembled. Although the outer surfaces can be cleaned and the equipment then cold-sterilised, it is impossible to reliably clean these instruments and therefore sterility cannot be guaranteed. Additionally, the plastic becomes brittle with repeated use and may unexpectedly break in use and the sharpness of any blade will rapidly diminish.

Reusable instruments have a higher capital cost but can be taken apart for cleaning and can be re-sterilised by autoclave. Complex instruments (and particularly those with a lumen) are only reliably sterilised in a vacuum (rather than gravity-displacement) autoclave, however. If they have a blade, it may be possible to re-sharpen or replace this.

Reposable instruments are less commonly used but offer a lower item cost than reusable items. The manufacturers specify guidelines that allow limited reuse when cleaned and sterilised according to their instructions. The instrument should be marked each time it is resterilised so that it is disposed off appropriately.

The laparoscopy team

Endoscopic surgery requires a coordinated team, of which nurses and technical assistants are an essential part. Their role is important not only for proper care and maintenance of the equipment, but for operating-room and equipment set-up, as anaesthesia and surgical assistants, and to identify and solve unexpected system failures.

To improve operating-room efficiency, training before the procedure is beneficial, as is the provision of written protocols for equipment set-up, use and cleaning. The operating-room team should also be able to anticipate urgent needs, such as rapid control of haemorrhage or conversion to an open procedure.

Before surgery starts, the team should ensure that all the required units (tower, suction, electrosurgery and irrigation systems) are available and functioning properly. All the equipment and the theatre trolley are prepared while the surgeons are scrubbing up; the fluid irrigation system is then connected to the lavage solution (lactated Ringer's solution or 0.9% saline). At the onset of the procedure the monitor, the tower and the powered equipment, if required, are switched on. The camera head and cable, if not sterile, are covered with a protective sterile sleeve and the telescope attached. The light cable is connected to the light source but is switched on only when the surgeon is ready. A dedicated anaesthetist – or a nurse in charge only of anaesthesia – is advisable in any endoscopic procedure, to monitor the patient properly and to allow the surgeon to concentrate only on endoscopy.

Endoscopic surgery often requires at least one scrubbed surgical assistant, to pass instruments and to hold either the endoscope or instruments during surgical procedures. This role is often taken by a veterinary nurse or technician. During arthroscopy, help in positioning the patient intraoperatively is also essential, in order to increase joint space and improve the visualisation of intra-articular structures. In most laparoscopic and thoracoscopic procedures, the primary surgeon cannot act also as laparoscope operator; consequently, a team of three people is necessary (surgeon, camera operator and trolley nurse). The assistant in charge of the laparoscope should attempt to maintain a constant view of the surgical field and the surgeon should be able to visualise instruments entering through the cannulae without the need to move the laparoscope from the surgical field.

After the procedure, the nursing staff is in charge of cleaning, sterilising and storing instruments and equipment. All the components and instruments need to be checked for correct function, and the operating-room staff communicate with equipment suppliers to obtain technical support and replacement if needed.

Further reading

Beale, B.S., Hulse, D.A., Schulz, K. and Whitney, W. O. (2003) *Small Animal Arthroscopy*. WB Saunders, Philadelphia, PA.

Chamness, C.J. (1999) Endoscopic instrumentation. In *Small Animal Endoscopy*, Tams, T.R. (ed.), pp. 1–16. Mosby, St Louis, MO.

Chamness, C.J. (2008) Instrumentation. In *BSAVA Manual of Canine and Feline Endoscopy and Endosurgery*, Lhermette, P. and Sobel, D. (eds), pp. 11–30. British Small Animal Veterinary Association, Gloucester.

Freeman, L.J. (ed.) (1998) *Veterinary Endosurgery*. Mosby, St Louis, MO.

Kudnig, S.T., Monnet, E. and Riquelme, M. (2003) Effect of one-lung ventilation on oxygen delivery in anesthetized dogs with an open thoracic cavity. *American Journal of Veterinary Research* 64, 443–448.

Kudnig, S.T., Monnet, E., Riquelme, M., Gaynor, J.S., Corliss, D. and Salman, M.D. (2004) Cardiopulmonary effects of thoracoscopy in anesthetized normal dogs. *Veterinary Anaesthesia and Analgesia* 31, 121–128.

Lhermette, P. and Sobel, D. (eds) (2008) *BSAVA Manual of Canine and Feline Endoscopy and Endosurgery*. British Small Animal Veterinary Association, Gloucester.

Magne, M.L. and Tams, T.R. (1999) Laparoscopy: instrumentation and technique. In *Small Animal Endoscopy*, Tams, T.R. (ed.), pp. 397–408. Mosby, St Louis, MO.

Mayhew, P.D. (2009) Advanced laparoscopic procedures in dogs and cats. *Veterinary Clinics of North America, Small Animal Practice* 3, 925–939.

McCarthy, T.C. (ed.) (2005) *Veterinary Endoscopy for the Small Animal Practitioner*. Elsevier Saunders, St Louis, MO.

Monnet, E. and Twedt, D.C. (2003) Laparoscopy. *Veterinary Clinics of North America, Small Animal Practice* 33, 1147–1163.

Quandt, J.E. (1999) Anesthetic considerations for laser, laparoscopy, and thoracoscopy procedures. *Clinical Techniques in Small Animal Practice* 14, 50–55.

Radlinski, M.G. (ed.) (2009) Endoscopy. *Veterinary Clinics of North America, Small Animal Practice* 39(3).

Rawlings, C.A. (2009) Diagnostic rigid endoscopy: otoscopy, rhinoscopy, and cystoscopy. *Veterinary Clinics of North America, Small Animal Practice* 39, 849–868.

Richter, K.P. (2001) Laparoscopy in dogs and cats. *Veterinary Clinics of North America, Small Animal Practice* 31, 707–727.

Sobel, D. and Lulich, J. (2008) An introduction to laser endosurgery. In *BSAVA Manual of Canine and Feline Endoscopy and Endosurgery*, Lhermette, P. and Sobel, D. (eds), pp. 220–227. British Small Animal Veterinary Association, Gloucester.

Stasi, K. and Melendez, L. (2001) Care and cleaning of the endoscope. *Veterinary Clinics of North America, Small Animal Practice* 31, 589–603.

Tams, T.R. and Rawlings, C.A. (eds) (2011) *Small Animal Endoscopy*, 3rd edn. Mosby, St Louis, MO.

Van Lue, S.J. and Van Lue, A.P. (2009) Equipment and instrumentation in veterinary endoscopy. *Veterinary Clinics of North America, Small Animal Practice* 39, 817–837.

Walton, R.S. (1999) Thoracoscopy. In *Small Animal Endoscopy*, Tams, T.R. (ed.), pp. 471–482. Mosby, St Louis, MO.

Weil, A.B. (2009) Anesthesia for endoscopy in small animals. *Veterinary Clinics of North America, Small Animal Practice* 39, 839–848.

References

Abel, F., Pierce, J. and Guntheroth, W. (1963) Baroreceptor influence on postural changes in blood pressure and carotid blood flow. *American Journal of Physiology* 205, 360–364.

Bailey, J.E. and Pablo, L.S. (1998) Anesthetic and physiologic considerations for veterinary endosurgery. In *Veterinary Endosurgery*, Freeman, L.J. (ed.), pp. 24–43. Mosby, St Louis, MO.

Duke, T., Steinacher, L. and Remedios, A.M. (1996) Cardiopulmonary effects of using carbon dioxide for laparoscopic surgery in dogs. *Veterinary Surgery* 25, 77–82.

Joris, J.L., Noirot, D.P., Legrand, M.J., Jacquet, N.J. and Lamy, M.L. (1993) Hemodynamic changes during laparoscopic cholecystectomy. *Anesthesia and Analgesia* 76, 1067–1071.

Mayhew, P.D. and Brown, D.C. (2007) Comparison of three techniques for ovarian pedicle hemostasis during laparoscopic-assisted ovariohysterectomy. *Veterinary Surgery* 36, 541–547.

Wilson, M.S. (1993) Non-surgical intrauterine artificial insemination in bitches using frozen semen. *Journal of Reproduction and Fertility, Supplement* 47, 307–311.

Wilson, M.S. (2001) Transcervical insemination techniques in the bitch. *Veterinary Clinics of North America, Small Animal Practice* 31, 291–304.

Chapter 2
Diagnostic Arthroscopy
Martin R. Owen

Introduction

In modern small animal veterinary practice, arthroscopic management for many manifestations of joint disease has become the preferred approach over traditional investigative studies and to open joint surgery. Arthroscopic techniques offer several advancements over historical methods of diagnosis and treatment of joint disease:

- the opportunity to see intra-articular structures and lesions, with great clarity and with magnification,

- the ability to recognise lesions not visible to the naked eye,

- the ability to probe and mechanically test intra-articular structures using magnified vision, enabling sensitive evaluation of their structural integrity,

- the ability to surgically treat intra-articular lesions accurately and with precision, with minimal morbidity.

Arthroscopic instrumentation

Arthroscope

Arthroscopes are fine-diameter telescopes comprised of a series of lenses that collect and transmit an image from the tip of the arthroscope along its shaft to the eyepiece. The lenses are surrounded by optic fibres which

Clinical Manual of Small Animal Endosurgery, First Edition. Edited by Alasdair Hotston Moore and Rosa Angela Ragni.
© 2012 Blackwell Publishing Ltd. Published 2012 by Blackwell Publishing Ltd.

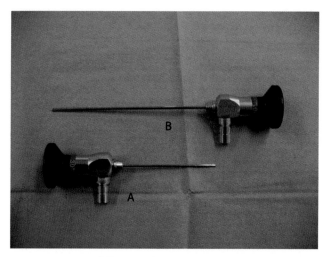

Fig. 2.1   A, 1.9 mm 30° oblique arthroscope; B, 2.4 mm 30° oblique arthroscope.

transmit light from a light source down the arthroscope shaft, illuminating the subject area captured at the tip. Arthroscopes are characterised by their diameter, their viewing angle and their working length.

Diameter

The most popular sizes of arthroscope used in small animal arthroscopy are the 1.9, 2.4 and 2.7 mm arthroscopes (Fig. 2.1). In large joints in giant-breed dogs, a 4 mm arthroscope can be usefully employed, since for all sizes the larger the diameter of the arthroscope used, the greater the field of view and the greater the illumination, hence the better the visualisation. Conversely, the smaller the arthroscope, the more limited the view and the greater the fragility of the arthroscope. For this reason great care must be taken when using the smaller arthroscopes to prevent damaging them during use and handling.

Lens angle and viewing angle

The lens angle is the angle between the axis of the arthroscope and the centre of image visible at the tip of the arthroscope. For most applications of small animal arthroscopy, it is helpful to use an arthroscope that has a 30° viewing angle, such that the centre of the image viewed is 30° away from 'straight ahead'. The 30° arthroscope facilitates a large area of view by rotation of the arthroscope about its length. In this way, a large area is viewed without changing the direction and position of the arthroscope within the joint. The field of view at the tip of the arthroscope is determined by the size of its objective lens, which is a function of the diameter of the arthroscope. Smaller-diameter arthroscopes have smaller lenses, with smaller fields of view. Consequently, there is a non-linear progressive decrease in visible area imaged as smaller arthroscopes are considered, and thus use of the smallest arthroscope requires considerable skill to locate intra-articular structures and instruments.

Working length

The working length describes the length of the shaft of the arthroscope. The working length of the arthroscope is generally a function of its diameter, since increased length increases the susceptibility to damage by bending and hence narrow arthroscopes tend to be short, with a 1.9 mm arthroscope being approximately 100 mm and a 2.4 mm arthroscope being approximately 110 mm in length. An arthroscope with a short working length allows the arthroscopist to 'finger brace' the arthroscope against the joint being examined, giving greater steadiness of hand. Longer working lengths can be useful for the shoulder joint and for the stifle joint, where greater depth of soft tissue must be penetrated to access the joint.

Arthroscope sheath and obturators

The arthroscope requires its own dedicated sheath which is protective against bending and facilitates administration of fluid into the joint, around the arthroscope tip, maintaining a clear view within the joint. The sheath has its own dedicated obturators to protect it during penetration of soft tissues and through the joint capsule, and to enable passage of the sheath through the soft tissues without the sheath becoming filled with soft tissue. The ensheathed obturator is always used to access the joint, replacing the obturator with the arthroscope once the joint cavity is entered. This prevents forceful damage to the fragile tip and shaft of the arthroscope. Both blunt and sharp obturators are available (Fig. 2.2). Sharp obturators penetrate the joint capsule readily but risk damage to structures within the joint following entry. Hence a blunt- or semi-blunt-ended obturator tip is preferable to prevent iatrogenic damage to intra-articular structures during sheath introduction into the joint. A locking system fixes the arthroscope or the obturator within the sheath when in use.

Light source and fibre-optic cable

Suitable light sources for arthroscopy include halogen and xenon, but a xenon light source is significantly preferable since the light from xenon is bright and a whiter light, giving better visual clarity and colour rendition. Lamp wattage varies from 100 to 400 W, with low wattage being satisfactory for small joints and the higher power being necessary if other endoscopic procedures are performed (e.g. laparoscopy) using the equipment. The lifespan of xenon bulbs is limited to approximately

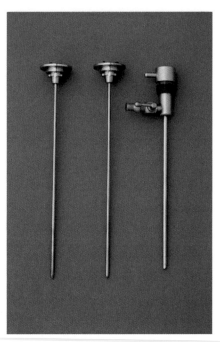

Fig. 2.2   Arthroscope cannula with blunt and sharp obturator.

500 h; some light units indicate remaining bulb life. Keeping a spare bulb is sensible, in case of bulb failure. Many light sources have automatic intensity control through feedback from the camera output, maintaining appropriate illumination and image quality during arthroscopy. Manual control of light intensity is also possible, enabling fine adjustment of the image by the arthroscopist.

Light is transmitted from the lamp unit to the arthroscope through a fibre-optic cable (Fig. 2.3), connected to the arthroscope light post. Each manufacturer's light source has its own connection mechanism coupling the source to the cable and the connections joining the fibre-optic cable to the arthroscope are also manufacturer-specific. Connection converters are readily available to couple most fibre-optic connector styles to each arthroscope make and model, allowing for suitable size matching between almost any fibre-optic cable and any arthroscope. Small arthroscopes require use of a thin light cable to prevent loss of light. The light cable comprises a bundle of flexible yet delicate glass fibres that break if the cable is bent or wound too tightly, hence the cable should be wound gently when stored or transported. Fibre breakage reduces the light transmission through the cable, eventually rendering the cable unusable. Although the fibre-optic cable delivers 'cold light' at the arthroscope tip (compared to historical systems utilising a bulb at the tip of the scope), the light cable can heat up during use and for this reason it should not be placed directly on the patient to avoid risk of thermal burn.

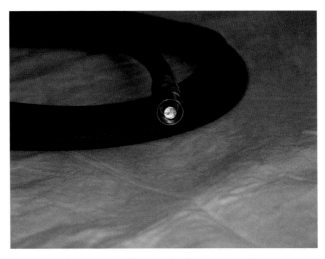

Fig. 2.3 Close-up image of a fibre-optic light cable. The cable should be wound gently to avoid breaking the delicate glass fibres.

Camera unit

The arthroscopic image is projected from the arthroscope eyepiece to the monitor via an endoscopic video camera system comprising a camera head, which clips onto the eyepiece, and a control unit. The camera head contains a light-responsive electronic chip that converts the image to an electronic signal, which is transferred to the camera controller, processed and exported as a signal recognised by the display monitor and recording device. Most camera controllers produce a number of export formats. Super VHS (s-VHS) output gives the highest-quality image reproduction but attention is required in the use of s-VHS-type cable connections since they are not robust. A composite video cable output is therefore a suitable alternative which is more resistant to damage during handling. A camera unit with multiple outputs of each type is ideal since it enables easy connection of additional devices such as recorders (DVD, camcorder, computer, etc.) in addition to maintaining the connection to the monitor.

Monitor

A medical-grade monitor is necessary to get the best reproduction of the arthroscopic image generated by the camera unit. The monitor needs to work on the same video signal as the camera unit (PAL in Europe and NTSC in North America); hence, when equipment is purchased or replaced, care should be taken to purchase equipment that runs on the appropriate video signal. Flat-screen technology has become the industry standard but a traditional high-quality colour medical-grade cathode-ray-tube monitor provides a perfectly good image. The monitor should accept s-VHS and composite signal inputs and similar output channels are extremely useful, for the purposes of connecting recording devices to the monitor, if necessary, to capture and keep images of the procedures performed. Basic image adjustment of contrast, brightness and colour can be helpful features to adjust the image quality during the arthroscopic procedure.

Records

Digital image capture has become the standard method of image collection and storage and a variety of hardware is available to achieve this, ranging from camcorders, DVD recorders, USB streaming and capture devices plugged in to either a personal computer or a dedicated medical digital-signal video-archiving device (Fig. 2.4). It is useful to make recorded video sequences when a procedure is of particular interest and a permanent record is required. For the most part, still images are adequate to provide a record of the arthroscopic findings, the procedure and the postoperative intra-articular appearance. Captured frames from video recordings are only of low resolution when viewed as still images hence a still-image-capturing device is required to generate good-quality still images.

Joint irrigation and distension

Steady and constant fluid flow through the joint during arthroscopy maintains a clear field of view, flushing away surgical debris and haemorrhage. Isotonic lactated Ringer's solution or sodium chloride are both suitable irrigation fluids. Fluid is passed through the arthroscope sleeve,

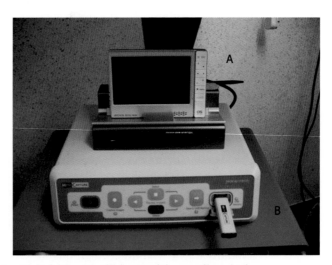

Fig. 2.4   Digital (A) and still-image (B) recording devices.

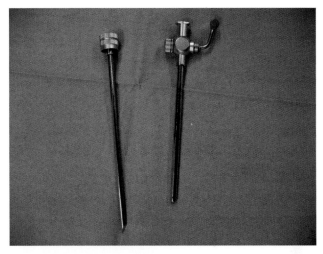

Fig. 2.5 Fenestrated cannula with trocar. A fenestrated cannula is particularly useful for stifle arthroscopy, when soft tissue can partially occlude the cannula; hence, multiple fluid-egress points are useful.

past the scope tip, ensuring the view is not compromised by particulate matter or haemorrhage, which is flushed away from the scope tip. To create fluid flow through the joint a constant outflow or egress is required. Without good egress, the fluid entering the joint tends to extravasate into the periarticular soft tissues and this progressively prevents fluid distension of the joint cavity, reducing the intra-articular space until the view is totally compromised. For small joints, a large-bore (22 gauge or larger) needle provides a suitable egress but for the shoulder joint, and certainly for the stifle joint, a fenestrated egress cannula is necessary for uninterrupted fluid outflow (Fig. 2.5). Efficient fluid flow requires a head of pressure and for small joints this can be achieved using a simple fluid compression bag in which the pressure is maintained with a hand pump (Fig. 2.6). With this system the fluid pressure and therefore the flow rate tend to be variable and erratic. Fluid pumps provide better-controlled pressure and therefore improved fluid flow. Pumps give precise control over intra-articular pressure and fluid flow rates, normally prioritising pressure over flow rate. Most pumps function using a peristaltic roller mechanism, giving accurate control of pressure delivery, which is generally set at between 40 and 100 mmHg. A fluid pump gives improved clarity of vision throughout arthroscopic procedures and this tends to reduce the duration of surgery (Fig. 2.7).

When high volumes of fluid are used, a collection system is useful to contain the wet area in the procedure room/operating theatre. Waste fluid can be directed via flexible tubing attached by Luer-lock to the egress cannula/needle into a collection bag or waste bowl. Alternatively, waste fluid may be allowed to flow onto an impervious patient drape and then to the floor, where it can be scavenged using a floor suction

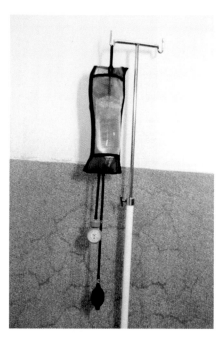

Fig. 2.6   Fluid compression bag with hand pump and manometer, useful for small joints.

device (Fig. 2.8). When fluid is collected via tubing connected to the egress cannula, care must be taken to ensure that the presence and weight of the tubing does not cause damaging impingement of the egress cannula/needle against articular cartilage. Simple and quick procedures which use a low volume of fluid can be performed using an adhesive drape with an integrated fluid-collecting pouch, although this technique requires careful setting up of patient position and draping to ensure that the fluid is effectively collected in the pouch (Fig. 2.9).

Arthroscopic surgical instruments

For arthroscopic surgery, a few basic surgical instruments are additionally required, including a scalpel blade and handle; and in case the operator wishes to convert an arthroscopic procedure into an arthrotomy, a routine set of traditional surgical instruments should be readily available. An arthroscopic procedure also requires a small selection of syringes (2, 5 and 20 ml) and injection needles (22–14 gauge).

Cannulae

In order to readily introduce arthroscopic instruments through peri-articular soft tissues with minimal difficulty and to induce the least peri-

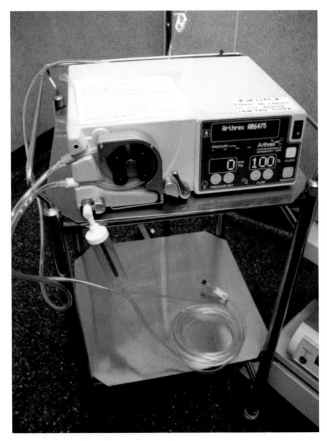

Fig. 2.7   Fluid pump for delivery of irrigation fluid. The improved clarity of vision provided by the pump allows reduced surgery times.

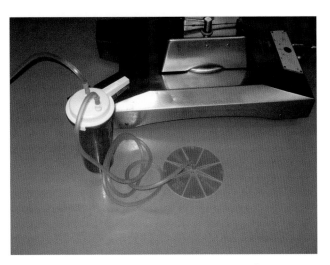

Fig. 2.8   Floor suction device connected to a vacuum line.

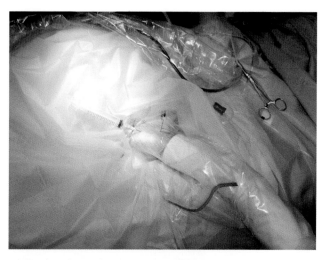

Fig. 2.9   Adhesive drape incorporating fluid-collecting pouch, used here for elbow arthroscopy.

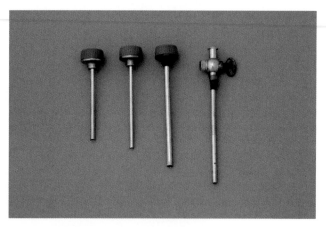

Fig. 2.10   Instrument cannulae with rubber diaphragms and (far right) a fenestrated cannula.

articular tissue damage, arthroscopic cannulae are used (Fig. 2.10). Instrument cannulae are available in different diameters and lengths and a selection of diameters should be available enabling selection of a suitably small-diameter cannula for small joints, and using the more convenient larger diameter cannulae in larger joints. Some cannulae are supplied with their own dedicated obturator (blunt ones are preferred) to enable introduction into the articular cavity. Some cannulae have a removable soft rubberised diaphragm that enables insertion and removal of instruments while limiting fluid loss from the joint. Use of instrument cannulae enables thorough flushing of the joint, with minimal extravasation of fluid into peri-articular soft tissues. This enables longer windows of operating time without collapse of the joint space, which is especially important for the novice arthroscopist.

Hand instruments

Arthroscopic hand instruments are fine enough to work within the confines of instrument cannulae and within the constraints of small articular spaces and yet they are manufactured to be sufficiently robust and stiff such that they resist bending or breakage during use within the joint. Some instruments are available in a blackened finish, which prevents glare and improves the surgical view. A basic set of instruments includes (see also Fig. 2.11):

- blunt probe,
- curette,
- meniscal knife (protected blade),
- 'banana' knife (unprotected blade),
- hooked knife,
- hand burr,
- grasping forceps,
- biopsy forceps.

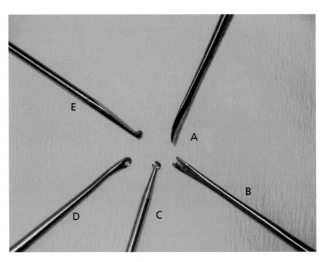

Fig. 2.11   Arthroscopy tools working tips. Clockwise from top: A, 'banana' knife; B, meniscal knife; C, hand burr; D, hand curette; E, blunt probe.

A right-angled blunt probe is useful for palpating articular cartilage to assess its mechanical integrity, to identify osteochondral lesions, to manipulate meniscal tears and to retract soft tissues. An arthroscopic curette is useful to debride osteochondral and subchondral bone lesions. A straight curette passes readily through the instrument cannula but an angled curette can be preferable in some applications to work on surfaces that are difficult to access. Knives are used to cut soft tissues such as the soft-tissue attachments of loose osteochondral fragments. The meniscal knife has a protected blade, making it useful for performing a combination of blunt and sharp dissection rather like the action of a periosteal elevator in open surgery. The meniscal knife is very useful for freeing osteochondral fragments of the coronoid process from its soft-tissue attachments. Sometimes the unprotected banana knife and hooked knife are necessary for cutting soft tissues and this is performed with care to avoid cutting tissue beyond the field of view. A hand burr is an efficient instrument for debriding and abrading lesions of bone and of cartilage. Although slower than a powered burr or shaver, a hand burr is inexpensive and its use does not require setting up of the additional equipment required with power instruments. Grasping forceps are modified alligator forceps that are fine and delicate in dimension (Fig. 2.12). Some models are resistant to mechanical failure in use through an 'overload protection' mechanism. Grasping surfaces with fine serrations are recommended to grip tissues with minimal risk of breaking the forceps through overzealous squeezing of the jaws. Some forceps have locking jaws which help protect against such misuse. In addition to grasping forceps, a pair of biting or biopsy forceps can be useful for taking biopsies of soft tissue and for debriding soft-tissue or meniscal lesions.

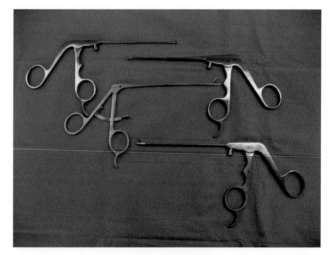

Fig. 2.12 Grasping forceps. The second pair from the bottom has a ratchet that allows the instrument jaws to be locked, preventing overzealous squeezing.

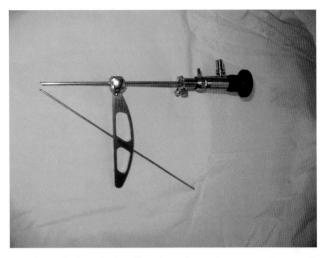

Fig. 2.13   Triangulation device fitted to the arthroscope sleeve. The sharp switching stick shows triangulation.

Aiming device

Introducing the instruments into the arthroscopic view is technically challenging for the novice arthroscopist and for each joint approached during the learning experience. Effective arthroscopic surgery requires achieving a suitable direction for the instruments that gives an arthroscopic view of the instrument tip enabling intuitive control, while enabling manipulation of the instrument handle without interference with the arthroscope. Initially it is challenging to achieve suitable placement of the instruments and an aiming device removes the error in this procedure. The aiming device clips onto the arthroscopic cannula sleeve and gives a fixed triangulation for the instrument (Fig. 2.13). It is necessary to attach the aiming device to the cannula at the correct height from the tip before the cannula is inserted into the joint to ensure that the scope tip and the instrument meet at the field of view.

Joint distractor

Improved access to small joints is facilitated by distraction or leverage of the joint, stretching tissues and opening the joint cavity. Distraction can be achieved by bracing the joint against a fulcrum, like a sandbag or a customised brace, while an assistant applies directed force to the distal limb. Distraction of the stifle joint can be also be achieved using a custom-made distraction device (Fig. 2.14) that engages percutaneously placed pins inserted into the subchondral bone on adjacent sides of the joint. The threaded rod of the distractor spans the joint and progressive tightening of the adjustment wheel tensions the soft tissues of the joint

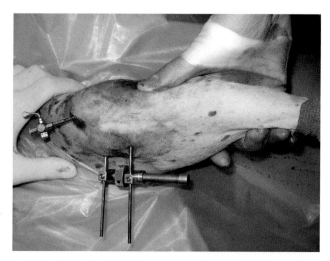

Fig. 2.14   Stifle distractor. In this case a custom-made distraction device is used.

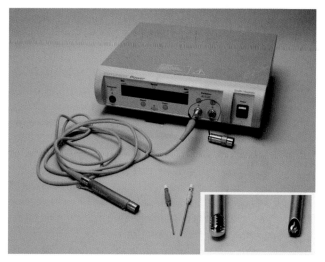

Fig. 2.15   Control unit and handpiece for motorised shavers and burrs. The tips are shown in the inset.

whilst distracting the articular surfaces, opening the joint space, improving the view and increasing the working space.

Power shavers/burrs

A motorised burr efficiently and rapidly removes bone and cartilage, enabling removal of large lesions in minimal time. The control unit for a power burr/shaver is hand- or foot-operated, enabling the operator to control the speed and the direction of the action of the handpiece (Fig. 2.15). Active suction is applied to the hand tip during its operation, to remove the debris and haemorrhage created during operative surgery. For the soft-tissue shaver, suction draws tissue into the shaver tip enabling efficient debridement of soft tissue. Each burr/shaver tip comprises two pieces: a rotating blade and an outer cannula. Numerous different styles of arthroscopic shaver and burr tips are available although relatively few are applicable for small animal arthroscopy. A protected or semi-protected burr tip is preferable for use in small joints to prevent iatrogenic damage to tissue juxtaposed to surgical lesions. Power shaver/ burr blades are sold as 'single use', but multiple use of each blade is possible in small animal arthroscopy because in a typical procedure the blade does relatively little work and hence it remains sharp for several procedures. Careful cleaning and re-sterilisation are required for safe reuse of the blades.

Electrocautery

Arthroscopic electrocautery or radiofrequency units include a control box and a connecting cable, with a handpiece or tip, of which there are several designs. Electrocautery/radiofrequency generates heat by creating molecular friction in tissues, which is useful for cauterising vessels and for ablating tissue, like proliferated synovium, diseased cranial cruciate ligament, damaged menisci and the fat pad of the stifle joint. Monopolar electrocautery directs electrical current from the instrument tip to the tissue surface, through the patient's body to the earth plate, while bipolar units create an arc of electrical energy that travels through the tissues and fluid at the instrument tip and back to the anode of the instrument tip. As a consequence, the zone of heated tissue is more controlled. The heat generated by arthroscopic electrocautery is potentially damaging to articular cartilage and care must be taken to avoid excessive heating of cartilage peripheral to the surgical lesion within the articular environment.

Arthroscopic tower

A wheeled trolley or tower is required to keep the camera control unit, monitor, light source, pressure pump, recording device, electrocautery unit and any additional equipment together and conveniently mobile to allow movement of the gear around the operating room. Arthroscopy towers are of sturdy construction so that they can comfortably withstand the weight of the various items of equipment (Fig. 2.16).

Equipment care

Arthroscopic equipment should be cleaned with a suitable mild detergent immediately following each arthroscopic procedure. Surgical instruments

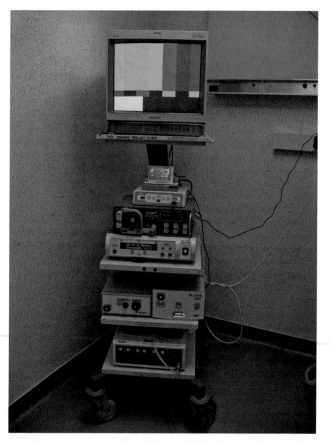

Fig. 2.16 Arthroscopy tower in which multiple items of equipment are housed; consequently, sturdy construction is important.

can be maintained using traditional methods for surgical instruments; for example ultrasonic cleaning with an enzymatic detergent product, prior to rinsing and steam sterilisation. The arthroscope, the camera and light cables should not be ultrasonically cleaned; they can be cleaned by wiping, then sterilised using ethylene oxide, or by cold sterilisation in glutaraldehyde solution immediately prior to use.

Principles of arthroscopic investigation and surgery

Arthroscopic investigation or treatment must be preceded by a thorough clinical and orthopaedic examination and, in most cases, a radiological study that localises disease to the joint or joints of concern.

While only a small region of skin requires clipping and aseptic preparation for arthroscopic surgery it is generally prudent for all but the most

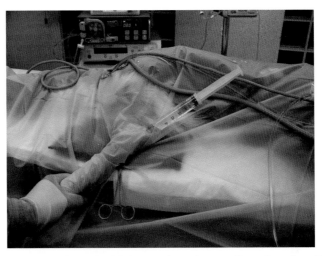

Fig. 2.17 Patient draped with impervious drape adhesed to the elbow joint using surgical adhesive spray.

routine of procedures to clip and prepare the limb as for open surgery, since sometimes it is necessary to convert the arthroscopic procedure to an open arthrotomy and it is preferable to have the patient suitably aseptically prepared for such an eventuality. To keep the patient protected from the arthroscopic irrigation fluids, an impervious drape should be applied to the arthroscopic approach surface of the joint, with the drape being large enough to prevent wetting of the patient. Either a self-adhesive drape or alternatively an adhesive spray should be used to retain the impervious drape on the surgical field (Fig. 2.17). Beyond the surgical field, clips or clothes pegs can be applied to fix the drape to the operating table, maintaining the slippery drape in its intended position.

Arthroscopy is a surgical procedure and penetrating the joint, and distracting and twisting the limb to open joint spaces, are painful events that require anaesthesia and appropriate analgesia. In addition to systemically administered analgesic agents and to inhalational anaesthetic agents, intra-articular administration of local anaesthetic (e.g. ropivacaine 0.75%, 1–2 ml) a few minutes prior to commencement of arthroscopy can improve intra-operative pain control. Similarly, postoperatively an intra-articular injection of a combination of ropivacaine (0.75%, 1–2 ml, not exceeding 2 mg/kg) and morphine (0.1 mg/kg) can augment the efficacy of the analgesic protocol used.

The operating room should be prepared with some thought, so that the surgeon, the patient and the arthroscopy tower are all aligned, with the surgeon looking directly beyond the patient at the monitor on the arthroscopy tower (Fig. 2.18). This alignment of patient and equipment is comfortable and it allows intuitive movements of the arthroscope and instruments. Once connected to the arthroscope, it is important to

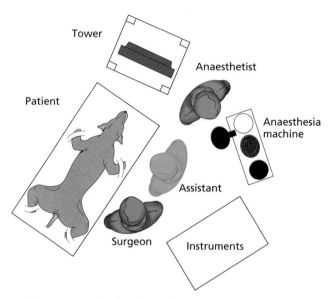

Fig. 2.18 Theatre organisation for arthroscopy. The surgeon, the patient and the arthroscopy tower are all aligned, with the surgeon looking directly beyond the patient at the monitor on the arthroscopy tower.

maintain the camera orientated correctly so that excursions inside the joint capsule correlate with the image viewed on the monitor. For this reason the camera is held in a fixed orientation (normally with the camera cable pointing towards the surgeon's midriff). To make use of the increased field of view facilitated by the 30° viewing angle, the scope is rotated on its axis by moving the light post and cable. A fully functional surgical operating table should be used to allow tilting and elevation/lowering of the table to facilitate easy access to all surfaces of the joint under investigation. Patient tilting is especially important for stifle arthroscopy, when positioning the dog in a reclined dorsal recumbency facilitates the most convenient arthroscopic examination. Positioning aids such as sandbags, vacuum beanbags and ties are necessary to position the patient prior to draping and to act as a fulcrum or to assist distracting a joint to improve arthroscopic access.

Prior to performing any preparatory procedure the light post is connected to the arthroscope sleeve and the light source is activated, the scope is inserted into the cannula and the camera head is fixed to the scope eyepiece. Focus is adjusted by directing the tip of the scope close up to a sterile surgical swab, brightness is adjusted at the light source and white balance is performed and confirmed while the swab is viewed. Once the equipment is set up and the image quality is satisfactory, the arthroscopic procedure can progress. Generally, the arthroscopic procedure proceeds with three preliminary steps, as described below.

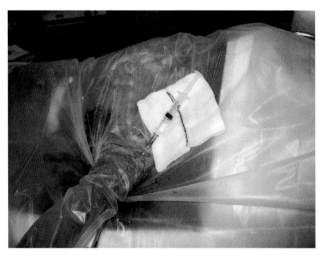

Fig. 2.19   Before injecting local anaesthetic, joint fluid is withdrawn and assessed.

- First, a needle (normally 22 or 19 gauge and 40–50 mm) is inserted into the joint and joint fluid is aspirated and retained for assessment (gross or cytologic) and the joint is distended by syringe with arthroscopic lavage fluid containing ropivacaine (dose as discussed above). Thumb pressure is maintained on the syringe to maintain distension of the joint while retaining the access to the joint cavity (Fig. 2.19).

- Second, the access point for the arthroscope is determined and confirmed by inserting a needle in the location and direction intended for the arthroscope. When the correct location and direction are identified, the needle enters the joint space, gliding between the opposing two articular surfaces. It can be helpful to maintain this 'locator' needle in position to ensure subsequent correct position and orientation of the arthroscope cannula and trocar. A stab incision is made in the skin that follows the needle down to the joint capsule and the arthroscope cannula with blunt trocar inserted is introduced into the joint, following the same path as the locator needle (Figs 2.20 and 2.21). Correct insertion of the cannula is confirmed when the trocar is removed and irrigation fluid egresses from the cannula. The arthroscope is carefully inserted through the cannula, the Luer lock is locked into position and irrigation fluid is connected to the scope cannula, making the needle the egress cannula (Fig. 2.22). The locator needle is removed, while the 'distension' needle is retained to allow egress of fluid. It is often helpful to replace or augment the distension needle with a larger needle (19–14 gauge) to provide a superior fluid egress.

- Thirdly, the instrument portal is identified by insertion of a needle at the appropriate location. Fluid egress occurs as the needle punctures

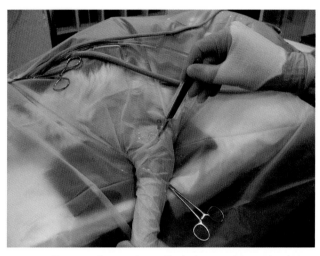

Fig. 2.20   A small-gauge 'locator' needle is inserted into the joint space and a soft-tissue tunnel is created with a no. 11 scalpel blade following the direction of the needle.

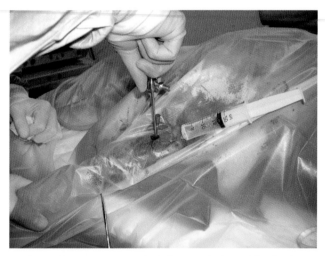

Fig. 2.21   The arthroscope cannula is inserted alongside the locator needle.

the joint capsule and correct direction of the needle is confirmed when the needle tip becomes visible in the arthroscopic field of view. Tri-angulation of the needle tip is usually achieved by inserting the needle parallel to and less than 1 cm from the arthroscope cannula, aiming to place the needle tip a few millimetres in front of the viewing angle of the scope tip, taking care to orientate the light post accordingly. The needle should be directed so as to avoid crossing the scope tip,

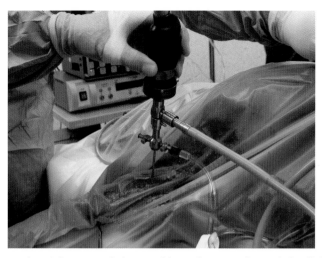

Fig. 2.22 The arthroscope is inserted into the cannula, and the fluid ingress is transferred to the arthroscope sleeve.

where the needle will not be visible through the arthroscope. Care should be taken to insert the needle sufficiently far from the scope such that when the needle is replaced with an instrument the surgeon's instrument hand does not interfere with handling of the scope. Once a suitable location and direction of needle is obtained, a stab incision is made along the path of the needle to the joint capsule and the instrument cannula with trocar is inserted along the needle path. The needle and trocar are removed and arthroscopic surgery commences through the instrument cannula.

Diagnostic arthroscopic investigations

Arthroscopic evaluation enables direct visualisation of intra-articular structures, generally giving a markedly superior assessment of the anatomy and any pathophysiological changes within the joint compared with the findings achieved from imaging techniques and traditional open arthrotomy. Using a systematic arthroscopic investigative approach, the majority of the articular space is directly visualised and the appearance of articular cartilage, synovium and intra-articular structures (e.g. intra-articular ligaments, tendons, menisci, etc.) can be accurately assessed. The detailed and magnified view obtained from a systematic examination of the joint enables the creation of a map or chart of the joint on which the integrity of articular structures, or pathological changes thereof, and their degree can be recorded. In addition, the functional integrity of intra-articular structures can be assessed by manipulation and by probing, which can identify pathological changes that are not immediately evident from visual inspection alone.

Recording the arthroscopic findings on a standardised chart (see Table 2.1) of the joint space enables a logical and reproducible method of documenting articular health and disease. A standardised recording chart for each joint enables comparison of arthroscopic findings within a single patient, when monitoring serial changes and for comparison between patients. Furthermore, the adoption and use of universally accepted charts for mapping the findings of arthroscopic investigations will facilitate exchange and sharing of information that is readily widely understandable.

Cartilage lesions are graded according to a modified Outerbridge system that has gained wide acceptance in veterinary orthopaedics (see Table 2.2).

Investigative arthroscopy of the elbow joint

A medial approach enables examination of the majority of the structures that are commonly affected in diseases of the elbow joint. A 2.4 mm arthroscope is suitable for large-breed dogs and for immature medium-sized dogs that have marked joint effusion and joint laxity, since the 2.4 mm scope can be inserted readily into these joints. A 1.9 mm scope is better suited for smaller dogs and for those without marked effusion and joint laxity. The ideal position for the arthroscope portal is distal and slightly caudal to the medial epicondyle (see Chapter 3 in this volume for more details), since this gives a good view of the entire medial side of the joint including:

- the anconeus,
- the ulnar trochlear notch,
- the coronoid (lateral, central and medial),
- the radial head (medial aspect),
- the medial aspect of the humeral condyle (cranial, central and caudal regions),
- the lateral aspect of the humeral condyle (axial region).

Following scope insertion into the joint and transfer of fluid ingress onto the arthroscope cannula it is helpful to establish a good egress, adjusting the position of the needle used for the initial distension of the joint, or replacing it with a larger gauge (19 gauge or larger). Once any bleeding resulting from insertion of the arthroscope has been flushed away, a systematic exploration of the joint can be performed. The camera is maintained in an upright orientation such that the proximal aspect of the joint is always at the top of the viewed image and a systematic

Table 2.1　Arthroscopic assessment of the elbow joint (reproduced with permission from James L. Cook, Sean Murphy, Noel Fitzpatrick and Keiichi Kuroki)

Indicate joint(s) scoped, portals used and position of limb, and document with images or video

	Appearance, functional integrity		
Medial compartment			
Medial coronoid	Normal	Abnormal	Comments:
Medial humeral condyle	Normal	Abnormal	Comments:
Synovium	Normal	Abnormal	Comments:
Proximal compartment			
Anconeus	Normal	Abnormal	Comments:
Ulnar notch	Normal	Abnormal	Comments:
Synovium	Normal	Abnormal	Comments:
Lateral compartment			
Radial head	Normal	Abnormal	Comments:
Lateral coronoid	Normal	Abnormal	Comments:
Lateral humeral condyle	Normal	Abnormal	Comments:
Synovium	Normal	Abnormal	Comments:

Articular cartilage (draw pathology, document size and grade according to modified Outerbridge scale)

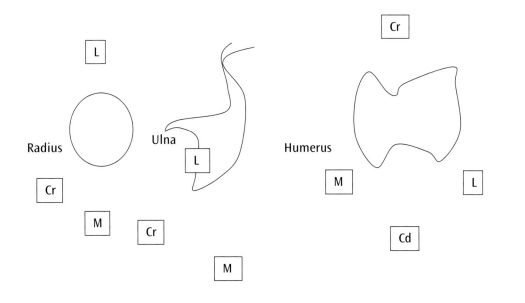

Table 2.2   Arthroscopic grades of articular cartilage lesions (modified Outerbridge scale)

Grade	Findings
0	Normal cartilage
I	Chondromalacic cartilage (soft and swollen)
II	Fibrillation
	Superficial fissuring or erosion or pitting of the cartilage surface
	Lesions do not reach subchondral bone
III	Deep fissuring that reaches subchondral bone or deep ulceration that does not reach subchondral bone
IV	Exposure of subchondral bone
V	Eburnated bone

examination of the joint normally follows the order of the structures outlined above. Hence, the light post is rotated craniodistally and the arthroscope is tilted craniodistally while the trochlear notch is maintained in view and followed proximally, leading to the anconeus. Reversal of this manoeuvre and continued tilting of the scope caudally with further caudal rotation of the light post enables examination of the distal ulnar trochlear notch and the caudomedial aspect of the radial head. Insertion of the scope slightly deeper into the elbow joint reveals the lateral coronoid and the axial edge of the lateral part of the humeral condyle. Tilting the camera further caudally brings the medial coronoid into view and the cranial and central parts of the coronoid are examined by inserting the scope slightly further into the joint.

The entire coronoid region is inspected for signs of cartilage damage and fragmentation of the craniolateral aspect of the medial coronoid. The medial aspect of the radial head should also be examined for signs of cartilage injury/disease. Progressive rotation of the light post distally while also tilting the camera distally enables inspection of the medial aspect of the humeral condyle, working from cranial, passing over the central region and finishing with the caudal portions of the condyle. The scope should be retained deep within the joint initially to inspect the axial component of the condyle, looking for evidence of the cartilage fissure that can occur with incomplete ossification of the humeral condyle in dogs of susceptible breeds. Gentle traction on the scope may be necessary to view the medial, abaxial condyle and care should be taken to avoid pulling the scope from the joint cavity during this manoeuvre. The central and cranial portions of the humeral condyle should be examined carefully since chondral lesions are common here, where the condyle articulates with the ulnar coronoid.

Following a visual assessment of the joint space an instrumented inspection of the structures may be indicated. The instrument portal is cranial to the arthroscope portal, in the region of the medial collateral ligament (see Chapter 3 for more details). The arthroscope is positioned to view the coronoid process and a needle (e.g. 22 gauge) is inserted almost parallel to the arthroscope aiming to place the needle tip into the

viewed region of the joint just cranial to the arthroscope tip. It is preferable to maintain the scope position and to manipulate the needle and
not the arthroscope until *triangulation* is achieved. A deep, 3 mm longitudinal incision is made adjacent to the needle, creating a soft-tissue
tunnel access to the joint, and a blunt trocar is directed down the soft-
tissue tunnel and into the joint cavity, passing parallel to and next to the
needle. Once the obturator is visualised by the scope, the needle is
removed. An instrument cannula is inserted into the joint over the obturator, followed by a blunt probe in exchange for the obturator. Once the
blunt probe is visualised, instrumented inspection of the joint begins.
Continued pronation of the distal antebrachium is essential to maintain
a working space within the medial aspect of the elbow joint.

The coronoid region is probed to assess the integrity of its overlying
cartilage and to determine if the coronoid region is stable or conversely
if fragmentation of the coronoid process is present. Probing of the cartilage may reveal abnormally soft cartilage, mild chondromalacia or
fissuring. If an unstable coronoid fragment is present, yellow avascular
bone is visible on the underside of the fragment and on the coronoid
bed. On occasions, a coronoid fragment remains *in situ* still covered with
a layer of cartilage, through which the yellowed avascular bone of the
fissure plane is visible. These fragments *in situ* may be easily displaced
in some cases by gentle probe pressure, or they may be rigid. Occasionally, a needle inserted into a fissure demonstrates fragment instability.

Most elbows affected by disease in the coronoid region also have
cartilaginous injury to the medial aspect of the humeral condyle. These
changes range from mild fibrillation through fissuring to flap formation
and eburnation with exposure of extensive areas of subchondral bone
(Grade 5 lesions). Mildly fibrillated or fissured chondral lesions should
be gently probed to assess the integrity of the cartilage to try to identify
loose cartilage flaps *in situ*. Examination of the humeral condyle may
identify the presence of a cartilage fissure consistent with incomplete
ossification of the humeral condyle. Confirmation of the presence of such
a fissure may be assisted by firm pronation of the antebrachium, which
can open the fissure making it more readily identifiable.

In addition to investigation of ulnar coronoid lesions (also known as
medial compartment disease), other indications for investigative elbow
arthroscopy include:

- assessment of articular cartilage integrity when there is ununited
  anconeal process (since this lesion often occurs in association with
  additional developmental pathology within the elbow),

- assessment of articular tissues, for example investigation of synovial
  disease (such as sepsis, immune-mediated disease or neoplasia),

- investigation of traumatic injuries to the articular surfaces and
  subchondral bone,

- investigation of unexplained elbow pain.

Investigative arthroscopy of the shoulder

A lateral arthroscopic approach enables a good-quality examination of all of the structures of the shoulder joint with the exception of the lateral aspect of the joint, the lateral joint capsule and the lateral collateral ligament. This is because the lateral arthroscopic approach reveals the lateral structures only at the periphery of the arthroscopic field and skill and considerable care are required for inspection of these structures because of the tendency to withdraw the arthroscope from the joint cavity while performing this manoeuvre.

The egress portal is established in the cranial compartment of the shoulder joint using an 18-gauge, 40 mm hypodermic needle. The needle is inserted caudomedially at 70° from the middle of the midpoint of the proximal ridge of the greater tubercle (see Fig. 3.12). Aspiration of joint fluid confirms intra-articular placement and once a sample of synovial fluid is obtained the joint is distended first with irrigation fluid containing 7.5% ropivacaine (1 mg/kg), then with a distending volume of irrigation fluid. When the needle is correctly placed, fluid is instilled easily and reverse pressure is detected on the syringe plunger when approximately 10 ml of fluid is instilled. Articular distension is maintained by thumb pressure on the syringe plunger by a scrubbed assistant. A few minutes are required for the onset of action of the local anaesthetic agent. The arthroscope portal is established by inserting a second needle directly vertical, just distal to the acromial process of the scapula. Fluid egress confirms intra-articular placement and the needle is advanced to the hub, confirming the correct line of penetration that travels between the articular surfaces of the humerus and of the glenoid cavity. Traction on the limb assists to widen the articular separation, facilitating this procedure. A 3 mm-long, deep incision is made into the skin and superficial soft tissues adjacent to and following the direction of the needle. The arthroscope cannula with the blunt obturator is inserted into the joint following the direction of the locator needle. Firm pressure is required to puncture the joint capsule and the index finger is placed against the shoulder to brace the scope against overinsertion into the joint while the cannula is pushed firmly through the joint capsule. The obturator is removed and fluid egress from the cannula confirms its intra-articular location. Free movement of the cannula in a craniocaudal direction but resistance to proximodistal tilting additionally confirm its location in the articular space.

When the arthroscope is inserted into the joint, the initial view generally shows the medial structures of the joint capsule. Gentle retraction of the arthroscope reveals the convex articular surface of the humeral head and the concave surface of the glenoid cavity of the scapula, enabling orientation. Continued distraction of the joint by the surgical assistant enables a systematic inspection of the structures of the shoulder joint.

In the distant foreground the cranial component of the Y-shaped medial glenohumeral ligament is visible (Fig. 2.23) adjacent to the sub-

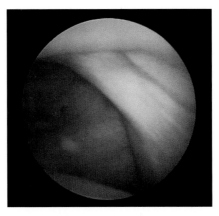

Fig. 2.23 Left shoulder, medial aspect. The cranial arm of the medial glenohumeral ligament is visible, with the subscapularis tendon of insertion in the background.

scapularis tendon of insertion; the medial aspect of the joint capsule occupies the background. The articular surface of the glenoid cavity is inspected by rotation of the light post ventrally and tilting of the arthroscope ventrally, with gentle retraction of the arthroscope, if necessary. Further rotation of the light post cranioventrally and tilting of the arthroscope cranioventrally brings the caudal glenoid cavity into view and reversal of this manoeuvre reveals the cranial glenoid cavity and the tendon of origin of the biceps brachii. Rotation of the light post further dorsally brings the tendon into view and the tendon can be followed as it enters the bicipital groove. Further caudal tilting of the arthroscope brings the arthroscope tip past the biceps tendon, allowing inspection of the cranial compartment of the shoulder joint as it surrounds this structure. Reversal of these manipulations enables a survey of the articular surface of the humeral head and brings the arthroscope back to the position of insertion.

Inspection of the caudomedial compartment of the joint is possible by cranioventral tilting of the arthroscope with rotation of the light post to view the caudal component of the medial collateral ligament. The integrity of the medial collateral ligament, the subscapularis tendon and the medial joint capsule can be further assessed by abduction of the limb. Only a small degree of abduction is normally possible and abduction is seen to tension the structures of the medial aspect of the joint. Insertion of the arthroscope over the humeral head with additional cranial tilting of the arthroscope reveals the caudal shoulder joint pouch and the caudal recess of the joint is viewed by judicious rotation of the light post.

The appearance of the articular cartilage should be evaluated using the modified Outerbridge scale (see Table 2.2), and where there are cartilage lesions it is helpful to catalogue these using a chart representing the joint surfaces (Table 2.3). Thickened cartilage or fissured cartilage

Table 2.3   Arthroscopic assessment of the shoulder joint (reproduced with permission from James L. Cook, Sean Murphy, Noel Fitzpatrick and Keiichi Kuroki)

Indicate joint(s) scoped, portals used and position of limb, and document with images or video

	Appearance, functional integrity
Cranial compartment	
Biceps tendon	comments:
Bicipital groove	comments:
Synovium	comments:
Supraglenoid tubercle	comments:
Supraspinatus insertion	comments:
Medial compartment	
Subscapularis tendon	comments:
Medial glenohumeral ligament	comments:
Synovium	comments:
Medial 'labrum'	comments:
Caudal compartment	
Caudal glenoid, 'labrum'	comments:
Synovium	comments:
Lateral compartment	
Lateral glenohumeral ligament	comments:
Synovium	comments:
Lateral 'labrum'	comments:

Articular cartilage (draw pathology, document size and grade)

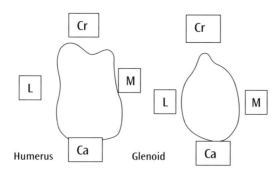

Cranial compartment:

Medial compartment:

Caudal compartment:

Lateral compartment:

should be further evaluated mechanically using an instrumented technique. The cranial aspect of the humeral head is most readily reached using an instrument placed cranially. Sometimes the ingress needle can be used for this purpose, despite the unfamiliar angulation of insertion, if triangulation has been achieved. If the ingress needle is readily visible and its direction is suitable, a cannulated instrument portal can be created following the same direction into the joint. Instrumented inspection of the middle and caudal aspects of the shoulder requires a caudally placed instrument portal. The optimal site for the caudal instrument portal is caudal and slightly distal to the tip of the acromion. In a middle-sized dog a needle is inserted into the shoulder joint approximately 2 cm caudal to the distal tip of the acromion, aiming to place the needle tip in the vicinity of the arthroscope tip, but avoiding crossing the arthroscope. For the novice arthroscopist, an aiming device is invaluable for this triangulation. Once triangulation is achieved, an instrument portal can be established following an identical path to the joint cavity. Thickened cartilage should be probed to evaluate its integrity and adhesion to underlying subchondral bone. If radiological investigation suggests the presence of an osteochondrosis lesion, arthroscopically visible fissures should be probed to check for the presence of an osteochondritis dissecans flap *in situ*.

Since shoulder disease is usually characterised by synovitis and synovial proliferation that affects the entire joint, it is rare that arthroscopic visual inspection detects only a single injured structure that is hyperaemic or fibrillated or covered in proliferated synovium and consequently identifiable as the only cause of a painful shoulder. Consequently, instrumented evaluation of the shoulder joint is also useful for assessing the integrity of the soft-tissue structures. When there is synovitis affecting the biceps tendon, instrumented probing and manipulation of the tendon can be helpful to reveal macroscopic tears in the tendon that are otherwise not visible on the surface most readily viewed. Arthroscopic inspection and probing may identify tearing of the tendon fibres or adhesion between the tendon and an inflamed and constricted bicipital groove. The blunt probe is also useful to assess the mechanical integrity of the other soft-tissue structures, including the glenohumeral ligaments and the subscapularis tendon.

Due to the risk of accidentally removing the arthroscope, inspection of the lateral aspect of the shoulder joint is performed at the end of the arthroscopy. The arthroscope is returned to its insertion position and slowly withdrawn from the joint while tilting caudally. Rotation of the light post towards the patient's shoulder joint directs the arthroscopic view laterally within the joint. The lateral aspect of humeral head and of the glenoid cavity are viewed and, in the background, the craniolateral joint capsule and caudolateral joint capsule can be inspected with careful manipulation of the arthroscope and light post. An alternative approach to the arthroscopic inspection of the lateral joint compartments uses an additional medially placed arthroscopic portal and a 'hanging limb' preparation. This technique requires a degree of experience and details are described elsewhere.

When the appearance of the soft tissue raises a suspicion of sinister disease, rather than indicating developmental, degenerative disease or traumatic injury, a biopsy forceps can be used through the instrument cannula in place of the blunt probe to obtain a tissue biopsy for his-topathological analysis and/or bacterial culture.

Investigative arthroscopy of the stifle

Current indications for investigative stifle arthroscopy include the inves-tigation of undiagnosed stifle pain or of stifle effusion of uncertain origin. Arthroscopy of the stifle joint requires some technical skill and successful arthroscopic experience in other joints is recommended prior to under-taking stifle arthroscopy. An assistant is invaluable in order to maintain the limb in a suitable position, to flex and extend the joint and to apply varus and valgus force when required during the procedure. Generally, with the patient in dorsal recumbency, a cranial parapatellar arthroscope portal is used, just lateral to the insertion of the patellar ligament. The stifle joint must be flushed with irrigation fluid throughout the arthro-scopic procedure to maintain a clear field of view because of the tendency for the intra-articular structures (fat pad and proliferated synovium) to obscure the arthroscope tip otherwise. A pressurised fluid pump is rec-ommended to achieve a constant delivery of fluid at steady pressure and a wide-lumen fenestrated egress cannula is necessary for fluid flow without extravasation into the peri-articular structures. Proliferative synovitis is commonly encountered in the stifle joint and a motorised shaver is necessary to remove excessive synovial villi and the normal fat pad from around the arthroscope tip to give a good intra-articular view. Once a clear visual path is created, which is normally several times the diameter of the arthroscope, a visual inspection of the joint is performed.

The principles of arthroscopic inspection follow the routine of inspect-ing the articular cartilage and grading cartilage lesions, where present, using the modified Outerbridge scale (Table 2.2), and recording the find-ings on a chart specific to the stifle joint (Table 2.4). The femoral con-dyles and the articular surface of the patella are viewed and inspected in a systematic manner. If osteochondrosis/osteochondritis is suspected from the diagnostic work-up, areas of thickened or fissured cartilage should be probed to identify regions of unstable osteochondritis disse-cans cartilage *in situ*.

Additionally, the integrity of the cranial and caudal cruciate ligaments is inspected visually, and by probing to establish functional integrity. The menisci are inspected for evidence of fibrillation or tearing. Obtaining a good view of the menisci is challenging, requiring coordinated valgus/varus stressing of the limb with directed rotation of the distal limb by

Table 2.4   Arthroscopic assessment of the stifle (reproduced with permission from James L. Cook, Floris Lafeber, Keiichi Kuroki, Denise Visco, Jean-Pierre Pelletier, Loren Schulz and Thomas Aigner)

Cranial cruciate ligament
- ☐ Intact, normal
- ☐ Intact, degenerative
- ☐ Partial tear, <25%
- ☐ Partial tear, 25–50%
- ☐ Partial tear, >50%
- ☐ Complete tear

Caudal cruciate ligament
- ☐ Normal
- ☐ Abnormal

Score and map articular cartilage, synovial, and meniscal pathology

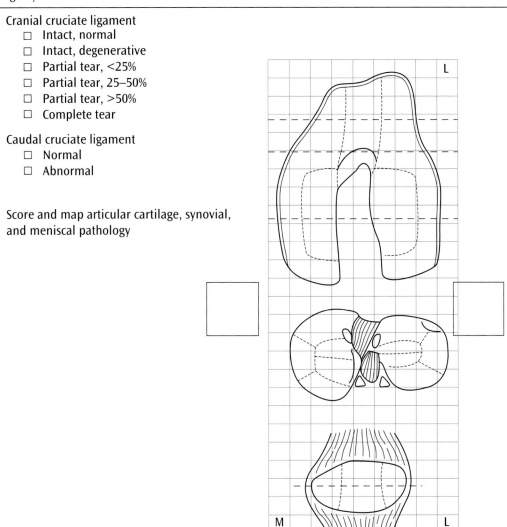

Score cartilage lesions using modified Outerbridge scale

Arthroscopic scoring of synovium
Score medial and lateral and put in boxes on diagram above

(Continued)

Table 2.4   (*Continued*)

Gross characteristics	Score
Normal: opal white, semi-translucent, smooth, with sparse, well-defined blood vessels	0
Slight: focal involvement, slight discoloration, visible proliferation/fimbriation/thickening, notable increase in vascularity	1
Mild: diffuse involvement, slight discoloration, visible proliferation/fimbriation/thickening, notable increase in vascularity	2
Moderate: diffuse involvement, severe discoloration, consistent notable proliferation/fimbriation/thickening, moderate vascularity	3
Marked: diffuse involvement, severe discoloration, consistent and marked proliferation/fimbriation/thickening, diffuse hypervascularity	4
Severe: diffuse involvement, severe discoloration, consistent and severe proliferation/fimbriation/thickening, thickening to the point of fibrosis, and severe hypervascularity	5

L, lateral; M, medial.

the surgical assistant in combination with ideal placement of the arthroscopic portal. Alternatively, a stifle distraction device (Fig. 2.14) can be used to obtain a good view of the meniscus and to increase the working space for instruments. Meniscal inspection is more readily achieved when the cranial cruciate ligament is ruptured and debrided prior to attempting to view the menisci. A blunt probe is useful to manipulate the meniscus at the same time as the cranial thrust manoeuvre is performed to identify non-displaced tears.

Investigative arthroscopy of the hip

Current indications for arthroscopic evaluation of the hip include the investigation of some forms of hip pain and the assessment of the hip joint prior to performing pelvic osteotomy surgery for hip dysplasia. With the patient in lateral recumbency, the arthroscope portal is created following the routine of first placing the locator needle to identify the joint space, followed by joint distension, and then placing the arthroscope portal at 12 o'clock with reference to the femoral head. An assistant applies traction to the limb to distract the joint space and facilitate insertion of the arthroscope. When the arthroscope is fully inserted, the soft tissues of the acetabular fossa and the round ligament of the head of the femur are initially viewed. Controlled retraction on the scope brings the acetabular cartilage into view and systematic tilting of the arthroscope with directed rotation of the light post, combined with manipulation of the limb by the assistant enables inspection of the articular surfaces of the femoral head and the acetabulum, the acetabular labrum and the joint capsule. Cartilage and soft-tissue health or disease should be recorded using a hip-joint-specific chart.

Investigative arthroscopy of the carpus and tarsus

Arthroscopic investigation and treatment of the small joints in dogs is less well established compared to the experience in the larger joints. In the carpus, investigations of arthropathies, intra-articular fractures, unexplained pain, neoplastic processes and joint instability are all current indications for investigative arthroscopy. For investigation of the carpus, the patient is positioned either in sternal recumbency or in dorsal recumbency with the limb drawn caudally, both positions giving ready access to the dorsal aspect of the carpus. Both a dorsolateral and a dorsomedial portal to the antebrachiocarpal joint are generally employed enabling both sides of the joint to be viewed. The dorsolateral arthroscope portal is located between the digital extensor tendons and the dorsomedial portal is located medial to the axial midline of the carpus, midway between the distal radial articular surface and the radial carpal bone. These two portals are used interchangeably as the egress/instrument portal and the arthroscope portal enabling examination of both the medial and the lateral components of the antebrachiocarpal joint. Inspection of intra-articular pathologies follows the normal principles of arthroscopic investigation, using joint-specific charting and performing instrumented evaluation of soft tissues and of articular cartilage to fully evaluate functional integrity of tissues.

Indications for arthroscopic investigation of the tarsus are similar to those of the carpus, including investigations of arthropathies, intra-articular fractures, unexplained pain, joint instability, neoplastic processes and investigation of osteochondrosis. Arthroscopic investigation of the entire tarsus requires the use of two dorsal portals and two plantar portals to fully evaluate the joint space but investigation for synovial biopsy or investigation of lesions localised to one side of the joint (as determined by diagnostic work-up) require only one or two portals. Patient positioning is important to ensure that the hind limb can be manipulated in all planes during the procedure because the tarsal joint space is small and obtaining a good view of the area of interest can be challenging. It is useful to position the patient with the distal limb hanging from the edge of the operating table to maximise excursions during arthroscopy. Arthroscopic inspection and evaluation are assisted by blunt probing to evaluate soft tissues and cartilage and biopsy/grasping forceps are invaluable for tissue sampling.

Further reading

Åkerblom, S. and Sjöström, L. (2006) Villonodular synovitis in the dog: a report of four cases. *Veterinary and Comparative Orthopaedics and Traumatology* 19, 87–92.

Åkerblom, S. and Sjöström, L. (2007) Evaluation of clinical, radiographical and cytological findings compared to arthroscopic findings in shoulder joint lameness in the dog. *Veterinary and Comparative Orthopaedics and Traumatology* 20, 136–141.

Bardet, J.F. (1998) Diagnosis of shoulder instability in dogs and cats: a retrospective study. *Journal of the American Animal Hospital Association* 34, 42–54.

Beale, B.S., Hulse, D.A., Schulz, K. and Whitney, W.O. (2003) *Small Animal Arthroscopy*. Saunders, Philadelphia, PA.

Case, J.B., Hulse, D., Kerwin, S.C. and Peycke, L.E. (2008) Meniscal injury following initial cranial cruciate ligament stabilization surgery in 26 dogs (29 stifles). *Veterinary and Comparative Orthopaedics and Traumatology* 21, 365–367.

Chow, J.C.Y. (2001) *Advanced Arthroscopy*. Springer Verlag, Berlin.

Cook, J.L. and Cook, C.R. (2009) Bilateral shoulder and elbow arthroscopy in dogs with forelimb lameness: diagnostic findings and treatment outcomes. *Veterinary Surgery* 38, 224–232.

Devitt, C.M., Neely, M.R. and Vanvechten, B.J. (2007) Relationship of physical examination test of shoulder instability to arthroscopic findings in dogs. *Veterinary Surgery* 36, 661–668.

Ertelt, J. and Fehr, M. (2009) Cranial cruciate ligament repair in dogs with and without meniscal lesions treated by different minimally invasive methods. *Veterinary and Comparative Orthopaedics and Traumatology* 22, 21–26.

Innes, J.F. and Brown, G. (2004) Rupture of the biceps brachii tendon sheath in two dogs. *Journal of Small Animal Practice* 45, 25–28.

Jardel, N., Crevier-Denoix, N., Moissonnier, P. and Viateau, V. (2010) Anatomical and safety considerations in establishing portals used for canine elbow arthroscopy. *Veterinary and Comparative Orthopaedics and Traumatology* 23, 75–80.

Kulendra, E., Lee, K., Schoeniger, S. and Moores, A.P. (2008) Osteochondritis dissecans-like lesion of the intercondylar fossa of the femur in a dog. *Veterinary and Comparative Orthopaedics and Traumatology* 21, 152–155.

Lapish, J. and Van Ryssen, B. (2006) Arthroscopic equipment. In *BSAVA Manual of Canine and Feline Musculoskeletal Disorders*, Houlton, J.E.F., Cook, J.L., Innes, J.F. and Langley-Hobbs, S.J. (eds), pp. 177–183. British Small Animal Veterinary Association, Gloucester.

Lehmann, M. and Lehmann, K. (2004) Modification of the triangulation technique for arthroscopy of the canine shoulder joint using a new target device. *Veterinary and Comparative Orthopaedics and Traumatology* 17, 1–8.

Martini, F.M., Pinna, S. and Del Bue, M. (2002) A simplified technique for diagnostic and surgical arthroscopy of the shoulder joint in the dog. *Journal of Small Animal Practice* 43, 7–11.

Meyer-Lindenberg, A., Langhann, A., Fehr, M. and Nolte, I. (2003) Arthrotomy versus arthroscopy in the treatment of the fragmented medial coronoid process of the ulna (FCP) in 421 dogs. *Veterinary and Comparative Orthopaedics and Traumatology* 16, 204–210.

Miller, J. and Beale, B. (2008) Tibiotarsal arthroscopy – applications and long-term outcome in dogs. *Veterinary and Comparative Orthopaedics and Traumatology* 21, 159–165.

Miller, M.D. and Cole, B.J. (2004) *Textbook of Arthroscopy*, vol. 355. Elsevier, Philadelphia, PA.

Mitchell, R.A. and Innes, J.F. (2000) Lateral glenohumeral ligament rupture in three dogs. *Journal of Small Animal Practice* 41, 511–514.

Olivieri, M., Ciliberto, E., Hulse, D.A., Vezzoni, A., Ingravalle, F. and Peirone, B. (2007) Arthroscopic treatment of osteochondritis dissecans of the shoulder in 126 dogs. *Veterinary and Comparative Orthopaedics and Traumatology* 20, 65–69.

Olivieri, M., Piras, A., Marcellin-Little, D.J., Borghetti, P. and Vezzoni, A. (2004) Accessory caudal glenoid ossification centre as possible cause of lameness in nine dogs. *Veterinary and Comparative Orthopaedics and Traumatology* 17, 131–135.

O'Neill, T. and Innes, J.F. (2004) Treatment of shoulder instability caused by medial glenohumeral ligament rupture with thermal capsulorrhaphy. *Journal of Small Animal Practice* 45, 521–524.

Person, M.W. (1989) Arthroscopic treatment of osteochondritis dissecans in the canine shoulder. *Veterinary Surgery* 18, 175–189.

Pettitt, J.F. and Innes, J.F. (2008) Arthroscopic management of a lateral glenohumeral ligament rupture in two dogs. *Veterinary and Comparative Orthopaedics and Traumatology* 21, 302–306.

Ridge, P. (2009) Feline shoulder arthroscopy using a caudolateral portal, a cadaveric study. *Veterinary and Comparative Orthopaedics and Traumatology* 22, 289–293.

Riener, S., Lehmann, K., Lorinson, D. and Skalicky, M. (2009) The cranial instrument port in arthroscopy of the canine shoulder joint. *Veterinary and Comparative Orthopaedics and Traumatology* 22, 295–302.

Saunders, W.B., Hulse, D.A. and Schulz, K.S. (2004) Evaluation of portal locations and periarticular structures in canine coxofemoral arthroscopy: a cadaver study. *Veterinary and Comparative Orthopaedics and Traumatology* 17, 184–188.

Schulz, K.S., Holsworth, I.G. and Hornof, W.J. (2004) Self-retaining braces for canine arthroscopy. *Veterinary Surgery* 33, 77–82.

Strobel, M.J. (2002) *Manual of Arthroscopic Surgery*. Springer Verlag, Berlin.

van Bree, H.J. and Van Ryssen, B. (1998) Diagnostic and surgical arthroscopy in osteochondrosis lesions. *Veterinary Clinics of North America, Small Animal Practice* 28, 161–189.

van Bree, H.J., Degryse, H., Van Ryssen, B., Ramon, F. and Desmidt, M. (1993) Pathologic correlations with magnetic resonance images of osteochondrosis lesions in canine shoulders. *Journal of the American Veterinary Medical Association* 202, 1099–1105.

Vandevelde, B., Van Ryssen, B., Saunders, J.H., Kramer, M. and Van Bree, H.J. (2006) Comparison of the ultrasonographic appearance of osteochondrosis lesions in the canine shoulder with radiography, arthrography, and arthroscopy. *Veterinary Radiology & Ultrasound* 47, 174–184.

Van Ryssen, B. (2006) Principles of arthroscopy. In *BSAVA Manual of Canine and Feline Musculoskeletal Disorders*, Houlton, J.E.F., Cook, J.L., Innes, J.F. and Langley-Hobbs, S.J. (eds), pp. 184–192. British Small Animal Veterinary Association, Gloucester.

Vermote, K.A.G., Bergenhuyzen, A.L.R., Gielen, I., van Bree, H.J., Duchateau, L. and Van Ryssen, B. (2010) Elbow lameness in dogs of six years and older. Arthroscopic and imaging findings of medial coronoid disease in 51 dogs. *Veterinary and Comparative Orthopaedics and Traumatology* 23, 43–50.

Werner, H., Winkels, P., Grevel, V., Oechtering, G. and Böttcher, P. (2009) Sensitivity and specificity of arthroscopic estimation of positive and negative radio-ulnar incongruence in dogs, an in vitro-study. *Veterinary and Comparative Orthopaedics and Traumatology* 22, 437–441.

Wiemer, P., van Ryssen, B., Gielen, I., Taeymans, O. and van Bree, H.J. (2007) Diagnostic findings in a lame-free dog with complete rupture of the biceps brachii tendon – a case report in a unilaterally affected working Labrador Retriever. *Veterinary and Comparative Orthopaedics and Traumatology* 20, 73–77.

Chapter 3
Operative Arthroscopy
Martin R. Owen

Arthroscopically assisted surgery of the canine elbow

Indications for arthroscopic surgery of the elbow include:

- medial compartment disease,
- ununited anconeal process,
- septic arthritis.

Whereas arthroscopic procedures probably have reduced risk of infection compared to open surgeries, perioperative antimicrobial therapy is recommended following standard surgical protocols. Elbow arthroscopy is routinely performed from the medial aspect of the elbow joint since most lesions affecting the elbow can be investigated and treated with access to the joint from the medial aspect. A 2.4 mm arthroscope is recommended for elbow arthroscopy in large-breed dogs since this scope gives a good field of view and the fluid flow rates are suitable to maintain a clear view during surgical procedures. A 1.9 mm scope is preferable in smaller elbow joints in order to access the joint without risking iatrogenic damage to articular surfaces and to navigate the articular space without interfering with the surgical instruments in the limited space. However, this small arthroscope yields a significantly reduced field and depth of view hence greater arthroscopic skill is required to perform procedures. The resistance to fluid flow rate of the standard 2.2 mm-diameter cannula surrounding the 1.9 mm scope requires a pressure pump and, even with pressurised fluid flow, achieving adequate fluid

Clinical Manual of Small Animal Endosurgery, First Edition. Edited by Alasdair Hotston Moore and Rosa Angela Ragni.
© 2012 Blackwell Publishing Ltd. Published 2012 by Blackwell Publishing Ltd.

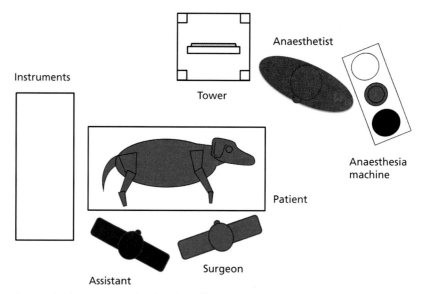

Fig. 3.1 Theatre organisation for elbow arthroscopy. The surgeon and the assistant are on the side of the laterally recumbent patient, and the arthroscopy tower is located on the opposite side.

irrigation can be problematic. A 3.5 mm-diameter high-fluid-flow cannula is available for the 1.9 mm scope which helps to maintain a haemorrhage-free view when performing surgery; this high-flow cannula is useful when allowed by the size of the joint treated.

The patient is positioned in lateral recumbency with the upper limb tied caudally along the side of the thorax and the surgical limb laid on the operating table, with the elbow joint positioned on a sandbag, near the edge of the operating table (Fig. 3.1). Prior to giving intra-operative analgesia, aspiration of joint fluid confirms intra-articular placement and allows sampling for analysis for conditions for which joint fluid analysis contributes to the diagnostic work-up. Intra-articular preoperative analgesia is delivered using a combination of 1–3 ml of 7.5% ropivacaine with 0.1 mg/kg morphine (Fig. 3.2). The injection needle is inserted into the joint space from caudal, alongside the olecranon, passing the needle under the medial epicondyle. Following injection, the needle and syringe are left in place. During the few minutes of onset of the analgesia, the theatre trolley is organised, the patient is draped using an adhesive fluid-impervious drape and the arthroscopy equipment is set up and prepared. This should include confirmation that the arthroscope is appropriately focused and white-balanced, the irrigation system is operating and the monitor and the recording equipment are functioning.

Surgically assisted elbow arthroscopy requires three portals: the egress, the arthroscopic portal and an instrument portal (Fig. 3.3). The egress portal is already established by the preoperative analgesia injection and transfer of syringes to a 10 or 20 ml syringe enables distension of the

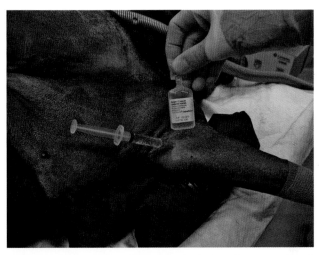

Fig. 3.2 Ropivacaine is injected intra-articularly prior to performing arthroscopic surgery.

joint with irrigation fluid (lactated Ringer's solution; Figs 3.4–3.6). Easy injection and detection of back pressure on the syringe plunger confirm correct needle location in the articular space. Maintenance of plunger pressure is helpful to keep the joint distended while making the arthroscope portal. The medial epicondyle of the humerus is palpated and the orientation of the long axis of the humerus is confirmed. With reference to a radiograph of the patient's elbow joint, the humero-ulnar joint space is estimated as it lies distal to the epicondyle. At this level, a point approximately 5 mm caudal to the medial epicondyle is used and a 'locator' needle is inserted perpendicular to the skin surface, dropping vertically into the joint space (Fig. 3.7). Fluid egress confirms puncture of the joint pouch, but placement between the articular surfaces of the humero-ulnar joint requires deeper penetration (Fig. 3.3). The soft-tissue tunnel arthroscope portal is created with a 2–3 mm skin incision made with a no. 11 or 15 blade (Fig. 3.8) and subsequently the arthroscope cannula and blunt obturator are inserted into the joint space directly following the direction of the locator needle. It is helpful for the assistant to distract the medial aspect of the joint space through a combination of pronation and valgus stress on the distal antebrachium. The surgeon braces the cannula against the skin surface of the elbow to avoid overzealous and deep penetration of the joint that can damage articular structures. Once the joint is entered, the trocar is removed and fluid escapes from the cannula, confirming correct placement. Vigorous flushing using the remaining fluid in the distension syringe expels bleeding created during scope insertion. The arthroscope is inserted and locked with a Luer-lock to the cannula and the pressurised fluid line is connected to the scope cannula, while the fluid egress is enlarged, if necessary, by placing a large-bore needle (14 gauge) alongside the needle used for

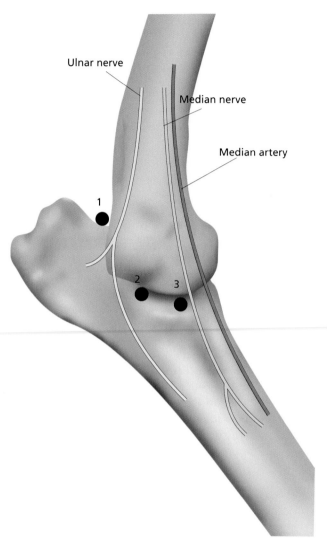

Ulnar nerve

Median nerve

Median artery

1

2   3

Fig. 3.3 Medial view of the elbow joint showing portal locations: 1, egress portal; 2, arthroscopic portal; 3, instrument portal.

distension of the joint. Using an irrigation pump, a fluid-ingress pressure of 70–100 mmHg with low flow (up to 20%) is recommended. A floor fluid-scavenging device should be positioned and suction turned on to collect waste irrigation fluid (see Fig. 2.8).

The joint should be systematically explored (see Chapter 2 in this volume) and the arthroscopic view is returned to the craniomedial compartment of the joint. Next the instrument portal is created as follows: approximately 10 mm cranial to the arthroscope portal a 22-gauge needle is inserted perpendicular to the skin and almost parallel to the scope, aiming to place the needle tip into the articular space, just cranial to the

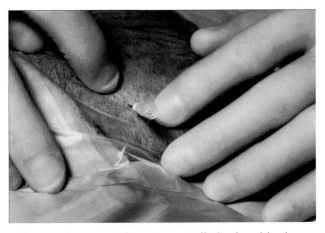

Fig. 3.4 Elbow arthroscopy. The egress needle is placed in the caudolateral joint pouch (right elbow, cranial to the right).

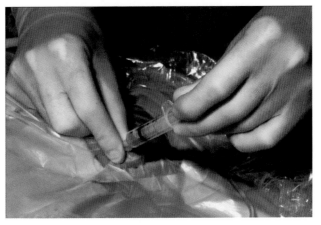

Fig. 3.5 Elbow arthroscopy. Joint fluid is aspirated to confirm intra-articular placement of the needle.

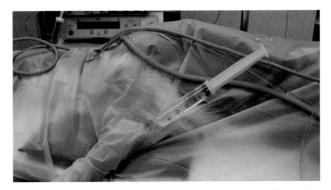

Fig. 3.6 Elbow arthroscopy. The joint is penetrated and distended with irrigation fluid.

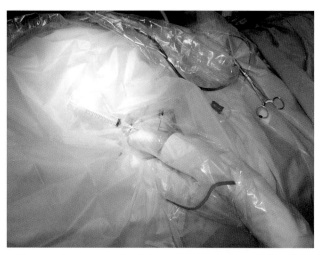

Fig. 3.7   Elbow arthroscopy. The locator needle is inserted to identify the joint line.

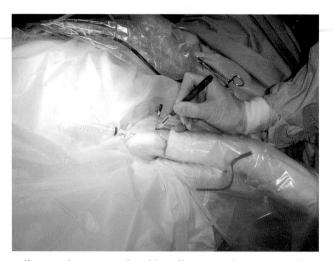

Fig. 3.8   Elbow arthroscopy. The skin adjacent to locator needle is incised prior to inserting the arthroscope sleeve with the obturator.

arthroscope tip. Attempts to puncture the joint too far cranially do not enable the needle tip to reach the arthroscopic view while placement too close to the scope results in too little working space to handle the arthroscopic instruments next to the scope. Once the joint space is located and the needle is inserted the most common reason for failing to view the needle tip is that the needle has been placed so as to cross the shaft of the scope. Redirecting the needle more parallel to the scope normally brings the needle into view. Redirection of the needle is more useful than moving the scope, since the latter is already correctly positioned and the former is not. Once *triangulation* is achieved, the instrument portal is created by incising the skin as previously described and inserting a blunt trocar directly along the path of the triangulation needle. The triangulation needle is removed and an instrument cannula is slipped over the trocar and into the articular space.

Arthroscopic investigation of dogs affected with elbow disease has contributed considerably to our current understanding of the lesions traditionally grouped together as 'elbow dysplasia'. The magnified view achieved arthroscopically has led to the recognition that lesions that were historically considered as isolated conditions often occur concurrently. This is especially true for lesions of the medial aspect of the humeral condyle and of the ulnar coronoid process and hence the term medial compartment disease has become popular to describe this common manifestation of elbow dysplasia. While in most clinical cases affected with either medial humeral condylar disease or ulnar coronoid disease it is probable that there is a degree of pathology in both areas, for the sake of clarity the following discussion will deal with each condition separately.

Arthroscopically assisted surgery of medial coronoid lesions of the ulna

A variety of appearances of the medial coronoid process of the ulna characterise different manifestations of its disease. The mildest arthroscopic appearance of disease shows softening of the articular cartilage while at the other end of the scale there may be eburnation of cartilage exposing subchondral bone, often with a completely separated fragment from the coronoid process (Fig. 3.9). When the arthroscopic changes appear mild, a blunt probe is used to palpate the surface of the coronoid process. The cartilage may appear softened, or there may be the impression of a linear indentation in the cartilage crossing the coronoid process due to a fissure line in the subchondral bone beneath. Firm pressure

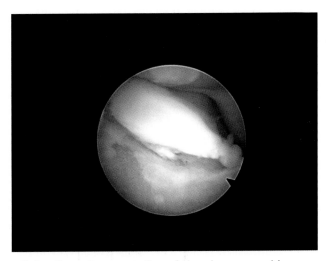

Fig. 3.9 Right elbow. Fragmentation of the ulnar coronoid process. The medial aspect of the radial head is visible in the background.

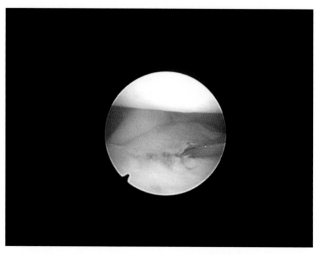

Fig. 3.10 A needle can be used to determine whether a coronoid fragment is unstable.

directed on the tip of such a lesion, away from or towards the arthroscope, may reveal an unstable coronoid fragment disguised by overlying cartilage (Fig. 3.10). Sometimes, directed pressure using a 'banana' knife or a needle into such a fissure line dislodges a fragment that is lying *in situ*. When the articular cartilage overlying a coronoid lesion looks normal, gentle probing easily identifies diseased cartilage as abnormally softened and gentle palpation of such cartilage often demonstrates its fragility, displacing it from the diseased underlying bone. Cartilage displacement or deliberate debridement reveals yellowed, relatively avascular subchondral bone. In such cases, current practice is to remove the abnormal cartilage and the yellowed avascular bone using a hand burr or a motorised shaver burr until healthy, bleeding subchondral bone is reached (Fig. 3.11). The debridement instrument may need to be removed intermittently and replaced with a probe while the joint is flushed to remove the debris and to maintain a clear field of view. Temporary arrest of irrigation enables evaluation of the subchondral bed to look for signs of healthy, bleeding subchondral bone. Once all the diseased coronoid subchondral bone is removed right up to the medial edge of the radial head and there is a healthy bed of bleeding subchondral bone, then healing takes the place through the formation of fibrocartilage which covers the exposed vascular subchondral bone.

Histomorphometric studies and bone mineral density studies performed on coronoid processes taken from dogs affected with coronoid disease indicate that injury extends throughout the medial coronoid process. Consequently, some workers advocate aggressive debridement of the coronoid process to the level of three or four widths of the burr (which is normally approximately 1 mm in diameter) below the height of the radial head, attempting to achieve an arthroscopic subtotal coro-

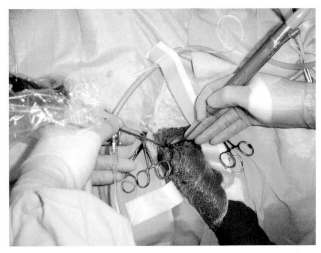

Fig. 3.11 Elbow arthroscopy. Diseased coronoid is removed using a motorised burr.

noidectomy. The efficacy of outcome of this more substantial coronoid debridement technique has not yet been objectively studied or reported despite widespread use of the technique. An arthroscopically assisted osteotome technique has been described to perform a subtotal ostectomy of the coronoid process, which may be indicated to remove the diseased coronoid tissue in its entirety. Clinical reports of efficacy or superiority of this technique are currently lacking. A large, modified instrument portal is used to insert an arthroscopic osteotome and following the osteotomy of the coronoid process the fragment is retrieved using large crocodile forceps. Some workers perform one or other of these more radical debridement procedures for the treatment of all of the arthroscopic manifestations of coronoid disease because the arthroscopic appearance does not seem to correlate with the extent of the disease in the underlying subchondral bone.

When the arthroscopic view, assisted by probing when necessary, reveals a separated fragment of the coronoid process, it is common practice to remove the fragment *en masse*. Soft-tissue attachments are severed using the meniscectomy tool, which is a protected knife, enabling safer cutting in the limited distant view. Soft-tissue attachments generally require severance cranial and lateral to the fragment. Once the fragment is loosened, grasping forceps are inserted and judiciously manipulated so that the fragment occupies the entire length of their jaws, thus maximising the grip on the fragment. The fragment is carefully retrieved using an initial twisting motion to tear remaining soft tissues prior to retrieval through the instrument cannula. When the fragment is large, resistance is detected as the open jaws of fragment holders impinge upon the cannula. Under such circumstances, the grip is maintained on the fragment and the grasping forceps are withdrawn concurrently with the cannula, drawing the fragment through the soft-tissue envelope. If the fragment is very large, it is necessary to increase the size of the instrument portal to accept sufficiently large grasping forceps for retrieval. In this circumstance it is preferable to work without using an instrument cannula to enable retrieval of a large fragment directly through the soft tissues. Large fragments can also be removed piecemeal by breaking off manageable fragments with the grasping forceps. Care should be taken to avoid damaging the delicate forceps when using this technique. A third method to remove a separated coronoid fragment is to burr the fragment using a hand burr or a power burr. Motorised burring has the advantage of being rapid; furthermore, the suction attached to the burr sleeve efficiently removes the osteochondral debris, maintaining a clear view and preventing loss of debris into the joint space. Some workers continue to debride the coronoid region to several burr diameters below the height of the articular surface of the radial head in an attempt to remove additional diseased bone from the coronoid process. The therapeutic value of this technique has not been assessed and the rationale behind this deliberate removal of subchondral bone from the coronoid bed is the highly variable outcome observed among clinical cases following simple retrieval of the coronoid fragment without additional treatment of the lesion. Following lavage of the joint to remove debris, remaining lavage fluid is aspirated using the egress needle and portals are closed with simple skin sutures. A repeat injection containing ropivacaine with morphine is given using the same doses as calculated for the preoperative administration to augment the postoperative analgesia protocol.

Arthroscopically assisted surgery of osteochondral lesions of the medial aspect of the humeral condyle

A change in the understanding of elbow dysplasia has led to a shift in the description of the lesions typically seen affecting the medial humeral condyle that were traditionally known as osteochondrosis. Histopathological analysis of these lesions has identified similar pathological changes to those seen in the 'transchondral fracture' that occur in traumatic injuries in adolescent human beings. Consequently, the term 'osteochondral' lesion is used to describe the flaps of cartilage and underlying subchondral bone seen affecting the medial aspect of the humeral condyle. These lesions often occur in association with arthroscopically visible disease of the coronoid process and they also occur in apparent isolation, although, in such circumstances, current opinion suggests that there is normally subchondral disease of the ulna, even if there is no grossly abnormal overlying cartilage.

The medial aspect of the humeral condyle is readily viewed and treated using the portals already described above, though sometimes it may be necessary to place the arthroscope portal a few millimetres further caudally to view the entirety of a large osteochondral lesion. The entire joint should be systematically inspected as described above for evidence of additional disease, prior to treating the humeral condylar lesion. Typically, medial humeral osteochondral lesions are visible upon insertion of the arthroscope. The caudoproximal extent of the lesion is determined by craniodistal tilting of the arthroscope with craniodistal rotation of the light post. The lesion is probed, if necessary, to identify a free edge of cartilage that can be grasped with grasping forceps. A large bite of cartilage is manoeuvred into the jaws of the grasping forceps and the cartilage is gently elevated from underlying bone. The flap is removed by gentle traction and tearing with judicious rotation of the grasping forceps to lift the flap from its attachment. Occasionally, the flap comes away as a single piece but more often multiple fragments are retrieved, revealing a crater-like defect in the subchondral bone in the condyle. Exchanging portals between the arthroscope and the instrument using a switching stick is helpful to view the lesion in its entirety and to obtain unimpeded access with the instruments. Remaining loose cartilage at the edges of the lesion is removed with a small curette, creating vertical edges. If denuded avascular bone lines the lesion without any evidence of healing fibrocartilage, stimulation of bleeding and of healing tissue may be indicated using the hand burr. Following debridement, the joint is thoroughly flushed to remove osteochondral debris and closure is routine. Prior to removal of the ingress/egress needle, intra-articular analgesia is administered using a combination of ropivacaine and morphine, as described above.

Arthroscopically assisted fixation of the ununited anconeal process

As for other manifestations of elbow dysplasia, objective outcome assessment for treatment of ununited anconeal process lesions is currently lacking. Present treatment recommendations advise re-attachment of the ununited anconeal process in skeletally immature dogs if radiological assessment indicates little evidence or only mild evidence of degenerative joint disease. Re-attachment of an ununited anconeal process is thought to provide joint stability and to decelerate progression of osteoarthritic degeneration of the joint. Ulnar osteotomy is necessary to relieve stresses acting on the anconeal process, facilitating fusion following fixation. Arthroscopic assistance of fragment re-attachment enables the surgery to be performed with less exposure to the joint compared to an open arthrotomy technique and this may result in lowered patient morbidity. The patient is positioned in dorsal recumbency and the affected limb is supported in an abducted position, allowing the surgeon maximum access to the caudomedial and caudal aspects of the elbow. Radiographs should be studied carefully prior to and throughout the procedure to assist accurate and correct implant placement. The anconeal fragment is re-attached using a lagged 3.5 mm bone screw and an anti-rotation arthrodesis wire, both of which are placed under arthroscopic guidance. Following attachment of the anconeal process, an oblique proximal ulnar osteotomy is performed in an open surgical manner using a caudal approach.

Arthroscopically assisted management of septic arthritis

Chronic septic arthritis generally requires aggressive treatment for successful resolution of infection and traditionally open surgery has been used to irrigate the joint and to mechanically agitate the synovium, perform subtotal synovectomy and to remove inspissated pus and fibrin clots. Septic arthritis should be investigated using routine laboratory protocols for bacterial culture and sensitivity, and antimicrobial treatment should be broad-spectrum, bacteriocidal and tailored to laboratory results. Arthroscopic surgical treatment of septic arthritis is effective using high volumes of pressurised fluid flow, preferably delivered by fluid pump and using a motorised shaver to agitate and to remove proliferative synovium. An instrument cannula or a wide-bore egress cannula is helpful to assist removal of fibrinous clots, blood and debris and intermittent occlusion of the egress cannula is helpful to distend the joint and elevate proliferative synovium from the field of view. Multiple portals may be necessary to access the joint thoroughly but excessive punctures should be avoided since these prevent distension of the joint and the working space is impaired. Following arthroscopic synovectomy, debridement and lavage, postoperative analgesia continues as necessary and antimicrobial treatment is generally continued for at least 4 weeks and generally for 1 week following resolution of clinical signs.

Arthroscopic surgery of the shoulder

Indications for surgical arthroscopy of the shoulder include:

- osteochondritis dissecans (or OCD),

- biceps lesions,

- treatment of glenohumeral ligament insufficiency,

- incomplete ossification of the caudal glenoid cavity,

- fracture reduction of the supraglenoid tuberosity,

- management of septic arthritis.

A standard 30° oblique arthroscope is ideally suited for shoulder arthroscopy. A 2.4 mm arthroscope is preferable for medium-sized breeds. In the giant breed, a long arthroscope is necessary to penetrate the joint through the lateral shoulder musculature and the longer length and strength of the 4.0 mm arthroscope is helpful. In small breeds, a 1.9 mm arthroscope may be better at avoiding iatrogenic damage to articular cartilage. A basic set of arthroscopic instruments is necessary for shoulder arthroscopy, comprising a blunt probe, grasping forceps, a hand burr, curettes and a switching stick. Additional instruments are necessary for some procedures, including a motorised shaver and an arthroscopic electrosurgery unit.

The patient is generally positioned in lateral recumbency, with the shoulder to be scoped uppermost. The shoulder should be aseptically prepared for open surgery in case the arthroscopic procedure must be abandoned and an open procedure performed. A hanging-limb preparation with free draping gives maximum access to the joint. First, the egress portal is established by placing a 40 mm 22–19-gauge needle into the cranial compartment of the shoulder joint. The shoulder is palpated and a point that is midway along the superior ridge of the greater tubercle of the humerus is identified. At this point, the needle is inserted caudomedially at approximately 70° from perpendicular, to penetrate the joint (Fig. 3.12). Following aspiration of joint fluid, which confirms correct

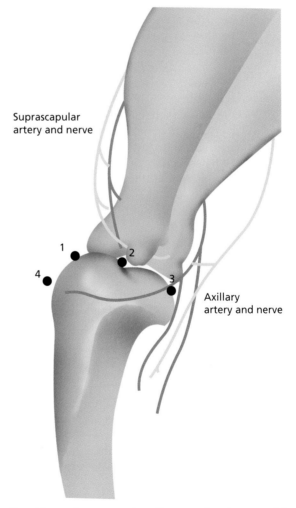

Suprascapular
artery and nerve

Axillary
artery and nerve

Fig. 3.12   Shoulder arthroscopy. Line diagram showing portal locations: 1, egress portal; 2, arthroscopic portal; 3, instrument portal; and 4, portal used to access the biceps tendon.

needle placement, the joint is distended with lactated Ringer's solution containing 2–3 ml of 7.5% ropivacaine (not exceeding 2 mg/kg) and 0.1 mg/kg morphine for a few minutes prior to further intervention. The arthroscope portal is located using a 22–19-gauge 40–50 mm needle inserted through the skin and soft tissues just craniodistal to the distal tip of the acromion, with the needle directed perpendicular to the skin and the long axis of the limb. The assistant applies traction to the limb to open the joint space easing this process and fluid egress from the needle confirms intra-articular placement. A small skin incision is created adjacent to the locator needle and the arthroscope cannula with blunt obturator is inserted firmly. A 'popping' sensation accompanies penetration of the joint capsule and fluid egress from the cannula following obturator removal confirms intra-articular insertion. During insertion of the arthroscope cannula, the surgeon's fingers brace the scope against the skin to prevent over insertion and damage to the shoulder. The arthroscope is inserted, the fluid-ingress line is connected to the scope cannula and fluid flow is activated. A 19-gauge or larger needle should be inserted, replacing the small-gauge needle used to distend the joint or, alternatively, an instrument cannula may be used as the egress portal. The entire shoulder joint should be investigated using a systematic approach, documenting pathological changes on the appropriate chart (see Table 2.3, arthroscopic assessment of the shoulder). Following thorough inspection of the joint space and intra-articular structures, the instrument portal is created approximately 1–3 cm from the arthroscope portal, depending on the size of the dog. A 40–50 mm 22–19-gauge needle is inserted into the articular space. The needle should be inserted almost parallel to the arthroscope, aiming to bring the needle tip just in front of the scope tip, which should be rotated with the view towards the needle. An instrument portal is created by incising the skin with a scalpel and inserting a switching stick and cannula through a soft-tissue tunnel adjacent to the locator needle or alternatively, following the skin incision, a soft-tissue tunnel is created by opening the tips of Metzenbaum scissors to create a large instrument portal.

Arthroscopically assisted surgery for OCD of the shoulder

In most cases, the cartilaginous flap is most evident caudally on the humeral head and has an attachment to normal cartilage at its cranial aspect (Fig. 3.13). The surgeon should decide between two surgical techniques: removal *en masse* or piecemeal removal. Smaller flaps are better suited to removal *en masse* whereas large ones tend to fragment and therefore are perhaps better suited to removal piecemeal using an instrument cannula.

The free edge of the flap is gently elevated with a probe or switching stick and a small area of attachment should be preserved to prevent the flap floating free. A large grasping forceps is inserted and the flap is firmly grasped along the length of the jaws of the forceps. Twisting the forceps

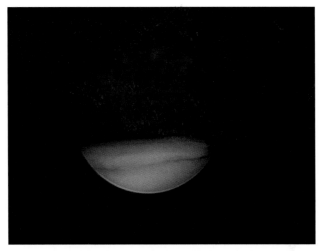

Fig. 3.13   Shoulder arthroscopy. OCD flap of the humeral head *in situ.*

along their axis while pushing the flap towards its remaining attachment frees the flap. The forceps are retrieved towards the instrument portal or cannula. If the fragment is larger than the portal, the flap is gently retained against the joint capsule and the portal is enlarged with Metzenbaum scissors prior to removal of the flap. If a cannula is employed it should be withdrawn at the same time as the forceps. If the fragment is very large it should be removed in small pieces. The fragment can be broken up using a hand burr or curette and pieces are retrieved using the graspers. Alternatively, a motorised shaver/burr can be used to break up the flap into tiny pieces of debris that are expelled from the joint by vigorous intermittent flushing.

Following removal of the flap, the edges of the cartilaginous defect are inspected and probed to check for stability and adhesion to underlying bone. Loose edges should be lifted as previously described and removed, creating vertical walls with normal cartilage surrounding the osteochondral defect. The surface of the defect created by the OCD lesion is inspected for evidence of vascularity and for fibrocartilagenous healing. According to some workers the latter is promoted by debridement of the subchondral bed using a burr with consequent creation of active bleeding. The clinical benefit of this procedure is not beyond debate and routine performance of this technique is not recommended.

Following retrieval of the OCD flap and treatment of the edge of the lesion, the joint is inspected for and cleared of loose debris and then flushed. The irrigation fluid is evacuated from the joint using the egress needle and the skin is sutured following removal of the instrument cannula and the arthroscope. An intra-articular combination of 7.5% ropivacaine (2 mg/kg) with morphine (0.1 mg/kg) is delivered through the egress needle prior to withdrawal.

Arthroscopically assisted surgery of the biceps tendon

Inflammation or injury to the biceps tendon causes shoulder pain and lameness. Examination of affected individuals may reveal shoulder pain but it is often difficult to localise which structures are the source of discomfort in a painful shoulder. Arthroscopic investigation is hence valuable in identifying biceps tendon pathology and discriminating biceps lesions from other shoulder problems. Biceps tendon pathology in dogs is still incompletely understood and direct trauma, indirect trauma and repetitive strain injury are each thought to be responsible for clinical cases of biceps disease. A degenerative process may pre-dispose the tendon to injury under physiological loading as observed in other tendon and ligament injuries in dogs. Direct trauma to the biceps tendon can lead to gross tearing of tendon fibres while indirect trauma due to compression from spinatus muscle tendonopathy and mineralisation can be responsible for damage to the biceps tendon in some cases. A diagnosis of biceps tendon pathology may be suggested by preoperative investigations but a definitive diagnosis requires arthro-scopic visualisation in most cases. Supportive investigative findings include radiological evidence of mineralisation of the biceps groove or the spinatus muscle tendons of insertion, or abnormal filling of the tendon sheath on shoulder arthrography. Ultrasonographic or magnetic resonance imaging may additionally show lesions affecting the spinatus muscles, or the substance of the biceps tendon or of the bicipital sheath.

Patient positioning for arthroscopic surgery of the biceps tendon is as described above. Generous clipping and aseptic preparation around the cranial and medial aspect of the shoulder joint are prudent in case of the necessary conversion of the procedure to an open approach. The shoul-der joint is routinely preoperatively analgesed with ropivacaine and distended with irrigation fluid. A good view of the cranial part of the shoulder joint is most readily achieved by placing the arthroscope portal slightly caudal (approximately 1 cm) to the tip of the acromion. Follow-ing insertion of the arthroscope, the entire shoulder joint is inspected and investigated for evidence of pathology and all findings are recorded. Biceps pathology is commonly identified in association with chronic synovitis and degenerative changes affecting other shoulder joint struc-tures. Care should be taken to fully evaluate the significance of patho-logical changes affecting the articular surfaces and structures of mechanical importance including the glenohumeral ligaments and the subscapularis tendon. The biceps tendon is inspected from its proximal origin on the supraglenoid tuberosity to the distal extent of the tendon in the distal recess of the biceps sheath. The tendon is evaluated for evidence of fibre tearing, inflammation and synovitis, while the biceps sheath is inspected for osteophyte formation, for synovial proliferation and for evidence of external compression of the sheath and tendon from spinatus tendonopathy. Synovial hypertrophy and proliferation are common in degenerative shoulder joints and not specific to a single structure within the joint itself. Consequently, synovial proliferation on the biceps tendon does not necessarily indicate primary disease of this structure. A blunt probe is useful to assess the integrity of the tendon and to assist visual inspection of the back of the tendon that is not readily visible. The probe is inserted through an instrument portal created just proximal and medial to the greater tuberosity (Fig. 3.12). A torn or diseased biceps tendon is transected close to its origin on the supraglenoid tuberosity. A sharp instrument (no. 11 scalpel blade, banana knife or meniscal knife) is inserted through the soft tissues of the instrument portal following the same direction as used for the blunt probe. The sharp instrument is used under direct arthroscopic guidance, transecting the tendon once the blade is in view. The tendon may also be sectioned using radiofrequency surgery (Fig. 3.14) where the equipment is available. Complete transection is confirmed when the free end of the tendon falls away into the biceps sheath upon elbow extension with shoulder flexion. Clinical reports suggest that it is not necessary to tenodese the biceps tendon.

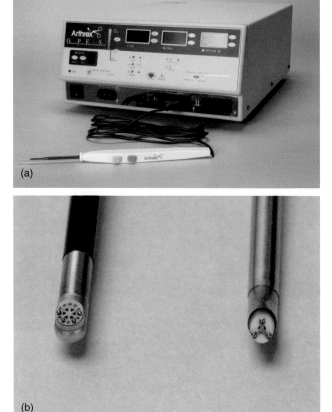

Fig. 3.14 (a) Bipolar radiofrequency unit with probe. (b) Detailed view of radiofrequency probe tips.

Severe restriction within the biceps tendon sheath is suggestive of spinatus muscle tendonopathy and when this arthroscopic finding is accompanied by supportive clinical findings and diagnostic imaging findings of spinatus tendonopathy the complex nature of the disease should be considered when planning treatment. When there is significant compromise to the integrity of the biceps tendon tenectomy is recommended. In some cases of spinatus tendonopathy shoulder pain and lameness appear to be attributable to the spinatus disease and not to indirect effects on the biceps tendon. Hence if the functional integrity of the biceps is not significantly compromised, arthroscopy should be completed, the biceps tendon should be left intact and the diseased spinatus tendon should be treated. Clinical reports indicate that spinatus tendonopathy can respond, in some cases, to intra-lesional injection with methylprednisolone and accompanied by strict rest. Surgical treatment is required for non-responders to medical treatment and a section of the spinatus tendon of insertion is excised by traditional surgery.

Arthroscopic treatment of glenohumeral ligament insufficiency

Shoulder pain and chronic forelimb lameness attributed to *shoulder instability* have become increasingly recognised following the introduction of arthroscopy to small veterinary orthopaedics because of the ability to visualise pathological changes in the support structures within the shoulder joint. Arthroscopic signs of 'wear and tear' are not uncommonly observed on shoulder arthroscopy in mature dogs and undoubtedly, because arthroscopy remains a relatively new modality, there is a risk of misinterpretation of the findings of shoulder arthroscopy. This leads to the potential for overdiagnosis of shoulder instability if arthroscopic findings are evaluated in the absence of supportive evidence from orthopaedic examination (Akerblom and Sjöström, 2007; Cogar et al., 2008). Increased shoulder abduction has been documented in sedated dogs affected with medial glenohumeral ligament insufficiency (Cook et al., 2005a) but the accuracy of the abduction angle test at correctly identifying dogs with shoulder instability has been subsequently questioned (Devitt et al., 2007).

The arthroscopic portals for investigating for shoulder instability are as described above. The medial joint capsule, the medial glenohumeral ligament and the subscapularis tendons should all be inspected along their length from their origin or most proximal extent to their insertion points and a blunt probe should be employed to investigate any signs of fibrillation or tearing to establish their significance. It can be helpful to stress the shoulder in abduction to evaluate the mechanical integrity of the medial support structures. Next, the lateral collateral ligament and the lateral joint capsule should be evaluated through controlled withdrawal of the arthroscope while at the same time tilting the scope cranially together with cranial rotation of the light post. Subsequent caudal tilting combined with caudal rotation of the light post allows examination of the structures caudal to the scope entry point. The lateral joint capsular structures are challenging to view because they are adjacent to the arthroscopic portal and care should be taken to avoid inadvertent removal of the scope during this examination.

Joint capsule and ligament tears may be partial or complete and the severity of a tear may influence the method of treatment for restoring joint stability. A partial tear may be treated by thermal contracture, using a radiofrequency probe (Fig. 3.14b) to contract the remaining intact but lengthened tissue adjacent to the tear (O'Neill and Innes, 2004; Cook et al., 2005b). Complete tears in the medial glenohumeral ligament have been treated by thermal contracture of the medial joint capsule, aiming to restore joint stability through capsular contracture alone. However, in such cases of marked laxity of the medial structures of the shoulder joint it is likely that extra-articular stabilising structures of the medial aspect of the shoulder are also compromised and the efficacy of treatment using intra-articular thermal shrinkage alone may be insufficient. Consequently, consideration should be given to performing open surgery, repairing torn or stretched structures. Imbrication of the subscapularis tendon of insertion and placement of prosthetic ligaments anchored to anatomic sites of origin and insertion have each been described for the successful management of medial instability of the shoulder joint (Pettitt et al., 2007). Biceps tendon transposition is also a useful and effective technique to restore medial shoulder stability. For radiofrequency-induced thermal capsulorrhaphy, different techniques for application of the heat source to the soft tissues are described, including 'spot welding', 'paint brushing' and 'grid lining'. Thermal shrinkage procedures risk thermal injury of articular cartilage and of peri-articular structures, hence radiofrequency surgery must be performed in a carefully controlled manner, following guidance specific to the model of equipment and for the radiofrequency probe used. High flow rates of irrigation fluid are indicated to try to prevent excess heating of the articular environment, since cartilage damage occurs at temperatures of 45°C and above (Horstman and McLaughlin, 2006).

Following thermal contracture, the treated tissues are mechanically weakened for at least 4 weeks and it is essential to prevent normal physiological loading of the tissues, which would risk stretching or tearing. Prevention of tissue loading during the recovery period is best achieved through using a non-weight-bearing sling or custom-made jacket that keeps the treated limb off the ground. Following removal of the non-weight-bearing device, re-introduction of limb use and of activity must be strictly controlled during the following weeks of the tissue remodelling and healing to prevent injury and stretching or tearing of the contracted tissues.

Lateral glenohumeral ligament injury and tears to the lateral aspect of the shoulder joint are encountered less frequently than injuries to the medial support structures. Resolution of shoulder pain and lameness has been reported following surgical stabilisation of the lateral aspect of the shoulder joint following the identification of injuries to the lateral support structures. The conventional open surgical technique uses bone anchors with suture to create prosthetic ligaments. More recently, arthroscopically placed sutures using a hanging-limb technique and a craniomedial portal to readily view the lateral aspect of the joint has been described for the management of lateral glenohumeral ligament rupture (Mitchell and Innes, 2000; Pettitt and Innes, 2008).

Following a stabilisation procedure for shoulder ligament insufficiency, the portals are closed prior to instillation with a morphine/ropivacaine combination (see above) for augmentation of the postoperative analgesia protocol.

Arthroscopically assisted surgery of the stifle joint

The patient is positioned in dorsal recumbency with the head up on a table tilted at approximately 30°. A vacuum beanbag secured to the table is used to keep the patient firmly positioned with the hind limbs able to hang over the end of the operating table. Following a routine aseptic hanging-limb preparation the joint is aspirated and instilled with 7.5% ropivacaine (2 mg/kg). The craniolateral portal is established at a landmark just lateral to the patellar tendon. Deep palpation identifies a bony protuberance on the proximal tibia that is just cranial to the long digital extensor tendon and a stab incision is made into the stifle joint just proximal to this landmark (Fig. 3.15). The stifle is held in extension and a blunt switching stick is inserted through the soft tissues and directed through the stifle joint, under the patellar ligament and the patella and pushed against the proximomedial pouch of the stifle joint. Firm pressure is applied and the skin is incised over the end of the switching stick. A fenestrated cannula is slipped over the switching stick (Fig. 3.16) into the stifle joint and the switching stick is removed. Maintaining the stifle in extension and keeping the tissues of the cranial part of the stifle lax, the cannula tip is directed over the medial trochlear ridge, settling the cannula in the medial recess of the stifle joint. Next, the arthroscope and blunt cannula are introduced through the lateral portal and advanced beneath the patella until the proximal joint pouch is detected by resistance. The obturator is withdrawn, the light post is attached, the arthroscope is inserted and motorised pressure-controlled fluid irrigation is started. The articular cartilage of the femoral trochlea, the trochlear ridges and the patella are systematically inspected and the synovium, the patellar ligament and the recesses of the stifle joint are evaluated, documenting pathological changes on a stifle-joint-specific chart. (see Table 2.4, arthroscopic assessment of the stifle)

The craniomedial portal is established, which will be used as an instrument portal. Prior to making the portal, the arthroscope is parked so that the tip lies within the intercondylar notch, viewing proximally. A

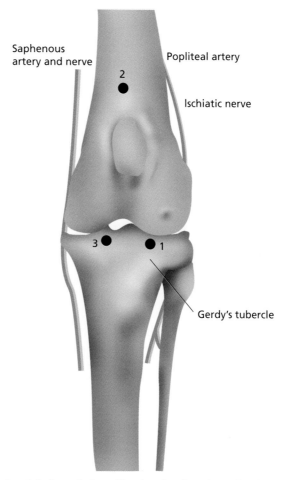

Fig. 3.15 Cranial view of the stifle showing location of arthroscopic portals: 1, arthroscopic portal; 2, egress portal; 3, instrument portal.

stab incision is made medial to the straight patellar ligament at the same proximodistal level as the lateral portal. A blunt obturator is advanced towards the intercondylar notch of the femur and passed into the arthroscopic view. Remembering the direction of insertion, the obturator is removed and replaced with a motorised shaver. The shaver blade is brought into view, with the protected surface directed towards the arthroscope tip to avoid damage to the arthroscope. Suction is activated and oscillatory shaving is performed to debride the fat pad and synovium, progressively enlarging the viewing window, sufficient to enable inspection of the cruciate ligaments and the menisci.

In human medicine, fat-pad debridement is associated with increased morbidity following arthroscopic surgery. If this is also true in veterinary patients, performing stifle arthroscopic surgery without performing fat-pad debridement may confer advantages. Using a stifle distractor

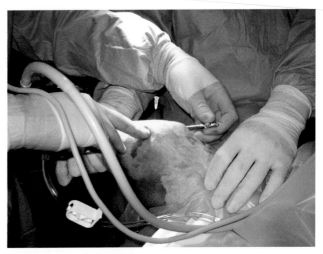

Fig. 3.16 Stifle arthroscopy requires use of a large-gauge fenestrated cannula to maintain fluid egress.

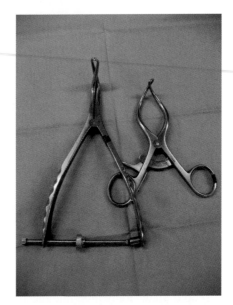

Fig. 3.17 Large and small stifle distractors. The overlapping tips enable insertion through a limited incision and distraction of articular surfaces.

originally designed for use in arthrotomies (Fig. 3.17) inserted through a mini arthrotomy enables arthroscopic inspection of the stifle joint and meniscal surgery without recourse to infrapatellar fat-pad debridement (Gemmill and Farrell, 2009). A purpose-made arthroscopic pin distractor provides sufficient view of the intra-articular structures to enable meniscal surgery without fat-pad debridement (Böttcher et al., 2009) and does not impede use of the arthroscopic instruments.

Arthroscopically assisted surgery of the cranial cruciate ligament and meniscal surgery

In dogs with cranial cruciate ligament insufficiency, currently the goals of surgery are:

- removal of the degenerate cranial cruciate ligament,

- inspection of the menisci and treatment of meniscal tears,

- restoration of stifle stability to prevent or minimise tibial subluxation during load-bearing.

Debate continues regarding the role of surgical excision of the degenerate cranial cruciate ligament in restoring stifle comfort and relieving pain in dogs affected with cranial cruciate ligament disease. Some authors claim that tibial plateau-levelling osteotomy (TPLO) surgery is protective of the diseased cranial cruciate ligament, arresting its progressive degeneration and breakdown. These authors advocate leaving a degenerate cranial cruciate ligament *in situ*, recommending solely debridement of the completely ruptured component of the ligament, preserving the intact portion of ligament. The proposed protective effect of TPLO on cranial cruciate ligament breakdown is based on reports of 'second-look' arthroscopy performed following TPLO. To date there are no histological studies that support the theory that degeneration of the cranial cruciate ligament is arrested by TPLO. In contrast, clinical evidence indicates that in many cases of cranial cruciate ligament disease failure to remove *en masse* the incompletely ruptured diseased cranial cruciate ligament results in ongoing lameness, hence the author currently recommends routine excision of diseased cranial cruciate ligament in its entirety in all cases. Removal of the diseased ligament appears to be more important when the ligament is only partially ruptured compared to when the ligament is already completely incompetent and broken down. Presumably, the process of ongoing rupture is associated with inflammation and pain and it would appear that this pain diminishes following severance or following final and complete naturally occurring rupture of the ligament. Debridement of the cranial cruciate ligament is most readily achieved using a motorised shaver.

Clinically relevant injury to the medial meniscus occurs predominantly in association with rupture of the cranial cruciate ligament. Meniscal lesions (medial and lateral meniscus) also occur in association with osteochondrosis lesions of the femoral condyle and as a consequence of traumatic injury to the stifle joint. Arthroscopic treatment of meniscal lesions is technically challenging and the surgeon should be prepared to convert the arthroscopic procedure to a limited arthrotomy in the event that the arthroscopic investigation/surgery proves unsatisfactory.

Following a systematic examination of the proximal compartment of the stifle joint, the cranial cruciate ligament is inspected visually and using a blunt probe. In most cases of cranial cruciate ligament disease grossly abnormal degenerative change, fibrillation, tearing and haemorrhage of the ligament are readily visible. Occasionally, in early disease, degeneration of the ligament may be appreciated only by careful probing, which identifies hidden torn fibres, or laxity of components of the ligament associated with fibrillation. Once a diagnosis of cranial cruciate ligament disease is made, if the lameness is not responsive to medical treatment, then surgical intervention, including removal of the degenerate ligament, meniscal surgery as required and a stifle-stabilisation procedure, are recommended to accelerate resolution of pain and lameness. The degenerate cranial cruciate ligament is debrided proximally and distally using a motorised shaver with a soft-tissue shaving tip, with the shaver in oscillating mode or using a radiofrequency probe (Fig. 3.14b), taking care to avoid excessive heating of the articular space. Care should be taken to avoid iatrogenic damage to the caudal cruciate ligament proximally and to the intermeniscal ligaments distally. Whereas cruciate ligament remnants are likely to remain, their role in promoting inflammation in the joint is no longer considered relevant.

Following removal of the cranial cruciate ligament, visualisation of the menisci is more readily achieved. The medial meniscus is inspected before the lateral meniscus since substantial lesions to the medial meniscus occur in association with cranial cruciate ligament injury and these are clinically significant. With the arthroscope tip in the intercondylar notch, the stifle is maintained in approximately 30° of flexion. The axial edge of the medial femoral condyle is followed towards the articular surface of the medial femoral condyle. The caudal pole of the medial meniscus is brought into view by controlled insertion of the arthroscope while maintaining the light post directed axially (at 3 o'clock for the right stifle and 9 o'clock for the left stifle) and the arthroscope is tilted laterally. A normal medial meniscus is pale and smooth, has a fine, smooth axial edge and there is a regular concavity to the upper surface. Fibrillation, roughening of the surface or presence of a thickened axial edge of meniscal tissue are all indicators of a probable meniscal tear (Fig. 3.18). A blunt probe is introduced through the medial portal and the functional integrity of the meniscus is assessed (Fig. 3.19). When a tear is present, the probe is used in tandem with careful visual inspection to evaluate its shape and type, since this influences the technique required for successful removal of the torn meniscal portion.

The most common substantial and significant meniscal injury that causes lameness and pain is the longitudinal vertical tear or 'bucket handle tear', in which a caudo-axial portion of the meniscus is crushed and torn such that a mid-body tear propagates in the substance of the meniscus. In the cranial cruciate-deficient stifle, continual and repeated subluxation of the tibia during the stance phase of gait pinches the medial meniscus. This creates the tear and pushes the torn portion of meniscus cranially. Continued crushing and tearing can fully sever the caudal attachment of the torn meniscal fragment, creating a large free meniscal

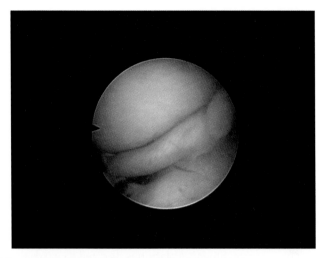

Fig. 3.18   Arthroscopic view of a meniscal tear.

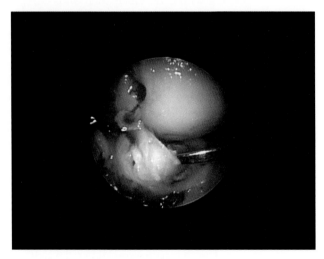

Fig. 3.19   Meniscal tear inspected with a probe.

flap that remains hinged cranially. Occasionally, other directions of meniscal tearing occur, resulting in radial tears and also in horizontal cleavage tears.

The treatment of bucket-handle tears is challenging and a sequential approach is recommended to enable removal of the lesion without its premature dislodgement, which compromises the arthroscopic view and subsequent safe and controlled removal of the torn fragment. Once the meniscal tear is visualised, prior to commencing removal, the arthroscopic window around the lesion should be evaluated and, if necessary, enlarged through additional shaving of proliferative synovium and fat pad. Once an unimpeded view is created, the torn portion is drawn cranially using a probe, and the mid substance of the fragment is firmly grasped with a grasper and maintained in mild traction by the assistant. Meniscal surgery is best performed using a radiofrequency surgery wand (Fig. 3.14b). Radiofrequency surgery produces heating of the articular environment and its injurious effect on articular cartilage should be minimised by maintaining high flow rates of irrigation fluid in the effort to prevent excessive intra-articular temperatures.

A fine-tipped tissue-ablation wand is inserted through the medial portal, proximal to the grasper and, while maintaining gentle traction on the grasper, the cranial and axial edges of the torn portion are ablated, progressing towards the normal peripheral meniscal tissue until the cranial extent of the torn portion becomes free. Inspection of the caudal attachment of the torn portion is facilitated by continued traction on the grasping forceps. Insertion of the ablation tip either proximal or sometimes distal to the grasping forceps enables severance of the caudal attachment. Ablation is directed towards the uninjured peripheral meniscal tissue with the intention of preserving maximal peripheral tissue by ablating with care. Once ablation is complete the wand is removed and the meniscal lesion is removed in the jaws of the grasper. Removal of the torn portion greatly improves the view of the remaining peripheral meniscal tissue and this is closely inspected visually; its functional integrity is determined using the probe. The cut edge of the meniscus is evaluated and additional ablation is performed, as necessary, to create a smooth axial contour to the remaining peripheral meniscus. The peripheral meniscus is probed carefully and the axial edge is gently tractioned with grasping forceps to check for additional longitudinal or horizontal tears and when such tears are identified they are treated by grasping, ablation and retrieval of the axial portion of damaged meniscus.

Following meniscal surgery the remaining peripheral meniscal tissue should be firm, the axial edge should have a smooth contour and gentle traction and probing of the meniscal tissue should confirm its functional integrity. Once medial meniscal surgery is complete the lateral meniscus is inspected. The arthroscope is tilted medially and the light post is rotated so that it remains directed axially, as mentioned previously. The inspection of the lateral meniscus commences at the caudal aspect of the joint and the caudal meniscofemoral ligament of the lateral meniscus is identified. Progressive medial tilting of the scope with controlled withdrawal enables a visual sweep over the lateral meniscus, progressing towards the cranial pole. Tiny radial tears are reported to occur, predominantly in the cranial horn and these are of unlikely clinical significance. Small longitudinal tears are also occasionally reported and because these may be of some clinical significance, when seen, they should be removed by ablation. Following meniscal surgery, the joint is irrigated copiously to remove surgical debris. Prior to the completion of surgery, if no additional regional local anaesthesia has been performed, an intra-articular injection of ropivacaine and morphine (see above) may be given to augment the postoperative analgesia protocol routinely employed.

When surgically managing cranial cruciate ligament disease in dogs, current opinion is divided as to the magnitude of any measurable clinical benefit to performing arthroscopic debridement of the cranial cruciate ligament and arthroscopic medial meniscal surgery prior to an open procedure such as TPLO. Proponents of arthroscopic investigation to treat the intra-articular component of cruciate disease in dogs suggest that the rate of occurrence of 'late' postoperative medial meniscal tears is lowered by arthroscopic investigation (Thieman et al., 2006). Other workers have not found evidence to support the benefit of arthroscopic inspection of the menisci when compared to instrumented meniscal inspection by limited arthrotomy (Fitzpatrick and Solano, 2010). It is likely that while stifle stabilisation is performed using traditional open procedures (such as TPLO), any potential for reduction in surgical morbidity through arthroscopic inspection and treatment of the joint is masked by the morbidity of the traditional open stabilisation procedure. In the future, as arthroscopically assisted minimally invasive approaches to stifle stabilisation of the cranial-cruciate-ligament-deficient stifle joint become established (Cook et al., 2010), the potential for reduced surgical morbidity through arthroscopic treatment of the stifle joint will be evaluated.

Arthroscopically assisted surgery of OCD of the stifle joint

OCD lesions occur can occur on both the lateral and the medial femoral condyle, although the lesions are observed more commonly on the lateral condyle. Affected dogs often have marked stifle effusion and pain. The arthroscopic portals used for arthroscopic surgery for OCD are as previously described and a stifle-distracting device is recommended to open the joint space, reducing the extent of fat-pad debridement required to inspect and work on the OCD lesion. For the surgical techniques, the reader is asked to refer to those described for shoulder OCD.

The meniscus beneath the OCD lesion should be carefully inspected visually, assisted with instrumentation, for signs of injury since meniscal tearing is not uncommon with stifle OCD. Tears should be treated by ablation as described above (Bertrand et al., 1997). Prior to completion of the arthroscopy, the opposite femoral condyle and underlying meniscus should be checked for evidence of disease and treated appropriately, if required. An intra-articular injection of ropivacaine (2 mg/kg) with morphine (0.1 mg/kg) should be given to augment the postoperative analgesia protocol.

Autogenous osteochondral grafting is an emerging treatment for osteochondral defects affecting the femoral condyle (Cook et al., 2008). The technique transfers dowels of articular cartilage with underlying subchondral bone from the non-weight-bearing sulcus terminalis of the medial and lateral femoral trochlear ridges into the OCD lesion in the femoral condyle. Currently the technique is performed using an open approach, but if long-term clinical results prove clinical efficacy then arthroscopically assisted autogenous osteochondral grafting may become the preferred method for this technique to reduce operative morbidity.

Arthroscopically assisted management of septic arthritis of the stifle joint

Management principles follow those described for the elbow.

Arthroscopically assisted surgery of the tarsus

Arthroscopic surgery of the tarsus is challenging due to the complex anatomy, and because of the limitations of the small intra-articular joint space. Arthroscopic assistance can be valuable in the surgical management of tarsal OCD, for obtaining surgical biopsies and for the management of septic arthritis. The reader is referred to the Further reading section at the end of this chapter for more details.

Postoperative care following arthroscopic surgery

Although arthroscopic surgery generally has lower surgical morbidity than traditional open joint surgery, control of postoperative pain remains an important aspect of care for the arthroscopic patient. Whereas the arthroscopic procedure often induces less surgical injury and pain than a comparable traditional arthrotomy, many of the conditions treated arthroscopically are of their own right painful. Patients consequently require postoperative analgesia that is appropriate and effective, and which is delivered with close monitoring in order to achieve good postoperative comfort. Routinely, postoperative analgesia should be assisted through the administration of intra-operative ropivacaine (0.5–1 mg/kg). This is best given prior to commencement of the arthroscopic surgery, since effective intra-operative analgesia reduces postoperative pain perception. At the end of the arthroscopic procedure an additional intra-articular injection is given (2 mg/kg), in combination with intra-articular morphine (0.1 mg/kg). The maximum total recommended dose of ropivacaine in dogs should not exceed 3 mg/kg, although in practice the quantity of drug given is limited in most cases by the volume of the 7.5 mg/ml solution that can be readily instilled into the intra-articular space, and doses approaching 1 mg/kg are more convenient given this limitation. Intra-articular analgesia contributes to postoperative pain management as part of a global approach to patient analgesia. Additional systemically administered analgesic agents should be given in the postoperative period, as necessary, to patients that are predicted to be or which are painful following the arthroscopic procedure.

Non-steroidal anti-inflammatory drug (NSAID) medication should be prescribed routinely for patients undergoing arthroscopic surgery. Under ideal circumstances, when clinical considerations permit, the NSAID is given intra-operatively to reduce the surgical nociceptive stimulus and is continued postoperatively for several days until the joint is comfortable. There is patient- and condition-associated variation in the duration for which there is musculoskeletal discomfort and for which NSAIDs provide a pain-relieving effect but, in general, NSAIDs should be administered for the duration for which discomfort is anticipated. For some patients, a 10-day period of treatment may be sufficient in duration, but many of the joint diseases treated arthroscopically are associated with marked and often chronic inflammation and pain, and resolution of discomfort does not occur rapidly following the arthroscopic procedure. For these patients, ongoing postoperative discomfort can be anticipated and a 2–4-week course of a licensed and safe NSAID may be required.

Some joint problems that are treated with arthroscopic intervention require considerable intra-operative manipulation and stressing of ligaments, causing intra-operative and postoperative pain. Some joint problems are associated with significant pain before the arthroscopic procedure and postoperative pain is anticipated. Such cases are indications for support in a compressive and supportive dressing which protects the joint from potentially painful movement in the early postoperative period. The compression from the dressing also helps to control the tendency for postoperative swelling. A supportive dressing may be maintained overnight following a procedure, or for several days, depending on the severity and controllability of the predicted postoperative pain. A supportive dressing prevents early postoperative movement and, in human beings, this promotes joint stiffness. However, it is not readily possible to achieve in animals the early postoperative ranges of joint motion achieved in humans with the use of continuous regional intravenous local anaesthetic infusions, combined with machine-delivered automated excursions of the operated joint. Consequently, the analgesic effect of a supportive dressing appears to offer the veterinary patient a better level of postoperative care than leaving the joint unsupported while attempting to perform passive range-of-motion activities that are markedly limited in terms of excursion by postoperative pain.

Some workers advocate the use of postoperative cold therapy applied intermittently using gel packs applied around the circumference of the arthroscopically treated joint. Cold therapy may be helpful in providing analgesia and in assisting resolution of swelling. In contrast to accepted wisdom regarding the beneficial effects of cold therapy, recent scientific evidence suggests that cold therapy may have adverse effects on tissue healing through interfering with the elevations in insulin-like growth factor that are important in tissue healing following injury (Lu et al., 2011).

Following surgery, once the patient is beginning to use the treated limb, if there is significant postoperative debility, a patient-specific rehabilitation programme should be implemented to encourage a gradual increase in function of the operated joint and gradually increasing weight-bearing with ambulation. The objective of the rehabilitation programme should be to restore the patient towards preoperative overground locomotory function in the most rapid and comfortable manner. Return of limb function may be assisted through promoting swimming, or wading through water in a water treadmill, or through activities on obstacle courses that encourage marked excursions of the treated diseased joint. Throughout the rehabilitation programme the progress of the patient should be closely monitored. Regardless of the rehabilitation methods used, the primary outcome measure should be an assessment of the function of the limb when the patient is walking and running, since ability to return to normal function in these important activities is the goal of the arthroscopic procedure and of the postoperative care.

Further reading

Bardet, J.F. (1998) Diagnosis of shoulder instability in dogs and cats: a retrospective study. *Journal of the American Animal Hospital Association* 34, 42–54.

Beale, B.S., Hulse, D.A., Schulz, K. and Whitney, W.O. (2003) *Small Animal Arthroscopy*. Saunders, Philadelphia, PA.

Burton, N.J., Perry, M.J., Fitzpatrick, N. and Owen, M.R. (2010) Comparison of bone mineral density in medial coronoid processes of dogs with and without medial coronoid process fragmentation. *American Journal of Veterinary Research* 71, 41–46.

Chow, J.C.Y. (2001) *Advanced Arthroscopy*. Springer Verlag, Berlin.

Danielson, K.C., Fitzpatrick, N., Muir, P. and Manley, P.A. (2006) Histomorphometry of fragmented medial coronoid process in dogs: a comparison of affected and normal coronoid processes. *Veterinary Surgery* 35, 501–509.

Fitzpatrick, N. and Yeadon, R. (2009) Working algorithm for treatment decision making for developmental disease of the medial compartment of the elbow in dogs. *Veterinary Surgery* 38, 285–300.

Fitzpatrick, N., Yeadon, R. and Smith, T.J. (2009) Early clinical experience with osteochondral autograft transfer for treatment of osteochondritis dissecans of the medial humeral condyle in dogs. *Veterinary Surgery* 38, 246–260.

Fitzpatrick, N., Smith, T.J., Evans, R.B., O'Riordan, J. and Yeadon, R. (2009) Subtotal coronoid ostectomy for treatment of medial coronoid disease in 263 dogs. *Veterinary Surgery* 38, 233–245.

Gielen, I., Van Ryssen, B., Coopman, F. and van Bree, H. (2007) Comparison of subchondral lesion size between clinical and non-clinical medial trochlear ridge talar osteochondritis dissecans in dogs. *Veterinary and Comparative Orthopaedics and Traumatology* 20, 8–11.

Kunkel, K.A. and Rochat, M.C. (2008) A review of lameness attributable to the shoulder in the dog: part one. *Journal of the American Animal Hospital Association* 44, 156–162.

Kunkel, K.A. and Rochat, M.C. (2008) A review of lameness attributable to the shoulder in the dog: part one. *Journal of the American Animal Hospital Association* 44, 163–170.

Lapish, J. and Van Ryssen, B. (2006) Arthroscopic equipment. In *BSAVA Manual of Canine and Feline Musculoskeletal Disorders*, Houlton, J.E.F., Cook, J.L.,

Innes, J.F. and Langley-Hobbs, S.J. (eds), pp. 177–183. British Small Animal Veterinary Association, Gloucester.

Miller, M.D. and Cole, B.J. (2004) *Textbook of Arthroscopy*, vol. 355. Elsevier, Philadelphia, PA.

Pucheu, B. and Duhautois, B. (2008) Surgical treatment of shoulder instability. A retrospective study on 76 cases (1993–2007). *Veterinary and Comparative Orthopaedics and Traumatology* 21, 368–374.

Strobel, M.J. (2002) *Manual of Arthroscopic Surgery*. Springer Verlag, Berlin.

Van Ryssen, B. (2006) Principles of arthroscopy. In *BSAVA Manual of Canine and Feline Musculoskeletal Disorders*, Houlton, J.E.F., Cook, J.L., Innes, J.F. and Langley-Hobbs, S.J. (eds), pp. 184–192. British Small Animal Veterinary Association, Gloucester.

References

Åkerblom, S. and Sjöström, L. (2007) Evaluation of clinical, radiographical and cytological findings compared to arthroscopic findings in shoulder joint lameness in the dog. *Veterinary and Comparative Orthopaedics and Traumatology* 20, 136–141.

Bertrand, S.G., Lewis, D.D., Madison, J.B., de Haan, J.H., Stubbs, W.P. and Stallings, J. (1997) Arthroscopic examination and treatment of osteochondritis dissecans of the femoral condyle of six dogs. *Journal of the American Animal Hospital Association* 33, 451–455.

Böttcher, P., Winkels, P. and Oechtering, G. (2009) A novel pin distraction device for arthroscopic assessment of the medial meniscus in dogs. *Veterinary Surgery* 38, 595–560.

Cogar, S.M., Cook, C.R., Curry, S.L., Grandis, A. and Cook, J.L. (2008) Prospective evaluation of techniques for differentiating shoulder pathology as a source of forelimb lameness in medium and large breed dogs. *Veterinary Surgery* 37, 132–141.

Cook, J.L., Renfro, D.C., Tomlinson, J.L. and Sorensen, J.E. (2005a) Measurement of angles of abduction for diagnosis of shoulder instability in dogs using goniometry and digital image analysis. *Veterinary Surgery* 34, 463–468.

Cook, J.L., Tomlinson, J.L., Fox, D.B., Kenter, K. and Cook, C.R. (2005b) Treatment of dogs diagnosed with medial shoulder instability using radiofrequency-induced thermal capsulorrhaphy. *Veterinary Surgery* 34, 469–475.

Cook, J.L., Hudson, C.C. and Kuroki, K. (2008) Autogenous osteochondral grafting for treatment of stifle osteochondrosis in dogs. *Veterinary Surgery* 37, 311–321.

Cook, J.L., Luther, J.K., Beetem, J., Karnes, J. and Cook, C.R. (2010) Clinical comparison of a novel extracapsular stabilization procedure and tibial plateau leveling osteotomy for treatment of cranial cruciate ligament deficiency in dogs. *Veterinary Surgery* 39, 315–323.

Devitt, C.M., Neely, M.R. and Vanvechten, B.J. (2007) Relationship of physical examination test of shoulder instability to arthroscopic findings in dogs. *Veterinary Surgery* 36, 661–668.

Fitzpatrick, N. and Solano, M.A. (2010) Predictive variables for complications after TPLO with stifle inspection by arthrotomy in 1000 consecutive dogs. *Veterinary Surgery* 39, 460–474.

Gemmill, T.J. and Farrell, M. (2009) Evaluation of a joint distractor to facilitate arthroscopy of the canine stifle. *Veterinary Surgery* 38, 588–594.

Horstman, C.L. and McLaughlin, R.M. (2006) The use of radiofrequency energy during arthroscopic surgery and its effects on intraarticular tissues. *Veterinary and Comparative Orthopaedics and Traumatology* 19(2), 65–71.

Lu, H., Huang, D., Saederup, N., Charo, I.F., Ransohoff, R.M. and Zhou, L. (2011) Macrophages recruited via CCR2 produce insulin-like growth factor-1 to repair acute skeletal muscle injury. *FASEB Journal* 25(1), 358–369.

Mitchell, R.A. and Innes, J.F. (2000) Lateral glenohumeral ligament rupture in three dogs. *Journal of Small Animal Practice* 41, 511–514.

O'Neill, T. and Innes, J.F. (2004) Treatment of shoulder instability caused by medial glenohumeral ligament rupture with thermal capsulorrhaphy. *Journal of Small Animal Practice* 45, 521–524.

Pettitt, J.F. and Innes, J.F. (2008) Arthroscopic management of a lateral glenohumeral ligament rupture in two dogs. *Veterinary and Comparative Orthopaedics and Traumatology* 21, 302–306.

Pettitt, R.A., Clements, D.N. and Guilliard, M.J. (2007) Stabilisation of medial shoulder instability by imbrication of the subscapularis muscle tendon of insertion. *Journal of Small Animal Practice* 48, 626–631.

Thieman, K.M., Tomlinson, J.L., Fox, D.B., Cook, C.R. and Cook, J.L. (2006) Effect of meniscal release on rate of subsequent meniscal tears and owner-assessed outcome in dogs with cruciate disease treated with tibial plateau leveling osteotomy. *Veterinary Surgery* 35, 705–710.

Chapter 4
Diagnostic Laparoscopy
Alasdair Hotston Moore and Rosa Angela Ragni

Diagnostic laparoscopy provides access to the abdominal cavity with a minimally invasive approach, and is therefore a safe alternative to conventional open surgery for evaluation of intra-abdominal structures and collection of biopsy samples. Rapid patient recovery and lower postoperative morbidity are a major advantage, especially when managing debilitated patients. At the same time diagnostic accuracy is greatly increased by magnification and excellent illumination of the field of view and by collection of biopsy samples of superior quality. All these characteristics have led to wide application of laparoscopy for diagnostic purposes.

Instrumentation

The basic kit required for diagnostic laparoscopy consists of a video system and a light source, which are the same used for many other endoscopic applications. In addition to this, specific equipment such as an insufflator and dedicated instruments are necessary to gain access to the abdominal cavity and perform the desired procedures.

The telescope is chosen according to the preference of the surgeon, and also depending on the possibility of having more than one available. Larger-diameter telescopes (5–10 mm) are preferred, because in the abdominal cavity there are no space restrictions and a large amount of light is absorbed; a 5 mm-diameter scope is adequate for most small animal procedures, and is recommended when only one scope has been purchased. The scope is introduced through the abdominal ports without

Clinical Manual of Small Animal Endosurgery, First Edition. Edited by Alasdair Hotston Moore and Rosa Angela Ragni.
© 2012 Blackwell Publishing Ltd. Published 2012 by Blackwell Publishing Ltd.

the need for an outer sheath; the cannula is sufficient to guarantee scope protection, and operative channels are not useful because of their limited diameter. Different viewing angles affect the visualisation of the operative field: although scopes with 0° viewing angle are the simplest to use, their field of view is the most limited. By rotating an angled telescope on its axis, the surgeon can obtain a wider field of view, which is very useful for examination of relatively inaccessible areas and for allowing more room for instrument manoeuvring.

However, spatial orientation with angled scopes is more challenging, and the instruments enter the field of view at different angles from what intuitively expected. To obtain a more 'anatomical' orientation, the light cable is held upwards, so that the angled view is facing down. A 30° viewing angle – a good compromise between size of the field of view and ease of spatial orientation – is usually preferred. Recently, a telescope has been devised which allows the possibility of changing the angle of view at the turn of a dial situated at the proximal end of the telescope (EndoCAMeleon®, Karl Storz GmbH and Co. KG, Germany).

A high-intensity (300 W) light source is recommended for laparoscopy, because of the need to illuminate a large cavity. The dark surfaces in the abdomen (liver, presence of blood) will also absorb light (Magne and Tams, 1999). Xenon light sources are preferred as they are considered to better reproduce the colours of the abdominal organs. If a less optimal light source is to be used, such as halogen, it is important to choose a high-quality camera, which will require less light (Magne and Tams, 1999).

For laparoscopy the endoscope is connected to a video camera, which sends the images to a monitor. This not only allows the operator to work more comfortably and to benefit from the help of assistants, but results in a superior image of the operating field, and is crucial for maintaining sterile conditions.

In order to visualise abdominal structures and interpose some space between the trocar-cannula units and the abdominal organs, an optical space needs to be created by insufflating the abdominal cavity with gas. Air is not advised for this purpose, as it could easily cause embolism; nitrous oxide is soluble in blood and could be employed, as long as energy-assisted devices are avoided, because nitrous oxide is highly combustible and spark ignition could occur. The gas most commonly used is carbon dioxide, which is non-combustible and readily absorbed in blood. These characteristics make carbon dioxide a safe choice, with very low risk of gas embolism, and not dangerous even when using energy-assisted devices. A minor disadvantage with carbon dioxide is the formation of carbonic acid on contact with peritoneal surfaces, which causes discomfort in the postoperative period (Magne and Tams, 1999).

Carbon dioxide is delivered by a dedicated insufflator. This is a computerised pump which controls gas flow rate and total volume of gas delivered, and maintains abdominal pressure at a preset value. The insufflator display also shows the total amount of gas delivered during the procedure, and the remaining pressure in the carbon dioxide cylinder.

The flow rate can usually be regulated between 1 and 20 L/min in 0.1 L increments. At the onset of the procedure insufflation rate should not exceed 1 L/min to allow the patient to slowly adapt to the increasing abdominal pressure. Once the desired abdominal pressure is reached the valve closes, stopping the delivery of gas. At this point the flow rate can be increased to allow inflation to be maintained despite ongoing leaks. An automatic insufflation feature will open the valve and restart gas flow if the intra-abdominal pressure falls below a predetermined value. This often occurs with insertion and removal of instruments, and particularly if suction is used.

To prevent a decrease in venous return and reduction in ventilating ability, intra-abdominal pressure should never exceed 12–13 mmHg in cats and 13–15 mmHg in dogs. These pressure levels are required for portal creation, as they allow a safe distance between the abdominal wall and the underlying structures. After all required portals have been established, an intra-abdominal pressure of 8–10 mmHg is usually sufficient to allow excellent visualisation.

Due to the large potential space of the peritoneal cavity, intra-abdominal pressure should be very low on the insufflator display at the beginning of the procedure. If at this point the intra-abdominal pressure is abnormally high, and all connections are in the open position, incorrect positioning of the cannula or Veress needle must be suspected.

Pneumoperitoneum is usually established with a Veress needle. This consists of a sharp outer trocar and a blunt hollow inner spring-loaded obturator, which retracts when the needle contacts the abdominal wall. As soon as the abdominal cavity is penetrated, the blunt inner stylet advances beyond the sharp tip, minimising the risk of injury to abdominal organs. The needle is equipped at the end with a Luer-lock adaptor, to which the insufflation tubing attaches. Veress needles can be disposable or reusable. Reusable needles are always sharp, and require less force to penetrate the abdominal wall. However, they are rarely used in veterinary medicine because of their cost. Re-sterilising and reusing disposable needles is possible, but it is not practical, as this would determine loss of sharpness and therefore defeat the purpose of their use.

Trocar-cannula units are used to introduce the telescope and operative instruments into the abdomen. They are available in different sizes, chosen accordingly to the diameter of the scope and instruments used: the cannula is usually 0.5–1 mm larger than the item inserted through it. Reducers are available to permit insertion of smaller instruments without loss of pneumoperitoneum.

Standard units consist of a hollow outer portion (cannula) and a sharp-pointed stylet (or trocar) protruding from the cannula. The stylet has a conical or pyramidal tip, and is used to penetrate fascia and muscles. Pyramidal tips are preferable for insertion in the closed manner, as they facilitate penetration. Once the abdominal cavity has been entered, the trocar is removed, and the cannula is used to introduce the scope and instruments. An automatic valve (a ball valve, trumpet valve or butterfly washer) seals the cannula when no instrument is present, thus preserving insufflation pressure.

A rubber washer seals around the instrument shaft when in place. A Luer-lock stopcock for gas insufflation is also usually present. Trocar-cannula assemblies can be reusable (made of stainless steel), disposable or hybrid. These can be re-sterilised a limited number of times. An advantage of reusable units is that the sleeves are usually made of hard clear plastic, thus allowing the operator to monitor progress of instrument insertion. In both disposable and reusable units the stylet becomes blunt with repeated use, and needs to be sharpened. Hybrid trocars can be a good solution, since they provide for easy replacement of components that wear easily. Opening the rubber seal manually when introducing the trocar also helps to prevent blunting. It is also important to check that the sharp tip is centrally placed, to avoid damage to the seal, which will result in gas leakage.

Cannulae are available with straight or threaded shafts: the latter are more difficult to insert, but the risk of their dislodgement during surgery is minimal. Innovative cannulae have recently been introduced to minimise the risk of trocar injury: some are equipped with optical viewing capability (optical trocars). In these trocars a distal viewing lens allows the light from the laparoscope to be seen, thus enabling the operator to follow the progress of the trocar during insertion. Other cannulae (Ternamian EndoTIP System®, Karl Storz) do not require a trocar, and are placed with a twisting motion after a small incision in the abdominal wall. Three trocar-cannula assemblies are typically required to perform laparoscopic interventions. This number can increase to four for more advanced procedures.

Although the essential kit for diagnostic laparoscopy consists of palpation probes, grasping forceps and biopsy forceps, a vast array of hand instruments are available, comparable to the ones for open surgery, with shafts of different lengths and diameters. General characteristics of the instruments to be considered are:

- the possibility of rotating the shaft and consequently the tip: instruments with an 'in-line' configuration allow easier rotation of the instrument around its axis, whereas instruments with a 'pistol-grip' configuration feel more stable in the operator's hand; the 'in-line' configuration is usually preferred for needle holders;

- the possibility of articulation of the instrument shaft; a knob on the shaft of the instruments causes the tip to angulate up to 90° when pushed; this reduces the need for additional portals, allowing the instrument to approach the tissue from various angles;

- the presence of a ratchet that allows the instrument to be locked onto tissue; this is especially important for grasping forceps, because if the instrument locks the operator can relax their grip;

- the presence of a single- or double-action mechanism at the effector end: in a single-action device only one jaw of the instrument is moving, whereas in a double-action instrument both jaws move when the operator's hand moves; this mimics more closely the movement of an open-surgery instrument, and is preferred when performing fine dissection;

- electrosurgical capability (mono- or bipolar, etc.).

Finally, advantages and disadvantages of disposable and reusable instruments have to be considered: disposable instruments are usually suitable for multiple uses as long as sterility and sharpness are preserved. Reusable instruments, although more expensive, are easier to clean, lubricate and sterilise. On the other hand, even reusable cutting instruments (e.g. scissors) need to be sharpened, more often if their electrosurgical capability is exploited.

Hand instruments are used for the following functions.

- Retraction: the simplest retractor is a blunt probe, which is used to move and 'palpate' organs; the probe is also used to apply pressure over a biopsy site to achieve haemostasis. The probe has 1 cm calibration markings along its shaft, for measurement of organs or lesions, which otherwise could prove difficult in the presence of magnification. Other types of retractor have projections that extend in a fan shape, thus providing a wide retracting surface.

- Tissue handling: as in open surgery, grasping forceps can be traumatic or atraumatic. Traumatic grasping forceps, such as laparoscopic Allis forceps, have teeth and are used to grasp only tissue to be removed. Atraumatic ones (e.g. laparoscopic Babcock and Debakey forceps) have fine serrations that hold tissue firmly but delicately. However, because of the loss of tactile feedback occurring in laparoscopy, even atraumatic forceps can damage tissues if too much force is applied. Avoiding the use of instrument ratchets helps the beginner in appreciating tissue friability. Grasping instruments are available in various shapes (blunt, curved, angled, duck-bill, dolphin-nosed), and may also be used with electrosurgery.

- Dissection: dissecting forceps (Maryland dissectors, Kelly and right-angle forceps, etc.) are used for blunt dissection. Curved and 'cherry' dissectors are useful for isolating blood vessels and delicate structures such as the cystic duct. Sharp dissection is usually carried out with scissors. Curved Metzenbaum scissors with 5 and 10 mm shafts are most commonly used; for very fine dissection straight scissors and micro scissors are available. Scissors can also be connected to electrosurgery, or other energy devices such as lasers and electronic scalpels can be used to accomplish dissection.

- Biopsy: oval cup (clamshell) biopsy forceps are the most versatile, and are commonly used for liver, spleen and lymph node biopsy, whereas punch biopsy forceps are preferred for biopsy of the pancreas. For kidney and deep-tissue biopsy core biopsy needles are required; for gall bladder aspiration specific long aspiration needles (or spinal needles) are employed.

- Haemostasis: different methods are available for controlling bleeding: clip application, sutures and use of energy-assisted devices. Vascular clip applicators are available in different sizes, and can be reusable or disposable. The clip is held in the applicator shaft and advanced until both tips are around the vessel, and the instrument is then closed on the tissue. Clamped tissue should fill approximately three-quarters of the internal diameter of a clip. Pre-tied loop ligatures are available for pedicles; alternatively, ligatures can be performed with several knotting techniques (extra- or intracorporeal). Extracorporeal knot-tying requires a 'knot-pusher', that allows to slide the knot tied outside of the body through the cannula and inside the body, up to the tissue being tied. Laparoscopic needle holders are instead used for intracorporeal suturing, and dedicated hook-type scissors are used to cut sutures. Energy-assisted devices are also commonly used for haemostasis. Electrosurgical units are the most economical, and therefore the most widespread in veterinary medicine; alternatives that can be used for careful dissection are diode and neodymium:yttrium-aluminium-garnet or Nd:YAG lasers and ultrasonic devices such as the Harmonic Scalpel® (Ethicon Endo-Surgery, Europe GmbH, Germany). The recent introduction of a bipolar electrothermal vessel sealer (LigaSure®, Valleylab, Tyco Healthcare UK), able to seal vessels up to 7 mm in diameter, has allowed a significant reduction in surgery times.

- Tissue removal: endoscopic staplers apply four or six 3–6 cm long staggered rows of staplers and cut between the middle rows, thus allowing easy removal of organ sections and anastomosis. Different cartridges are available (as in open surgery) depending on the thickness of the tissue to be resected. Morcellators cut tissue into smaller pieces, thus facilitating removal; specimen-retrieval bags are used to remove infected or neoplastic tissue. Commercially available bags usually come on a 10 mm applicator; for smaller samples, bags can be made inexpensively from a sterile surgical glove.

- Irrigation and suction: aspiration/irrigation units are available with various tips such as Poole or Yankauer; most devices combine suction and flushing capabilities, and some are also equipped with a monopolar dissection probe. They are designed to carry out suction and irrigation without significant loss of insufflation.

Anaesthetic considerations

Laparoscopy is usually performed under general anaesthesia. Special anaesthetic considerations and complete understanding of the physiological changes caused by abdominal insufflation and patient position are necessary to minimise potential complications related to anaesthesia. Patients should be thoroughly examined before undergoing general anaesthesia, and appropriate tests performed (complete blood count, biochemistry panel including electrolytes, urinalysis and other tests as necessary). Any dehydration or acid–base abnormalities should be corrected before the procedure, and the anaesthetic protocol should be individually tailored.

Current recommendation for animals undergoing general anaesthesia is that food should be withheld for 6 h in adult dogs (for shorter periods in immature animals), and water for 1 h before anaesthesia (Savvas et al., 2009). The nutritional status of the patient should be taken into account, and the insertion of a feeding tube anticipated.

A dedicated member of the team should be available to monitor the patient throughout the procedure; pulse oximetry, capnography and electrocardiography (ECG), together with an oesophageal stethoscope, should be used for assessing normal physiological parameters. Patients in critical conditions will benefit from invasive blood-pressure monitoring; this will also consent easy blood-gas sampling. Non-invasive methods, such as Doppler or oscillometric monitors, are sufficient for elective procedures. Mean arterial pressure should be maintained higher than 60 mmHg in small animal patients.

Crystalloid fluids should be administered to patients undergoing general anaesthesia, regardless of the anticipated amount of blood loss, as inhalant anaesthetics cause vasodilation and decreased venous return. Administration of colloids may be beneficial in selected cases.

In particular, induction with barbiturates is best avoided for laparoscopy, because of induced splenomegaly and consequent increased risk of splenic puncture. Nitrous oxide should not be used during procedures in which there is the risk of pneumothorax.

Hypothermia may also occur during laparoscopy, especially in small patients, as the insufflation gas is below room temperature and of low humidity, both of which cause significant patient cooling. Monitoring of patient's temperature and use of heating devices are important, particularly in long procedures.

Another important consideration is related to the increased intra-abdominal pressure consequent to insufflation, which compresses the vena cava, depressing venous return. The degree of haemodynamic change depends on the animal's intravascular volume, with more severe hypotension in hypovolaemic animals. Increased intra-abdominal pressure also causes cranial displacement of the diaphragm, which will decrease tidal volume and encourage atelectasis with associated increase in ventilation-perfusion mismatch. Respiratory and metabolic acidosis and hypoxaemia may result, especially in obese patients, or in those with pre-existent cardiopulmonary disease.

Assisted ventilation may be therefore necessary in obese or older patients, and is recommended in all procedures over 30 min duration to provide pulmonary support and reduce development of atelectasis. Positive-pressure ventilation minimises the effects of pneumoperitoneum, and normocapnia can be maintained by increasing the tidal volume and keeping the respiratory rate low (Quandt, 1999). The minimal amount of intra-abdominal pressure necessary to perform the procedure should also be used, and values in excess of 15 mmHg have to be avoided. A pressure of 8–10 mmHg allows excellent visualisation in most cases.

As carbon dioxide is the insufflation gas of choice, end-tidal carbon dioxide monitoring and pulse oximetry are important to detect hypoxaemia and hypercarbia. Diffusion of carbon dioxide across the peritoneal membrane will lead to significant increase in $PaCO2$ and decrease in $PaO2$, even in patients receiving mechanical ventilation (Duke et al., 1996). End-tidal carbon dioxide should be between 35 and 45 mmHg and $SpO2$ greater than 95%. Hypercarbia contributes to myocardial depression and increase in sympathetic tone, which may produce cardiac arrhythmias. Sinus tachycardia, ventricular arrhythmias and asystole are most commonly seen, especially in conditions of light anaesthesia. Bradycardia can instead develop as a consequence of peritoneal distension (Quandt, 1999). Another effect of hypercarbia is increase in intracranial pressure, mediated by increased cerebral blood flow. Thus, laparoscopy should be used with caution in patients with head trauma.

Body position of the patient during the procedure may also adversely affect the cardiovascular and respiratory systems. Inhalant anaesthetics depress the baroreflex, with consequent diminished reflex control of circulation following changes in body posture (Bailey and Pablo, 1999; Joris et al., 1993). The head-down tilt (Trendelenburg position), especially accompanied by abdominal insufflation, decreases ventilation and cardiac output. The risk of passive gastric reflux is also increased. The reverse Trendelenburg position, or head-up tilt, leads instead to reflex vasoconstriction, with increased heart rate and blood pressure (Abel et al., 1963). To prevent complications, more than 15° of tilt of the patient in a cranial or caudal direction should be avoided. Patients at higher risk of gastric reflux, such as those with gastric outflow obstruction, hiatal haernia or obesity may benefit from preoperative administration of metoclopramide, antacids and H2 blockers. An orogastric tube may be placed if the stomach appears enlarged (Quandt, 1999).

Early detection of complications (haemorrhage, pneumothorax, puncture of an organ and carbon dioxide embolism) is important to improve the outcome. Serial measurements or estimations of blood loss rather than serial determinations of packed cell volume or total protein levels are useful for selecting the type of fluid for resuscitation. The former will in fact not become evident for several hours, as volume expansion with fluid shifted from the extravascular space takes approximately 4 h, and splenic recruitment of red blood cells offsets the fall in packed cell volume even longer (Villiers, 2005). When the blood loss is less than 20%, crystalloids will suffice, whereas if the blood loss is between 20 and 30% colloids are necessary. Blood transfusion should be considered if the blood loss approaches 30%, as physiological mechanisms are no longer able to compensate.

Carbon dioxide embolism presents with a severe and sudden drop in blood pressure, development of a heart murmur, cardiac dysrhythmias and cyanosis. A rapid and transient rise in end-tidal carbon dioxide as the gas embolises is followed by a steep decline in this parameter, due to reduction of blood delivery to the pulmonary circulation (Staffieri et al., 2007). Capnography, together with ECG and blood-pressure monitoring, will assist in rapidly detecting carbon dioxide embolism.

An accidental perforation of the diaphragm, or a pre-existent congenital or acquired defect, may cause pneumothorax, which manifests itself with a change in ventilator pattern, accompanied by cyanosis, drop in $PaO2$ and caudal bulging of the diaphragm. Due to the positive peritoneal pressure, a tension pneumothorax will develop, which may be fatal if not rapidly recognised and treated. Increase in the minute ventilation, evacuation of the gas from the thorax with a thoracostomy tube, and abdominal desufflation are able to reverse the physiological effects while the laceration in the diaphragm is repaired. Conversion to open surgery is often necessary.

Postoperative care of animals undergoing laparoscopy includes multimodal analgesia, with parenterally administered opioids, and non-steroidal anti-inflammatory agents whenever possible. Although the discomfort after laparoscopy is mostly due to formation of carbonic acid on serosal surfaces, causing peritoneal inflammation and phrenic nerve irritation rather than incision-related pain (Magne and Tams, 1999), injection of local anaesthetic agents at the port sites at the beginning or at the end of the procedure is considered beneficial. Long-acting local anaesthetic agents such as bupivacaine or ropivacaine are always used; as their onset of action is delayed, a cocktail with lidocaine is preferred when the block is carried out at the end.

In preparation for laparoscopy the bladder should be emptied to minimise the risk of accidental puncture with the Veress needle or a trocar. The stomach and occasionally colon may need to be evacuated if they are distended. Distended viscera will also decrease visualisation of the surrounding areas.

The animal should always be clipped liberally, from 5 cm cranial to the xiphoid process to the pubis. Laterally, the patient is clipped as for a traditional open coeliotomy, and the whole clipped area is prepared aseptically. This will enable conversion to an open procedure should the necessity arise. This may happen because of technical difficulties or complications, or in case a surgically correctable lesion is encountered.

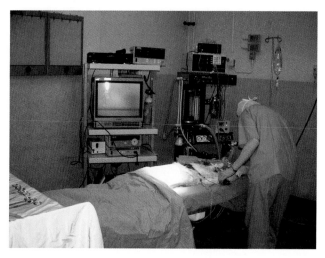

Fig. 4.1   Dog positioned in left lateral recumbency for laparoscopy through the right flank. The tower is positioned across the animal from the surgeon's position.

Positioning of the patient and surgical approach depend on the procedure performed, and on the organs examined. The two most commonly used approaches are the right lateral and ventral midline. The right lateral approach (Fig. 4.1) allows diagnostic evaluation of most of the liver (approximately 85%), gall bladder and extrahepatic biliary tree, descending duodenum, right limb of the pancreas, right kidney and right adrenal gland, and is therefore recommended for biopsy of these organs (Magne and Tams, 1999). This approach can also be used for laparoscopy-assisted gastropexy (Freeman, 2009), whereas other surgeons prefer for this procedure a modified ventral approach (Fig. 4.2).

The ventral midline approach offers a more extensive visualisation of the abdominal cavity and its content (Fig. 4.3), and is thus chosen for most surgical procedures (Twedt and Monnet, 2005; Monnet et al., 2008). For this approach the telescope portal is placed on midline, caudal to the umbilicus. In this location the falciform fat may interfere with visualisation of the cranial abdomen, especially in obese animals. However, withdrawal and manoeuvring of the telescope usually allows its positioning beyond the caudal border of the falciform ligament.

A left lateral approach is occasionally performed for visualisation and biopsy of the spleen, left kidney, left adrenal gland and left-sided liver masses, but since the spleen lies directly underneath the typical entry sites there is a high risk of puncturing it when positioning the trocar.

Portal entry sites can be more cranial or caudal in any of the above approaches, depending on the size of the animal and on the procedure to be performed, in order to ensure adequate organ visualisation and sufficient working space.

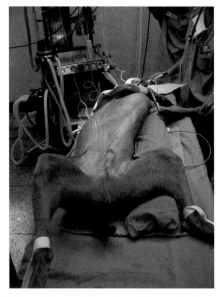

Fig. 4.2 Dog positioned in semidorsal position, tilted to the left, for laparoscopy-assisted gastropexy.

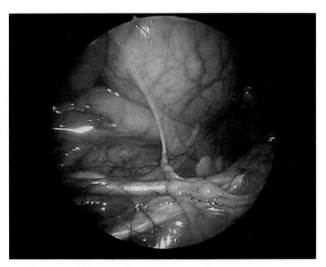

Fig. 4.3 View from the umbilicus into the left inguinal region during laparoscopy of a normal dog. The bladder is dorsal and the iliac arteries are seen ventrally.

Surgical technique

The first step in laparoscopy is induction of pneumoperitoneum. This can be achieved with the use of either a Veress needle (closed technique) or a Hasson trocar (open or paediatric technique). Palpation of the abdominal cavity is recommended before needle insertion, in order to identify underlying organs – most commonly the spleen – which must be avoided. The Veress needle is usually inserted at the same site as the first telescope portal; this is often located caudolateral to the umbilicus, where the abdominal wall is consistently thin (Kolata and Freeman, 1999a). A 1 mm skin incision is performed at the selected site, and the abdominal wall is lifted and tented by grasping it with forceps. The Veress needle is then inserted directed caudally at an angle with the skin, thus avoiding the spleen and the falciform ligament. Other measures directed at minimising risk of iatrogenic organ damage are placing the animal with the head slightly down (Trendelenburg position), and resting the heel of the non-dominant hand on the abdominal wall, to control the needle entry.

The Veress needle is grasped by the hub during abdominal wall insertion, thus allowing retraction of the inner blunt stylet. Once the abdominal cavity is entered, and no more resistance is encountered, the outer trocar retracts, and the spring-loaded blunt stylet protrudes, minimising the risk of trauma to the abdominal organs. After insertion, the needle is gently swept in a circular pattern against the abdominal wall, thus freeing it from any adhesions or omentum.

To verify appropriate intra-abdominal placement, the 'hanging drop test' is performed. This entails attaching a syringe partially filled with saline to the hub of the Veress needle. After having applied gentle suction to confirm the absence of blood or fluids, a drop of saline is placed into the hub of the needle, and the abdominal wall is tented. If the needle is properly placed in the peritoneal cavity the negative pressure present in the abdominal cavity aspirates the drop into the needle hub. Correct placement is extremely important, as placement into an organ, vessel or mass causes haemorrhage, which interferes with visualisation, and can also result in a fatal embolism.

The needle can also be incorrectly placed into the subcutaneous tissue, or into the omentum or falciform ligament. Subcutaneous placement results in subcutaneous emphysema, which will greatly increase the difficulty of the procedure. Subcutaneous emphysema will resolve in approximately 48 h. Similarly, insufflating carbon dioxide below the omentum or within the falciform ligament causes expansion of these structures, and consequent obscuration of the field of view.

Once correct placement of the needle is confirmed, the Luer-lock attachment at the hub of the needle is connected to the insufflation tubing, and pneumoperitoneum is established (Fig. 4.4). The pressure within the abdominal cavity should be initially low (2–3 mmHg), and carbon dioxide should be delivered at a rate of at least 1 L/min. Greater intra-abdominal pressure, or a flow rate close to zero, are suggestive of

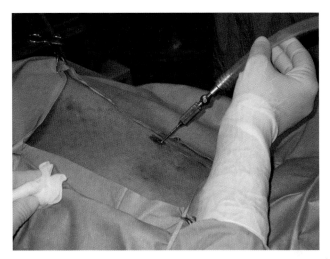

Fig. 4.4 Insufflating the abdomen by a Veress needle placed in the midline slightly cranial to the umbilicus.

occlusion of the needle tip (due to placement against a viscus, within the omentum or in a subcutaneous position). In this instance, the needle should be gently manipulated in and out of the abdomen to dislodge the occlusion, avoiding lateral movements in order to prevent injury to nearby structures. If the pressure remains elevated, re-placement of the needle is required. The abdomen at this point can be slowly insufflated up to a pressure of 13–15 mmHg (12–13 mmHg in cats); this can be reduced to 8–10 mmHg after port placement. When sufficiently distended, the abdomen becomes tympanic upon palpation, and the experienced operator can assess adequate separation between organs and abdominal wall by ballottement. Overdistension is best avoided, as it leads to decreased venous return and impairment in ventilation.

The trocar-cannula unit for the laparoscope can now be placed. The entry site is chosen, and a skin and subcutaneous tissue incision adequate for the size of the trocar is performed. Using an imprint of the cannula tip on the skin as a template helps in ensuring the correct diameter of the incision. This is very important, as an exceedingly large incision will cause gas leakage around the cannula, and may also lead to cannula dislodgement during instrument insertion or withdrawal. On the other hand, with a skin incision too small the force required to penetrate the abdominal wall will be increased, thus causing the trocar tip to get very close to viscera. A haemostat can be used to bluntly separate the muscle layers, to check incision size and minimise trauma to the abdominal wall.

If a threaded cannula is used, the skin incision should be slightly larger than the diameter of the cannula, which could otherwise get caught in the thread during cannula insertion. The fascial layer of the abdominal wall need also to be incised when using a cannula without trocar, which is introduced in the abdomen using a clockwise screw

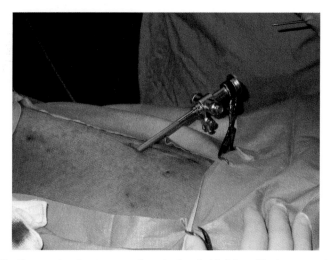

Fig. 4.5 Trumpet valve trocar placed after initial insufflations, ready for the scope to be introduced.

motion. A traditional trocar-cannula unit is passed through the abdominal wall with a controlled thrusting/twisting motion of hand and wrist, and is directed caudally to avoid the spleen. The upper end of the cannula is held firmly against the heel of the hand, and a finger is placed against the shaft, to limit penetration into the abdomen; the Luer-lock connection is closed, to avoid gas escape.

Soon after abdominal penetration the trocar is removed, to prevent organ trauma, and the cannula can be inserted further into the abdomen (Fig. 4.5). A valve present inside the cannula closes when the trocar is removed, thus preventing insufflation loss; when an instrument is introduced this valve opens automatically. Alternatively, the valve can be opened manually to avoid damage to a delicate instrument, as is the case with the laparoscope. The gas insufflation tubing is now connected to the Luer-lock attachment of the cannula, and the Veress needle is removed.

The open technique to achieve pneumoperitoneum was devised by Hasson to avoid injuries to intra-abdominal organs during needle placement. This technique requires a small incision through skin and abdominal wall, large enough to ensure that the abdominal cavity has been entered. Placing a stay suture through the abdominal wall fascia prior to the final incision is helpful to apply countertension and reduce the risk of organ damage. A blunt obturator-cannula is then inserted and sutured in place. If necessary, a gas-tight seal is achieved by tying stay sutures to a special cone ('olive') fitted over the cannula, or by placing a purse-string suture around it. This cannula is now used as the primary port. With this technique there is an increased risk of subcutaneous emphysema, due to gas leaking through the relatively large incision. The recent introduction of cannulae that do not require a trocar (Ternamian EndoTIP System, Karl Storz) has minimised the risk of injury to underlying structures without the disadvantages of an open technique. Furthermore, as these cannulae are placed with a twisting motion after a small incision in the abdominal wall, they are less easily dislodged during instrument insertion or removal.

Since the cold glass of the telescope lens tends to cause condensation of peritoneal moisture, the telescope should be warmed before insertion to prevent lens fogging. This is usually achieved by placing its tip into warm (40°C) sterile saline for 1–2 min, or holding it in the palm of the hand for a few moments. Anti-fogging solutions are also commercially available, or a povidone-iodine solution can be wiped across the distal lens. However, warming techniques are usually preferred, as the layer of solution can sometimes cause image distortion. Directing the carbon dioxide flow away from the endoscope also helps in avoiding the problem; in some cases gas inflow may need to be moved to an operative port. If fogging occurs during the procedure, gently touching the laparoscope tip on a serosal surface is usually sufficient to clear the lens. However, sometimes it is necessary to withdraw the telescope and clean it with a moist swab.

The light cable is then connected to the telescope, and its other end is handed to an assistant to be attached to the light source. The video camera is attached to the telescope, and the video system is turned on. Before entering the abdomen, the camera is 'white-balanced' by pointing it towards a white surface (this makes monitor colours more accurate) and focused until the image is sharp. The telescope can now be advanced trough the cannula and into the abdomen.

In order to facilitate precise localisation of lesions, and operative procedures, the camera is positioned so that the image on the monitor has the same orientation of the abdominal contents. To achieve this, the cable attached to the camera head always has to be directed towards the table. Once the telescope is in the abdomen, adequacy of pneumoperitoneum and presence of adhesions are verified, and the puncture sites (Veress needle and trocar-cannula unit) are inspected for damage to underlying organs. Occasionally the omentum can be draped over the scope on abdominal entry, interfering with visualisation. In this event, the omentum can be removed by positioning the scope slightly inside the cannula, and slowly withdrawing the cannula itself from the abdomen, until the omentum detaches.

The sites of insertion of secondary ports can now be chosen, depending on the procedure to be performed and on the anatomy of the patient. The selected locations must provide optimal access to the organs interested by the procedure, and have to be distant enough from the laparoscope (and from the organs themselves) to allow instrument manoeuvring without interference (Fig. 4.6 shows the triangulation technique). In situations where only one secondary portal is used it is usually placed on the side of the telescope of the operator's dominant hand (Fig. 4.7). The telescope and operating instruments also have to point towards the monitor, and the surgeon stands behind the camera, facing the monitor. When using telescope and secondary portals of the same size, it is sometimes convenient to switch locations between them.

Insertion is accomplished under direct visualisation. The proposed entry site is transilluminated with the telescope, thus identifying any large vessel present, and the skin depressed with a finger. This allows

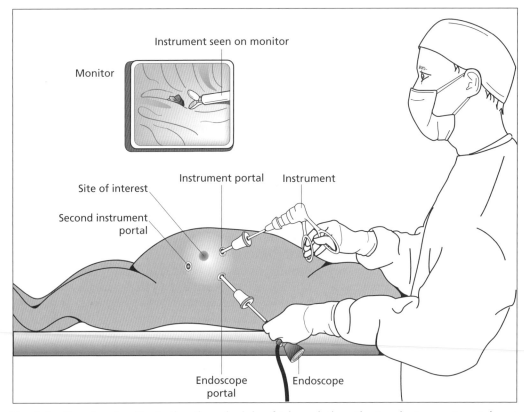

Fig. 4.6 Line drawing illustrating the principle of triangulation: the two instrument portals are placed on either side of the scope portal so that all three converge on the area of interest. The monitor is placed across the patient from the surgeon.

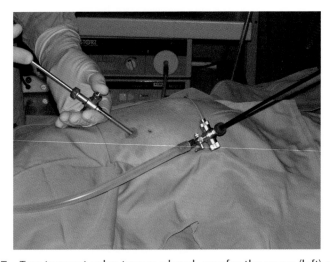

Fig. 4.7 Two trumpet valve trocars placed, one for the scope (left) and one for an instrument (right).

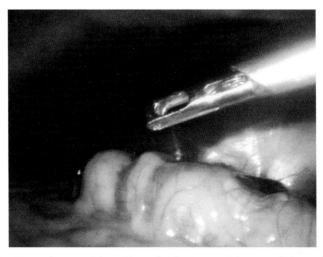

Fig. 4.8 Secondary port insertion: the instrument is passed through the secondary trocar under direct observation. Photograph courtesy of Mr P.J. Lhermette.

localisation of the entry site on the video monitor. The second port is established with the technique previously described, and the surgeon monitors the entry into the abdomen with the telescope (Fig. 4.8). This ensures that the trocar will not cause trauma to underlying organs. Similarly, instruments are never blindly inserted into the abdomen but directed towards the area of interest under visual monitoring. The telescope is positioned so that the tip of the cannula is in the field of view, and the instrument is inserted, closed, while its movement to the operative site is followed on the monitor. Only when the operative site is reached are the jaws of the instrument opened. Attention must be paid not to withdraw cannulae from the abdomen, as this would cause difficulties in maintaining the pneumoperitoneum, and consequently in reinserting them. This may occur more frequently in smaller patients, or when the abdominal wall is particularly thin.

Systematic examination of the abdomen is then performed, to detect any abnormalities. A blunt calibrated probe (5 mm in diameter, with 1 cm marks along the shaft) is usually employed to aid in manipulating organs and retract omentum. Retraction can be also achieved by tilting the table or rotating the animal on one side. This allows gravity to shift viscera away from the field of view and improves visibility. The table should never be tilted more than 15° to prevent complications.

If a significant amount of ascites is present, at the beginning of the procedure as much fluid as possible is removed. This is accomplished with fenestrated suction probes introduced through a secondary portal. However, abdominal fluid is best drained preoperatively, as the presence of fluid, often cloudy, greatly compromises visualisation of intra-abdominal structures. Furthermore, abdominal organs will also float on the fluid surface, increasing the risk of iatrogenic damage when inserting the Veress needle and the primary trocar and cannula. This risk is minimised by using a threaded cannula and an open technique to induce pneumoperitoneum.

Haemostasis is of paramount importance in minimally invasive surgery. Due to magnification, even small haemorrhages obscure the field of view and are therefore best prevented. Energy-assisted devices are preferred to dissect through vascular tissue planes.

In the event of haemorrhage, severed vessels are not easy to isolate, and using pressure to control bleeding can be difficult. After suction, clamping the tissue with grasping forceps allows temporary control, and once the vessel is identified, vascular clips, sutures or electrosurgical devices are used to achieve haemostasis. Persistent haemorrhage may require conversion to an open procedure.

At the end of the procedure, the abdominal cavity is inspected to rule out trauma to the viscera, haemorrhage or other complications. Insufflation pressure is best reduced to 4–6 mmHg to inspect ligature sites, as higher pressure may prevent bleeding (Kolata and Freeman, 1999b). If there is concern about active bleeding, it may be necessary to irrigate the site or lavage the abdomen and aspirate the fluid.

The instruments and telescope are then removed, and the pneumoperitoneum is evacuated by discontinuing insufflation and opening the valves of the cannulae. Gentle pressure is applied onto the abdominal wall while the cannulae are slowly removed. The puncture sites are inspected for bleeding, then sutured with interrupted sutures on the body wall and skin. Entry sites for small cannulae (less than 10 mm) require only skin suture. Finally, a long-acting local anaesthetic such as bupivacaine is infiltrated at the port sites.

Although it has been demonstrated that laparoscopic procedure are associated with less postoperative pain and a more rapid recovery (Magne and Tams, 1999), multimodal analgesia is necessary in the postoperative period, for as long as required by the individual patient. The patient needs to be monitored for insurgence of hypotension, as after desufflation the abdominal pressure decreases, with a consequent drop in vascular resistance. Patients that are haemodynamically stable usually tolerate hypotension well, but hypovolaemic animals, or those with cardiocirculatory compromise, may decompensate.

Exploratory laparoscopy and organ biopsy

In many cases, laparoscopic evaluation of intra-abdominal structures offers many advantages compared to exploratory laparotomy. Enhanced visualisation and opportunity to obtain reliable tissue samples allow the surgeon to acquire useful information also in animals with advanced disease, or in the work-up of challenging medical cases. Gastro- or enteral feeding tubes can also be inserted during the procedure. The surgeon can also perform laparoscopy in view of converting it to open surgery if the indication arises, for example in case of resectable disease. The shorter postoperative recovery time is beneficial in critically ill animals, and in cancer cases chemotherapy can be started sooner than with open procedures.

Hepatobiliary disease

One of the most common indications for laparoscopic examination and biopsy is hepatobiliary disease. Although many liver diseases are non-surgical, tissue samples are often required to obtain a diagnosis. Fine-needle aspirates cannot define lobular liver architecture and even core biopsy techniques often do not provide large enough samples to allow evaluation of liver architecture.

Laparoscopic liver biopsy allows excellent evaluation of the organ, and consequent precise sampling of the desired areas. Acquisition of larger pieces of tissue and a greater number of samples than those obtained with percutaneous needle biopsy increases the chance of a correct diagnosis. Percutaneous biopsy is also associated with an increased risk of inadvertent organ perforation. Visual confirmation of haemostasis – and the possibility to deal with haemorrhage directly – are of further advantage.

Before obtaining a liver biopsy coagulation parameters should be evaluated. Platelet count, prothrombin time (PT), partial prothromboplastin time (PPT) and mucosal bleeding time should be included. Although coagulopathies are a relative contraindication of laparoscopic liver biopsy, evaluations *in vitro* do not accurately predict the occurrence of bleeding after biopsy. Consequently, the administration of vitamin K or blood products before laparoscopic liver biopsy in patients with coagulation parameter abnormalities is usually not necessary.

When multiple organ examination and biopsy is required, the animal is placed in dorsal recumbency and a subumbilical telescope port is used. With the animal in a head-up position, the convex surface of the liver is easily visualised, although in obese patients the midline structures can be obscured by the falciform ligament. If the stomach is distended, an orogastric tube needs to be placed to aspirate gastric fluid to improve access to the liver. To provide access to the concave surface of the liver the animal has to be in a Trendelenburg position (with the head down). Tilting to the side instead increases visualisation to the contralateral liver lobes. The first instrument port is placed under direct visualisation in a paramedian position in either the right or left cranial quadrant of the abdomen, taking care not to place the cannula cranial to the last rib. This could in fact lead to entry in the thoracic cavity, with consequent pneumothorax. The minimum number of instrument portals that will provide access to all organs to be biopsied are created; the liver can be accessed through the same instrument portals used for the other laparoscopic procedures planned. In most cases two or three instrument ports are sufficient. A second port is usually placed on the contralateral side. In cases where a focal lesion is present the instrument port should be placed on the ipsilateral side.

In case of diffuse liver disease, if only liver evaluation and biopsy are required a right lateral approach is preferred by some laparoscopists. With this approach approximately 85% of the liver surface can be visualised, together with the extrahepatic biliary system and the right limb of the pancreas. The telescope portal is placed in the caudo-dorsal abdominal wall, just ventral to the lumbar muscles, approximately halfway between the caudal border of the ribs and the iliac wing. In patients with a small liver, or in large dogs, the entry site is positioned more cranially. Conversely, in small patients or in patients with hepatomegaly a more caudal entry site allows for increased working space for the scope and instruments. A second port is positioned again in the region of the paralumbar fossa, but midway between the spine and ventral midline. A single instrument port is often adequate.

Once the accessory port has been created, a blunt probe is inserted to manipulate the liver. The tip of the probe has always to be in the field of view, and is initially used to shift the omentum in a caudal direction. The liver is evaluated for size, texture, colour, margins, and presence of adhesions, mass lesions or nodules. Liver lobes are then individually lifted with the probe and inspected. The normal liver should be uniform, smooth, dark red in colour, with sharp margins, and should not tear or bleed when manipulated (Fig. 4.9).

The gall bladder and biliary system are now examined by retracting the scope slightly and elevating the right lateral and right middle liver lobes with it. While the liver lobes are elevated the gall bladder is palpated with the probe, and its size and turgidity are noted. Fig. 4.10 shows the appearance of a normal gall bladder. By elevating the gall bladder is then possible to examine the cystic, hepatic and common bile ducts and follow them to the duodenal insertion. This can be difficult in an obese

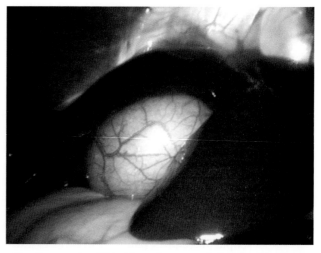

Fig. 4.9   The liver and gallbladder of a normal dog, in dorsal recumbency. Photograph courtesy of Mr P.J. Lhermette.

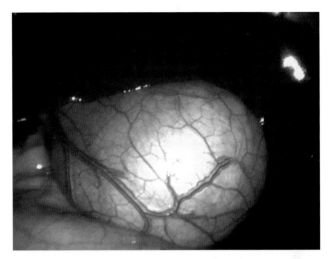

Fig. 4.10 Close-up view of a normal gallbladder. Photograph courtesy of Mr P.J. Lhermette.

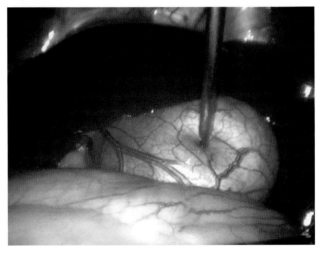

Fig. 4.11 Spinal needle introduced into the gallbladder for cholecystocentesis. Photograph courtesy of Mr P.J. Lhermette.

patient, and the probe is used to move fat and omentum out of the view. It is important to assess dilation and patency of the biliary system. The normal gall bladder is soft and fluctuant on palpation and the biliary tract is not distended. If obstruction is noted, its level and cause (mass, stricture) should be determined. The portal vein and caudal vena cava can be seen at the level of the insertion of the cystic duct into the common bile duct. At this level it is also sometimes possible to find extrahepatic portosystemic shunts.

Laparoscopy-guided cholecystocentesis (Fig. 4.11) can also be performed, using a 20- or 22-gauge needle. The gall bladder is punctured either with a long needle (such as a 20-gauge 5 cm spinal needle) placed percutaneously, or using a 5 mm laparoscopic needle tipped cannula through a standard operating port. In some instances, due to the increased viscosity of the abnormal bile, aspiration can prove difficult. The bile collected is submitted for cytology and aerobic and anaerobic culture. To prevent leakage after the procedure as much bile as possible is aspirated. Biliary centesis is not recommended if biliary obstruction is present because of the increased risk of leakage from the puncture site. Although aspirates can be taken directly through puncture of the exposed surface of the gall bladder, some surgeons prefer to place the needle across liver parenchyma into the gall bladder to reduce the risk of leakage.

Different techniques can be used to obtain liver biopsies. The preferred method is to use 5 mm laparoscopic cup biopsy forceps; this allows harvest of relatively large samples from the edge or the surface of the lobes with minimal tissue trauma and bleeding (Barnes et al., 2006; Vasanjee et al., 2006). Some biopsy forceps are also equipped with electrocoagulation capability. However, retrieval of biopsy samples using electrocoagulation is best avoided, as it may cause thermal injury to the sample. The areas to be biopsied are selected depending on the disease present: in case of focal lesions, biopsy samples have to be obtained not only from the affected areas, but also from areas with normal appearance. Areas of necrosis or areas characterised by increased vascularity and/or distended bile ducts are best avoided. Several samples are taken (usually five or six unless excessive bleeding occurs), from different liver lobes, and submitted for histopathology and aerobic and anaerobic culture. The large size of the samples obtained with 5 mm cup biopsy forceps (Fig. 4.12) allows acquisition of deep tissue, thus minimising the risk of non-representative biopsies when sampling areas close to the liver edge. Increased fibrous tissue is in fact present in subcapsular areas, and

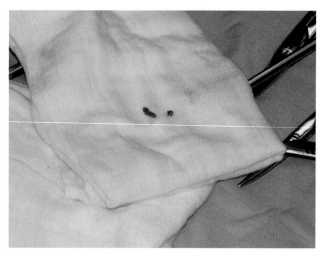

Fig. 4.12   Typical size of laparoscopic liver biopsies.

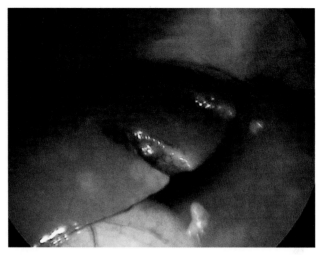

Fig. 4.13   Margin of liver after removal of two biopsies. Note that almost no bleeding has occurred.

therefore small samples taken at the edge of the lobes may not reflect deeper lesions.

The biopsy forceps are inserted through the operating port, directed toward the area to be sampled, and the tissue is grasped. The forceps are kept in position for 15–30 s, and then the tissue is gently twisted and pulled to retrieve the sample. In this way haemostasis is produced, diminishing the haemorrhage from the biopsy site. The area is closely monitored until haemorrhage stops (Fig. 4.13). This usually occurs within 2–3 min; if bleeding is more than expected, pressure can be applied to the biopsy site using the palpation probe or the tip of the laparoscope. If the haemorrhage persists, a haemostatic agent such as absorbable gelatine felt can be applied into the tissue defect and pressure applied for approximately 1 min.

Using a pre-tied loop ligature or extracorporeally assembled loop ligature to obtain biopsy samples is recommended in case haemorrhage is anticipated, such as in patients with coagulopathies, severe hepatic failure or highly vascular lesions. This technique requires one additional operating port for introducing the loop, which is manipulated around the biopsy site (usually the tip of a lobe). With a blunt probe or grasping forceps the liver lobe is elevated, so the loop can be positioned and tightened. The friable liver parenchyma is crushed, and the knot securely ligates the blood vessels and bile ducts, thus allowing the sample to be collected with laparoscopic scissors from the liver tissue distal to the loop.

A needle-core biopsy technique can also be used to obtain samples of the liver, but due to the restricted amount of tissue obtained this method is most often used to obtain samples of focal vascular liver masses. The biopsy needle can be inserted percutaneously through a small puncture just lateral to the xiphoid cartilage and manipulated under direct visualisation.

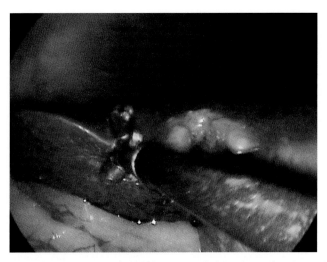

Fig. 4.14 Typical laparoscopic appearance of chronic canine hepatitis. The liver is mottled, sometimes described as having the appearance of sliced nutmeg. One biopsy has already been taken and the forceps are about to collect a second.

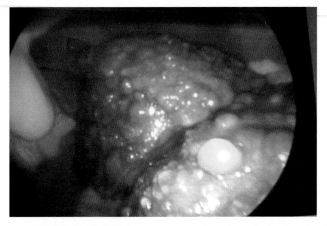

Fig. 4.15 Typical laparoscopic appearance of canine cirrhosis. The liver is pale and the surface nodular.

Examples of laparoscopic appearances of liver disease or abnormalities are seen in Figs 4.14–4.18; however, histology is essential to confirm the diagnosis.

The pancreas

Laparoscopy is also useful for evaluating the pancreas and differentiating pancreatitis from other extrahepatic biliary disease. This is particularly true in cases of chronic recurring pancreatitis with secondary biliary tract involvement. When pancreatic and liver evaluation and biopsy are

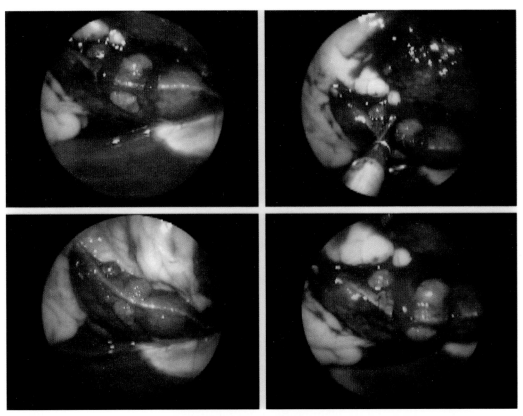

Fig. 4.16 A set of images obtained during biopsy of a cirrhotic liver with obvious nodular regeneration.

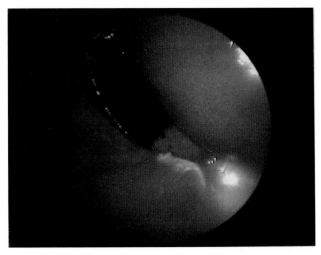

Fig. 4.17 Laparoscopic appearance of hepatic infarct in a dog (unknown cause). Note the clear-cut demarcation between normal liver and a much darker area of infarct.

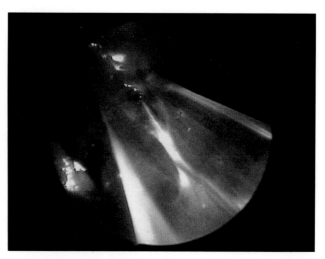

Fig. 4.18 Adhesion to the liver following previous open surgery and liver biopsy.

performed together a right lateral approach is used. This approach allows good visualisation of the right limb of the pancreas, but limited access to the left limb. To examine the whole pancreas, or when pancreatic exam/biopsy is performed at the same time as biopsy of other organs, a ventral midline approach is used, and the pancreas is accessed from the ports positioned for the other biopsy procedures. The animal is rotated to the left and the blunt probe or grasping/Babcock forceps are used to lift the duodenum and expose the right lobe of the pancreas. The right limb of the pancreas is followed beginning from the distal end as far to the left as possible. The left lobe, situated in the omental bursa, is visualised by elevating the greater gastric curvature and applying cranial traction to the omentum. Blunt dissection of the greater omentum caudally to gastro-epiploic vessels allows surgical access to it. The normal pancreas is pale cream in colour, with a lobulated appearance (Fig. 4.19). In cases of pancreatitis irregular firm tissue, fat necrosis and adhesions are often evident close to the pancreas, and may prevent its visualisation.

Punch biopsy forceps or, less commonly, cup biopsy forceps are used for pancreatic biopsy; with these instruments only one accessory port is needed. However, a second instrument port permits insertion of an instrument (such as a blunt probe or Babcock forceps) to hold the pancreas in place, and is necessary when manipulation of the surrounding organs is needed to obtain an unobstructed view of the pancreas. A second instrument port also allows use of a vessel-sealing device or a ligature biopsy technique.

Biopsies are collected from the lobe periphery, avoiding the body, where pancreatic ducts cross the gland to enter the duodenum together with the common bile duct. The area at the tip of the right pancreatic limb is also best avoided, as here the caudal pancreaticoduodenal vessels enter the gland.

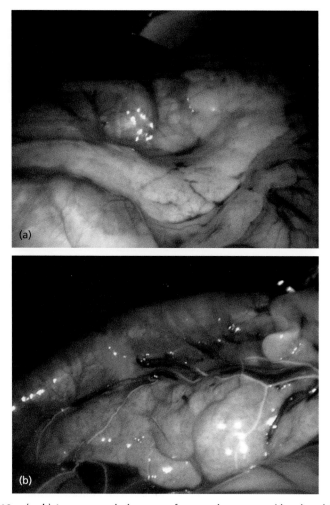

Fig. 4.19 (a, b) Laparoscopic images of normal pancreas (duodenal limb). Panel b shows a close up. Photographs courtesy of Mr P.J. Lhermette.

Haemorrhage from the biopsy site is addressed as for liver biopsies; alternatively, pre-tied loop ligatures or haemostatic clips placed in a V shape around the biopsy site can be used. Recently, a study evaluated the use of the Harmonic Scalpel for collecting biopsy samples in dogs (Barnes et al., 2006), comparing it with standard endoscopic instruments. Using the Harmonic Scalpel resulted in less haemorrhage but significantly greater inflammation.

In general, laparoscopic pancreatic biopsy has been demonstrated not to induce significant pancreatic injury or inflammation in normal dogs. However, minimising manipulation greatly decreases the risk of iatrogenic pancreatitis. One or two samples are usually harvested from the pancreas; liver biopsies are always collected at the same time, due to the high incidence of concurrent liver disease.

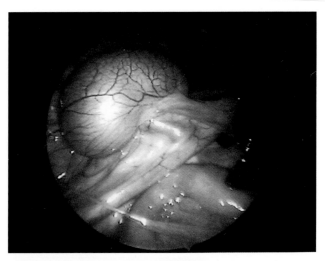

Fig. 4.20   Normal kidney seen via right-flank laparoscopy (note: this was a greyhound with minimal intra-abdominal fat; in other breeds, fat is likely to be covering the hilar vessels to a greater extent).

The kidneys

Laparoscopy allows excellent visualisation of the kidneys (Fig. 4.20) and collection of renal biopsies under direct visual guidance and magnification. This, in comparison with percutaneous ultrasound-guided biopsy technique, consents harvest of samples from desired areas and minimises the risk of injuries to adjacent organs or renal vessels. The possibility of monitoring the sampling site for haemorrhage, and to use pressure to induce haemostasis, also greatly decreases the risk of postoperative complications.

Before renal biopsy it is recommended to evaluate renal architecture with an ultrasound scan: hydronephrosis, cysts and ureteral obstruction are all contraindications to this procedure. Ultrasound scan also allows detection of focal lesions, important in selecting the area to be biopsied.

When a renal biopsy is planned it is also important to avoid the use of drugs that increase the renal blood flow, such as dopamine, to minimise haemorrhage from the biopsy site. Usually biopsies are taken from the right kidney, unless a unilateral lesion of the left kidney is suspected. The right kidney is less mobile, making sample collection easier; in addition, cannula placement on the left side is more difficult, due to the presence of the spleen directly under the entry site. The right lateral approach used for liver biopsy is therefore preferred, and the same trocar entry sites can be used.

Before biopsy the kidney is evaluated for position, contour and colour: the right kidney should be caudal and close to the right caudate process of the caudate lobe of the liver, whereas the left kidney is located just lateral to the spleen head. Often the kidneys are covered with omentum, which has to be shifted away in a caudal direction with a blunt probe. To visualise the right kidney it is also necessary to push the duodenum away. The presence of perirenal fat often hinders kidney visualisation in obese patients. The normal kidney is a pale purple colour, smooth and oval-shaped, with evident blood vessels.

The preferred way to obtain renal specimens is with the use of a Trucut® biopsy needle. Although this technique does not strictly require any instrument port, since the biopsy needle is inserted percutaneously, it is preferable to have one instrument port available for insertion of a palpation probe to provide haemostasis at the biopsy site. The probe is positioned near the kidney, and the location for needle insertion is determined. Palpation of the abdominal wall over the caudal border of the kidney is observed through the endoscope, thus avoiding the diaphragm, and allowing sampling of the renal poles. A 2 mm skin incision is performed at the entry site, and a 15 cm 14- or 16-gauge automated Trucut or similar biopsy needle is introduced under direct visualisation into the abdomen caudal to the diaphragm. The needle is inserted at a shallow angle to the capsule, directed away from the hilus, to avoid the corticomedullary junction, where the large arcuate vessels are located. Insertion of the needle parallel to the long axis of the kidney may prove difficult due to the angle of insertion of the needle through the body wall. The needle can alternatively be inserted at the poles, perpendicular to the long axis of the kidney. In particular, biopsy samples are more easily obtained from the cranial pole of the kidney, which is larger than the caudal pole. In any case, the aim is to obtain mostly the renal cortex with little medulla, to maximise the number of glomeruli recovered (Rawlings and Howerth, 2004) (Fig. 4.21). The surgeon must provide a

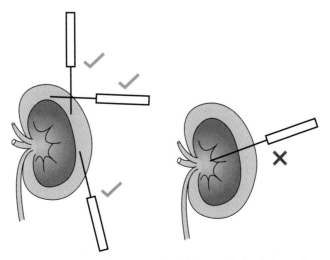

Fig. 4.21 Line drawing of a core needle biopsy of the kidney illustrating the correct possible paths of the needle to avoid entering the medulla.

sample that includes a minimum number of intact glomeruli, renal arterioles and cortical interstitium (Freeman, 2009).

Once properly seated into the kidney parenchyma, the needle is activated to cut the biopsy, and the sample is recovered. Two to three samples are usually collected. Following biopsy, pressure is applied for a few minutes to the renal surface with the palpation probe to control haemorrhage. Haemostatic foam application can be used if necessary. Postoperative haematuria, usually self-limiting, is a common sequel to any method of kidney biopsy.

The small intestine

For examination of the intestine two instrument portals are required. The procedure is usually performed with the patient in dorsal recumbency, with a standard ventral midline approach. The two instrument portals are located a few centimetres lateral to the scope on each side. Two pairs of Babcock forceps are used to grasp the intestine and 'run' as much of it as possible. The intestinal surface, blood supply and lymph nodes are evaluated. Small intestinal biopsies are usually obtained using a laparoscopy-assisted technique. This entails exteriorising the selected portion of intestine through a small incision in the abdominal wall. Pneumoperitoneum is lost during the procedure, and therefore intestinal biopsies are performed after other procedures. When the location for the biopsy is selected, the antimesenteric border of the intestine is firmly grasped with Babcock forceps and gently pulled up slightly inside the cannula. The intestine and forceps are then removed from the abdomen together with the portal. In order to easily exteriorise the intestine, it is often needed to enlarge the incision by 2–4 cm. This is carefully accomplished by cutting away from the cannula with a blade, under direct visualisation. For this procedure the use of a 10 mm port should be considered, as this is less likely to require enlargement and makes the procedure easier. Gelpi retractors can also be positioned in the incision, to keep it open and decrease compression of the mesenteric root.

Once a 3–4 cm section of the intestine has been exteriorised, stay sutures are placed on its antimesenteric border, and the biopsy is carried out in a standard fashion. After the biopsy is completed local lavage can be performed away from the abdominal incision site, and the intestine is gently replaced into the abdominal cavity. Care should be taken not to exteriorise too large a loop of intestine, as it can then be difficult to return it to the abdomen. In this case, the Babcock forceps inserted in the other instrument port can be used to gently pull the loop back into the abdominal cavity.

If multiple intestinal biopsies are required, the cannula needs to be reintroduced into the abdomen, and the pneumoperitoneum re-established. In order to create a sufficient seal to maintain insufflation of the abdomen, a purse-string suture can be placed around the operative port. Reinsufflation is also needed if inspection of biopsy sites for haemorrhage is necessary.

An alternative technique employs a laparoscopic wound-retraction device (Alexis Wound Retractor®, Applied Medical UK), which keeps a small circular orifice open into the abdomen. In this way the intestine can be exteriorised through a wider incision, avoiding the risk of compression of the mesenteric roots. The wound-retraction device is also useful in performing biopsy of other structures such as lymph nodes, and in various laparoscopy-assisted surgical procedures.

Mesenteric lymph nodes

Samples from small lymph nodes are usually obtained with an excisional biopsy. The lymph nodes are identified laparoscopically and carefully dissected from the surrounding tissue, preferably using the Harmonic Scalpel or other power-assisted device. Grossly enlarged lymph nodes can be biopsied with cup forceps, often following dissection of overlying mesentery to expose the surface. A right flank approach may be useful to improve exposure of the mesenteric lymph nodes.

Other abdominal organs

Laparoscopic biopsies can also be obtained from the spleen and the adrenal glands. Cup biopsy forceps are commonly employed, and the technique is the same as for liver biopsy. Care should be taken with splenic or adrenal biopsy, because significant haemorrhage is common.

In addition, laparoscopy is useful for staging and biopsying abdominal tumours. The excellent visualisation of vascular changes in tissue is very helpful in identifying metastatic disease: lesions less than 1 mm in diameter can be detected on the liver or peritoneal surface. This is particularly valuable in cases of unexplained ascites or suspected mesothelioma.

Complications

In addition to complications that may be encountered with any surgery (such as anaesthesia-related complications, haemorrhage, infection, wound dehiscence, adhesion formation, etc.), specific complications associated with laparoscopy generally arise from Veress needle and trocar insertion and abdominal insufflation. Insufficient or malfunctioning equipment, together with operator inexperience, play a major role in the insurgence of most operative complications, and consequently careful planning helps in minimising their occurrence.

Complications resulting from Veress needle or trocar insertion include major vessel injury and damage to underlying organs, which in turn can lead to mechanical organ damage and/or gas embolism. Abdominal-wall penetration may in fact injure the superficial or deep epigastric vessels, and also major abdominal vessel may be reached, especially in small patients. Although the organ more commonly injured during needle or trocar insertion is the spleen, because of its size and position, perforation of hollow viscera such as stomach, intestine and bladder has also been reported.

Various preventative measures are recommended to avoid these iatrogenic complications. Transillumination of the body wall before insertion of accessory portals allows identification of abdominal wall vessels; similarly, placement of secondary portals under visual inspection decreases the risk of damage to underlying organs. A controlled trocar insertion is also important, and the non-dominant hand may be placed onto the abdominal wall to act as a stop. Alternatively, the middle finger of the hand manoeuvring the trocar can be extended along the trocar shaft, to limit the depth of insertion. Other safety measures include emptying the bladder (and the stomach in case of overdistension) before the procedure, ensuring an adequate degree of pneumoperitoneum and placing the patient in a slight Trendelenburg position. The latter two steps are directed at increasing the distance between organs and insertion site. Finally, the Veress needle and the first trocar, which are inserted blindly, must be aimed away from the spleen.

Abdominal insufflation with the Hasson (open) technique has also been shown to significantly diminish the frequency of complications (Twedt and Monnet, 2005); alternatively, the use of optical trocars allows the passage of the endoscope into the lumen of the cannula during insertion, so that the trocar's progress can be monitored visually.

Early detection of complications is also essential to minimise damage: the areas of Veress needle insertion is explored as soon as the primary port is established, and the whole abdomen is inspected again before closure. Perforation of a hollow viscus is usually readily apparent, as urine or gastrointestinal contents are aspirated; Veress needle injuries are often self-limiting, whereas trocar-induced damage needs to be repaired. In this case, as in cases of significant haemorrhage due to spleen injury, conversion to open surgery is usually necessary. Damage to viscera may also occur during organ manipulation and biopsy, due to unexpected findings (biopsy of vascular tumours, abscesses, hydronephrosis), coagulopathies or inappropriate biopsy technique.

Complications secondary to insufflation are related to penetration of air in areas other than the abdominal cavity: subcutaneous emphysema, peritoneal tenting (air insertion between the muscle layer and the peritoneum), insufflation of the omentum, pneumothorax and gas embolism. Subcutaneous emphysema and peritoneal tenting are considered minor complications, but can create problems for continuing the procedure. The emphysematous space may in fact be so deep that the tip of the needle or trocar cannot easily reach the peritoneum. If this occurs, pneumoperitoneum must be established with the open technique; alternatively, the procedure is abandoned and can be repeated as soon as emphysema resolves, usually less than 48 h when carbon dioxide is the insufflation gas. With insufflation of the omentum (or mesentery), visualisation of the abdominal cavity is hindered, and the abdomen needs to be allowed to desufflate before continuing. If the needle is inappropriately inserted into and insufflates the falciform ligament, more lateral reinsertion usually allows continuation of the procedure.

A serious complication associated with insufflation is pneumothorax. This, together with pneumomediastinum and pneumopericardium, may occur consequently to inadvertent perforation of the diaphragm during laparoscopy, in the presence of diaphragmatic haernia or rupture, or may be due to overinsufflation (Twedt and Monnet, 2005). The positive pressure of pneumoperitoneum causes tension pneumothorax, which must be rapidly recognised and resolved. The abdomen should be promptly desufflated, and a thoracostomy tube inserted. After thoracic air evacuation the procedure can sometimes be continued laparoscopically, but more often conversion to open surgery is necessary.

Gas embolism is a potentially life-threatening complication occurring when gas is insufflated into the circulatory system following accidental placement of the Veress needle into a vessel or the spleen. Carbon dioxide continues to be absorbed during the recovery period and consequently embolism can occur even in the early postoperative period. However, the occurrence of embolism with carbon dioxide is relatively uncommon, as carbon dioxide is highly soluble in blood, and penetration of small amounts into the systemic circulation is usually without consequence. Large amounts of gas travelling to the right ventricle cause cardiocirculatory collapse, with sudden and profound decrease in blood pressure, insurgence of heart murmur and cardiac arrhythmias, and changes in end-tidal carbon dioxide (Quandt, 1999). Gas embolism must be treated quickly to avoid cardiac arrest; the animal should be placed in left lateral recumbency with the head down (Freeman, 1999; McClaran and Buote, 2009), and ventilated with 100% oxygen.

The cardiopulmonary effects of pneumoperitoneum are well tolerated in healthy animals (Duke et al., 1996); however, hypoxia and/or hypercarbia may develop in animals with pre-existing cardiac or pulmonary compromise. Insufflation of room temperature gas may also cause hypothermia, especially in long procedures.

Port site metastasis is a complication to be expected in cancer patients. Although different theories are advocated to explain their development, such as direct implantation during sample retrieval, exfoliation of cells during tumour manipulation, and dispersion following carbon dioxide insufflation or by haematogenous spread (McClaran and Buote, 2009), the use of specimen retrieval bags for removal of tumour samples is recommended. Commercially available retrieval bags usually come on a 10 mm applicator, and therefore require a large portal site; to obviate the problem, in case of smaller samples, bags can be made inexpensively from a sterile surgical glove.

Conversion to laparotomy cannot be considered a complication. However, patients undergoing conversion of the procedure often have increased requirements for intensive care. Conversions may be elective, due to poor exposure (as in case of adhesions, obesity or aberrant anatomy) or operator inexperience, or may be decided when a large resectable mass is found. Emergency conversions are usually consequent to uncontrollable haemorrhage or rupture of a hollow viscus, or are related to anaesthetic complications precluding continuation of carbon dioxide insufflation (hypercarbia, hypoxia). A conversion rate of 23% has been reported (McClaran and Buote, 2009) and it is therefore important for the patient and the operating team to be ready for it, should the necessity arise.

Further reading

Freeman, L.J. (ed.) (1999) *Veterinary Endosurgery*. Mosby, St Louis, MO.

Lhermette, P. and Sobel, D. (eds) (2008) *BSAVA Manual of Canine and Feline Endoscopy and Endosurgery*. British Small Animal Veterinary Association, Gloucester.

Mayhew, P.D. (2009) Techniques for laparoscopic and laparoscopic-assisted biopsy of abdominal organs. *Compendium: Continuing Education for Veterinarians* 31, 170–177.

McCarthy, T.C. (ed.) (2005) *Veterinary Endoscopy for the Small Animal Practitioner*. Elsevier Saunders, St Louis, MO.

Melendez, L. (ed.) (2001) Endoscopy. *Veterinary Clinics of North America, Small Animal Practice* 31(4).

Monnet, E. and Twedt, D.C. (2003) Laparoscopy. *Veterinary Clinics of North America, Small Animal Practice* 33, 1147–1163.

Radlinski, M.G. (ed.) (2009) Endoscopy. *Veterinary Clinics of North America, Small Animal Practice* 39(3).

Tams, T.R. and Rawlings, C.A. (eds) (2011) *Small Animal Endoscopy*, 3rd edn. Mosby, St Louis, MO.

Twedt, D.C. (1999) Laparoscopy of the liver and pancreas. In *Small animal Endoscopy*, Tams, T.R. (ed.), pp. 409–418. Mosby, St Louis, MO.

References

Abel, F., Pierce, J. and Guntheroth, W. (1963) Baroreceptor influence on postural changes in blood pressure and carotid blood flow. *American Journal of Physiology* 205, 360–364.

Bailey, J.E. and Pablo, L.S. (1999) Anesthetic and physiologic considerations for veterinary Endosurgery. In *Veterinary Endosurgery*, Freeman, L.J. (ed.), pp. 24–43. Mosby, St Louis, MO.

Barnes, R.F., Greenfield, C.L., Schaeffer, D.J., Landolfi, J. and Andrews, J. (2006) Comparison of biopsy samples obtained using standard endoscopic instruments and the harmonic scalpel during laparoscopic and laparoscopic-assisted surgery in normal dogs. *Veterinary Surgery* 35, 243–251.

Duke, T., Steinacher, S.L. and Remedios, A.M. (1996) Cardiopulmonary effects of using carbon dioxide for laparoscopic surgery in dogs. *Veterinary Surgery* 25, 77–82.

Freeman, L.J. (1999) Complications. In *Veterinary Endosurgery*, Freeman, L.J. (ed.), pp. 92–102. Mosby, St Louis, MO.

Freeman, L.J. (2009) Gastrointestinal laparoscopy in small animals. *Veterinary Clinics of North America, Small Animal Practice* 39, 903–924.

Joris, J.L., Noirot, D.P., Legrand, M.J., Jacquet, N.J. and Lamy, M.L. (1993) Hemodynamic changes during laparoscopic cholecystectomy. *Anesthesia and Analgesia* 76, 1067–1071.

Kolata, R.J. and Freeman, L.J. (1998a) Access, port placement, and basic endosurgical skills. In *Veterinary Endosurgery*, Freeman, L.J. (ed.), pp. 45–60. Mosby, St Louis, MO.

Kolata, R.J. and Freeman, L.J. (1998b) Minimally invasive surgery of the liver and biliary system. In *Veterinary Endosurgery*, Freeman, L.J. (ed.), pp. 151–159. Mosby, St Louis, MO.

Magne, M.L. and Tams, T.R. (1999) Laparoscopy: instrumentation and technique. In *Small Animal Endoscopy*, Tams, T.R. (ed.), pp. 397–408. Mosby, St. Louis, MO.

McClaran, J.K. and Buote, J.B. (2009) Complications and need for conversion to laparotomy in small animals. *Veterinary Clinics of North America, Small Animal Practice* 39, 941–951.

Monnet, E., Lhermette, P. and Sobel, D. (2008) Rigid endoscopy: laparoscopy. In *BSAVA Manual of Canine and Feline Endoscopy and Endosurgery*, Lhermette, P. and Sobel, D. (eds), pp. 158–174. British Small Animal Veterinary Association, Gloucester.

Quandt, J.E. (1999) Anesthetic considerations for laser, laparoscopy, and thoracoscopy procedures. *Clinical Techniques in Small Animal Practice* 14, p.50–55.

Rawlings, C.A. and Howerth, E.W. (2004) Obtaining quality biopsies of the liver and kidney. *Journal of the American Animal Hospital Association* 40, 352–358.

Savvas, I., Rallis, T. and Raptopoulos, D. (2009) The effect of pre-anaesthetic fasting time and type of food on gastric content volume and acidity in dogs. *Veterinary Anaesthesia and Analgesia* 36, 539–546.

Staffieri, F., Lacitignola, L., De Siena, R. and Crovace, A. (2007) A case of spontaneous venous embolism with carbon dioxide during laparoscopic surgery in a pig. *Veterinary Anaesthesia and Analgesia* 34, 63–66.

Twedt, D.C. and Monnet, E. (2005) Laparoscopy: technique and clinical experience. In *Veterinary Endoscopy*, McCarthy, T. C. (ed.), pp. 357–385. Elsevier Saunders, St Louis, MO.

Vasanjee, S.C., Bubenik, L.J., Hosgood, G. and Bauer, R. (2006) Evaluation of hemorrhage, sample size, and collateral damage for five hepatic biopsy methods in dogs. *Veterinary Surgery* 35, 86–91.

Villiers, E. (2005) Disorders of erythrocytes. In *BSAVA Manual of Canine and Feline Clinical Pathology*, 2nd edn, Villiers, E. and Blackwood, L. (eds), pp. 33–57. British Small Animal Veterinary Association, Gloucester.

Chapter 5
Operative Laparoscopy
Lynetta J. Freeman

Although there are a number of ways to approach operative laparoscopy, patient factors, skill of the endoscopist, available equipment and owners' desires guide the selection of approach for each animal. The wise veterinarian will select the technique that offers the greatest benefit with the least risk to the animal. Laparoscopists must have the skill to perform the procedure using the available equipment. In some cases, although a procedure is technically feasible, performing a totally laparoscopic approach requires so much more surgical time that it may not be in the best interest of the animal. Minimally invasive techniques are infrequently used in veterinary medicine, so decision-making regarding the approach is based more on the surgeon's opinion and experience than on outcomes of published studies. The purpose of this chapter will be to discuss totally laparoscopic, laparoscopy-assisted and hand-assisted laparoscopic for traditional operative laparoscopy, and to introduce two newly emerging approaches, called SILS™ and NOTES®, that may be applicable to veterinary minimally invasive surgery in the future.

Definitions

Totally laparoscopic procedures are performed exclusively through small incisions to introduce trocars into the abdominal cavity, as was discussed in the previous chapter. Usually *multiple ports* are placed, one to introduce the laparoscope for viewing the abdominal contents and one or two working ports for operative equipment. The multiple ports are arranged such that the surgeon can triangulate instruments to approach the target

Clinical Manual of Small Animal Endosurgery, First Edition. Edited by Alasdair Hotston Moore and Rosa Angela Ragni.
© 2012 Blackwell Publishing Ltd. Published 2012 by Blackwell Publishing Ltd.

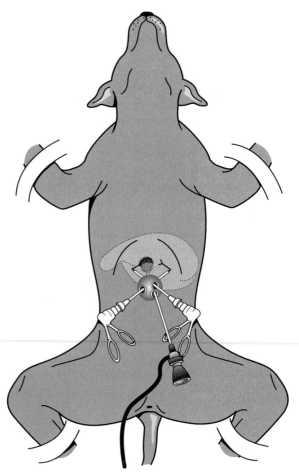

Fig. 5.1   Line drawing of single-incision laparoscopic surgery (SILS). A single port containing two working channels and the laparoscope is placed at the umbilicus. Articulating instruments are used to allow triangulation at the operative site.

area of interest. *Single-port* procedures are performed through only one incision in the abdominal cavity, usually at the umbilicus. They may be performed with an *operating laparoscope* (a rigid laparoscope containing a working channel) for viewing and coaxial introduction of instruments. In human surgery, specialised instruments are becoming available to enable what is known as single-incision laparoscopic surgery (*SILS*). A three-channel trocar (Fig. 5.1) is placed at the umbilicus and a rigid endoscope containing a flexible portion is introduced into one of the channels for operative viewing. Specially designed articulating instruments are introduced through the other two channels to enable triangulation of instruments on the target of interest. A complex procedure can then be performed through only one port and cosmetic outcomes are excellent since the incision is hidden in the naval folds. *Hand-assisted*

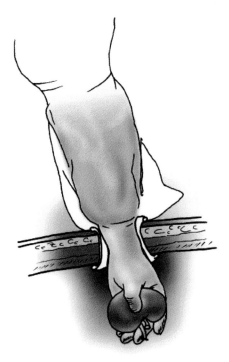

Fig. 5.2 Line drawing of hand-assisted laparoscopic surgery. From Rudd and Hendrickson (1999), Fig. 12.9. Reproduced with permission from Elsevier.

laparoscopy (HALS) is performed using a totally laparoscopic approach with a single large port (Fig. 5.2) that enables the surgeon to insert a hand into the abdominal cavity and maintain insufflation by providing a seal around the arm. These techniques are popular in human surgery for removing an intact kidney in donor nephrectomy procedures and whenever manipulation or removal of large organs such as the spleen or colon is anticipated.

Lap-assisted procedures are commonly performed in veterinary medicine for prophylactic gastropexy, intestinal biopsy, feeding-tube placement and cystotomy procedures. The lap-assisted procedure begins as a laparoscopic approach with placement of multiple trocars and, at the appropriate time, one of the trocars is removed and a mini-laparotomy is performed to expose tissue that needs inspection or suturing. In animals, the lap-assisted procedure is commonly performed because the body wall is thinner than human patients, making the mini-laparotomy less invasive, with less risk of dehiscence and wound infection than if the procedures were performed in people. The optical cavity in small animals is much smaller than in human patients, making endoscopic suturing and tissue manipulation more difficult. In addition, in veterinary medicine it is far more economical to suture, rather than use stapling devices, which are widely used in human surgery. The veterinary surgeon should always be prepared for conversion to an open procedure. Each laparoscopy case is prepared as if conversion will take place and the owners are informed of this risk when giving their consent for laparoscopy. When the initial examination suggests an involved procedure is warranted, or when traditional laparoscopy does not provide adequate and safe exposure, the surgeon may elect to perform *conversion to 'open' celiotomy*. The umbilical port is extended cranially and caudally along the linea alba, retractors are placed, and the procedure is converted from a laparoscopic to an open approach.

Anaesthesia and preoperative preparation

Anaesthesia and preoperative preparation proceed in a standard fashion as if the surgical procedure were going to be performed by open technique. Additional concerns for anaesthesia include increased abdominal pressure and absorption of carbon dioxide from pneumoperitoneum. With increased abdominal pressure there is reduced tidal volume, so assisted ventilation may be necessary. Carbon dioxide absorption leads to elevated P_aCO_2, warranting monitoring of pulse oximetry and end-tidal carbon dioxide (Weil, 2009). Positioning the animal for laparoscopy is critical to ensure that the procedure proceeds expediently. An operative table that is capable of being tilted head up or down and to the right or left simplifies the operative set-up. Having a monitor at both the head and foot of the table minimises the need to re-arrange the room during a procedure. It is very important to ensure that the animal is securely positioned and that it will remain so when the table is tilted. Very large animals have a tendency to slide down the table when the head is elevated or when tilted to the side if they are not properly secured.

General operative procedures

A well-trained surgical team is essential for smooth functioning of the operative procedure. While the animal is being draped the instruments for laparoscopy are opened and assembled on the back table. As the camera, light guide cable and insufflation tubing require connections to the endoscopy tower, a non-sterile operating room assistant trained in operation and trouble-shooting of the equipment and in capturing video images is essential. Each procedure usually involves a camera operator, the surgeon and an assistant to manage the back table of supplies and equipment. The surgical field is widely draped. After the field drape is applied and the video connections are made, the camera is white-balanced and the operation begins.

Access and visualisation

Primary port placement is safely achieved using the open technique for placement of a blunt-tipped Hasson trocar. A small incision is made

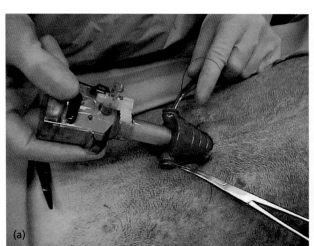
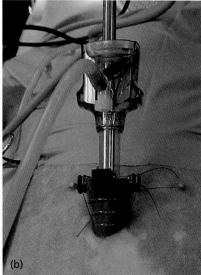

(a)

(b)

Fig. 5.3 Photographs of a Hasson trocar showing retention sutures secured to the olive plug. (a) Side view. Each suture is wrapped around the tying posts of the olive plug. (b) Top view. The insufflation tubing has been attached to the stopcock and the laparoscope is inserted.

through the skin and subcutaneous tissue down to the linea alba. Once this landmark is visualised the external sheath of the rectus abdominis muscle is elevated and an incision is made through the linea alba with a scalpel blade. After confirming entry into the peritoneal cavity, a suture is placed through the linea alba on each side of the incision and is tied to the olive plug of the trocar. The olive plug ensures a good seal between the trocar and the abdominal incision. The sutures hold the trocar in place during manipulation (Fig. 5.3). In cats and some dogs a portion of the falciform ligament must be removed to properly place the primary port and prevent smudging of the laparoscope when it is inserted. The carbon dioxide tubing is attached to the stopcock of the trocar and insufflation to 12 mmHg is begun. The obturator is removed and the laparoscope is inserted to perform a visual inspection of the abdominal cavity. To prevent laparoscope fogging during insertion into the warm abdominal cavity, prior warming or an anti-fog solution may be used.

Tissue manipulation and retraction

Depending on the operation, secondary ports are inserted under direct visualisation in a location to triangulate on the region of interest. The fingertip is used to indent the body wall and identify the site for port placement. Following a small skin incision, a sharp trocar is inserted, keeping the tip in the centre of the field of view at all times. When the trocar cannula is seen the sharp obturator is removed and the cannula is secured. Some trocars have threads on the outside of the cannula which are very helpful in keeping the cannula secure during the procedure. A blunt probe is useful for tissue manipulation. If tissue needs to be elevated, blunt grasping forceps can be utilised. If it is necessary to expose an organ, endoscopic Babcock forceps are useful in grasping and elevating tissue and viscera, such as the stomach or urinary bladder. Retraction is almost always achieved by positioning the animal and letting gravity assist in moving organs out of the field of view; however, fan-shaped retractors are available and are sometimes necessary to enhance exposure. When 5 mm-diameter instruments are inserted through 10 mm ports, a reducer cap is necessary to prevent loss of pneumoperitoneum.

Haemostasis

To maintain an adequate field of view, excellent haemostasis must be achieved or the operative field will become too dark for proper visualisation. A number of devices are used for haemostasis and each has advantages and disadvantages. For single, well-isolated pedicles, laparoscopic ligating clips may be used and, depending on the source, may be relatively inexpensive. Haemostasis of the ovarian pedicles and uterine body is most easily achieved with ultrasonic energy delivered by the Harmonic® Scalpel (Ethicon Endo-Surgery; Fig. 5.4) or by bipolar electrocoagulation delivered with the LigaSure™ vessel-sealing device (Valleylab). The author prefers the Harmonic Scalpel for safety and precise dissection; however, the water vapour generated during the pro-

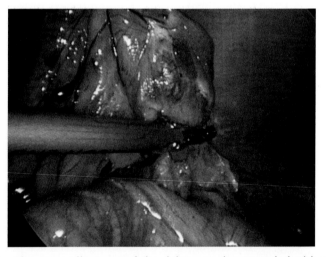

Fig. 5.4   The proper ligament of the right ovary is suspended with a percutaneous suture as the 5 mm Harmonic Scalpel device is positioned on the suspensory ligament and ovarian pedicle. There is minimal lateral thermal damage.

cedure must be vented to prevent obscuring the operative field. For large pedicles where precise dissection is not needed, I prefer the LigaSure or ENSEAL® (Ethicon Endo-Surgery) devices as they are capable of bipolar coagulation of vessels up to 7 mm in diameter. Pre-tied loop ligatures, such as the ENDOLOOP, can also be used when there are two operating ports and the tissue can be grasped through the loop (Fig. 5.5). As an alternative, sutures that are tied outside the body with a Roeder knot can be advanced into the cavity to perform secure ligation.

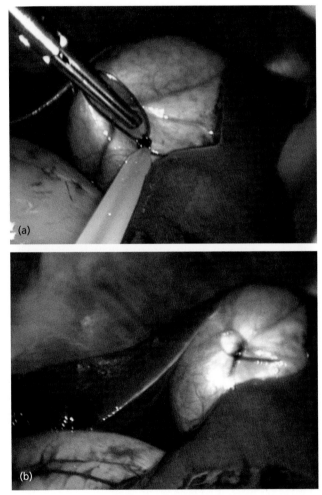

Fig. 5.5 A pre-tied loop ligature is being positioned and tightened to prevent bile leakage from the gall bladder after obtaining a bile sample for culture. Two working ports are required: (a) grasping forceps are inserted through the centre of the loop to grasp the tissue around the opening in the gall bladder; (b) final appearance after the loop has been tightened and the suture cut.

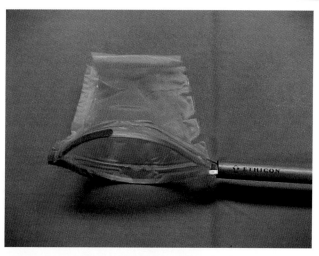

Fig. 5.6   Ethicon specimen-retrieval bag. The wire band assists in holding the specimen-retrieval bag open for insertion of tissue.

Tissue retrieval

Most of the time, tissue retrieval is simply facilitated by removing the trocar with the tissue, releasing the pneumoperitoneum and enlarging the incision. For retrieval of friable tissue or to ensure that contamination does not occur, a tissue specimen bag (ENDOPOUCH® Retriever™, Ethicon Endo-Surgery) may be used. The tissue is placed inside the bag and the top is closed. The tissue is then removed while in the bag (Fig. 5.6).

Inspection and closure

Final inspection of the operative site and abdominal viscera should be performed prior to closure to ensure that there is no active bleeding and no evidence of iatrogenic tissue injury. If necessary, the abdomen can be lavaged with sterile saline and the fluid aspirated. It can be quite difficult to remove all of the lavage fluid without loss of pneumoperitoneum, and therefore there is almost always some residual fluid left in the abdomen. I prefer to remove the secondary ports while the abdomen is still insufflated. The tissue layers are grasped as the trocar is removed because in this way they are best aligned and most easily visualised. Each tissue layer is closed in succession with one or two absorbable sutures. The Hasson trocar is removed last. The sutures are used to elevate the body wall and ensure that all of the excess carbon dioxide is allowed to escape. The linea alba, subcutaneous tissue and skin are then closed routinely. A 5% lidocaine patch (Endo Pharmaceuticals) may be cut and applied around each of the port sites to provide regional analgesia without systemic effects (Fig. 5.7).

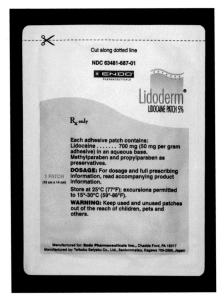

Fig. 5.7   A 5% lidocaine patch can be adhered to the skin and used for local analgesia around port sites.

Follow-up and aftercare

Postoperative recovery is managed very similar to open surgery. Postoperative analgesia is managed effectively with injectable opiod pain medication and/or non-steroidal anti-inflammatory medication.

Specific procedures

Ovariectomy, ovariohysterectomy

Surgical techniques for performing laparoscopic sterilisation of small animals have evolved over the past 20 years. Early procedures involving uterine horn occlusion were attempted as a tentative technique to prevent conception but resulted in accumulation of fluid in the uterine horns (Wildt and Lawler, 1985). In the early 1990s, when laparoscopy started to expand in human surgery but equipment was limited, up to five ports were placed to enable pre-tied surgical ligatures to be used effectively in performing the procedure (Freeman et al., 1992). As clients began to demand laparoscopy for its reduced postoperative pain and faster return to normal activity for their pets, the field expanded. New equipment for ligation of the ovarian pedicles became available (bipolar electrocoagulation, ligating clips, laser, Harmonic Scalpel) and techniques were revised to reduce the number of operative ports and improve operative time. Other workers studied a laparoscopy-assisted technique that involved enlarging a caudal midline incision for ligation of the uterine body using extracorporeal ligatures (Devitt et al., 2005). Simply performing an ovariectomy was advocated by veterinary surgeons in Europe, citing their experience with no increased rate of complications following ovariectomy in open procedures (van Goethem et al., 2006). When techniques for percutaneous suspension of the ovarian pedicle were reported and utilised effectively, the number of operative reports and operating time were reduced further. More recently there have been randomised studies demonstrating that dogs undergoing laparoscopic ovariohysterectomy required less postoperative analgesia than those undergoing an open procedure (Davidson et al., 2004; Devitt et al., 2005; Hancock et al., 2005). Another study demonstrated less decrease in postoperative activity levels with laparoscopic approaches in small dogs compared to open surgery (Culp et al., 2009). Currently, bilateral ovariectomy is commonly performed with an energy modality and one or two operating ports using the technique that will be described below.

Surgical procedure

Following general anaesthesia and positioning in dorsal recumbency the animal is aseptically prepared and widely draped. As a general guideline, in cats and very small dogs a 2.7 mm rigid scope is used, for dogs of less than 25 kg a 5.0 mm rigid laparoscope is used and a 10 mm rigid laparoscope is used for dogs of more than 25 kg. The size of the animal dictates the size of the Hasson trocar, which is placed on the midline just caudal to the umbilicus. After initial port placement, insufflation and examination of the abdominal cavity, a second 5 mm port is placed on the midline for insertion of a second instrument. The location of the second port depends on the animal's size, but approximately 5 cm caudal to the camera port in an average-sized dog seems to work well. Next, 5 mm grasping forceps are inserted to identify and retract the left uterine horn. To aid in visualisation the animal is tilted 30° or more to the right, towards the surgeon. The grasping forceps are used to trace the uterine horn proximally, to grasp the proper ovarian ligament, and to elevate the ovary to a convenient location on the abdominal wall for percutaneous suspension. The location must be inside the sterile field. By palpating the abdominal wall while elevating the ovary the appropriate site is selected. A laparoscopic spay hook (Fig. 5.8) or a large curved needle is inserted percutaneously through the body wall until the tip is visualised. The grasping forceps are then used to drape the ovary over the needle or hook to ensure that the ovary remains elevated away from underlying viscera. The needle or hook is then rotated to secure the tissue. If a needle and suture are used, the needle is removed from the body and forceps are applied to the suture outside the body. The laparoscopic spay hook has a weighted handle that, once rotated, maintains the hook in a fixed

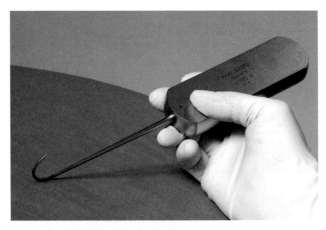

Fig. 5.8   The laparoscopic spay hook has a weighted handle. The sharp tip is inserted percutaneously and used to suspend the ovary from the body wall during laparoscopic ovariectomy.

location. Occasionally, there may be minor bleeding associated with this step; however, it is self-limiting as the ovary is subsequently removed. The grasping forceps are removed and the energy modality device is inserted in its place.

For rapid vessel occlusion of the ovarian pedicles, an energy system is required. A bipolar vessel sealing system such as the LigaSure or the ENSEAL can be used. The LigaSure system has a function that monitors tissue impedance while energy is being applied. When coagulation is complete the impedance rises, meaning that the tissue is dessicated and no additional energy is flowing through it; the system detects it and gives an audible signal or adjusts energy output to create the desired tissue effect. A separate trigger is then activated to transect the tissue. The ENSEAL system has a special design that includes a polymeric compound in the jaw of the device that is responsive to temperature. When the temperature of the polymer reaches 100°C, the conductive particles in the polymer expand to disrupt the flow of electrical current. The result is minimal lateral thermal spread, and reduced tissue scarring and sticking of tissue to the electrodes. The tissue is then cut by applying a second trigger. The technique for using both of these instruments is similar. The blade is positioned across tissue, energy is applied and then the trigger is pulled to cut the tissue.

The Harmonic Scalpel uses electrical energy to vibrate a piezoelectric crystal in the handpiece of the instrument. Ultrasonic energy is transmitted down the shaft of the instrument which then causes the blade to vibrate rapidly at 55 000 cycles per second (cps, or Hz). When tissue is captured between this active blade and the Teflon pad, heat from the friction of the moving blade is transmitted to the tissue, disrupting hydrogen bonds and resulting in the collagen molecules in the tissue adhering

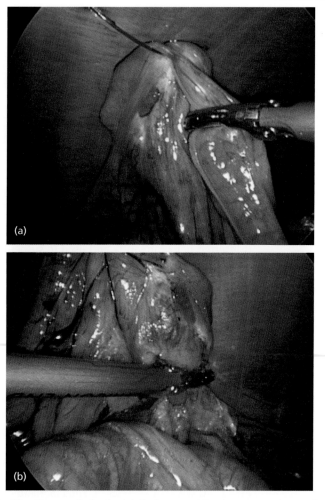

Fig. 5.9 The Harmonic Scalpel is being used for laparoscopic ovariectomy. (a) Transection of the left proper ovarian ligament. (b) Transection of the right ovarian pedicle and suspensory ligament.

to each other and forming a 'sticky coagulum' at low temperatures (Thompson and Potter, 1999). When energy is applied for a longer time, the temperature in the tissue continues to rise and protein is denatured, resulting in tissue coagulation. Tissue is stretched during the coagulation process and the blade cuts through it, resulting in haemostasis with minimal lateral thermal damage (Fig. 5.9). The technique for using the Harmonic Scalpel is slightly different from that used with bipolar devices. The jaws are applied across the tissue and, as energy is applied, slight traction is placed on the device to enhance tissue dissection.

During laparoscopic ovariectomy the ovarian pedicle and suspensory ligament are ligated and transected first. Transection of the fallopian tube and proper ovarian ligament or the proximal portion of the uterine horn follows. The ovary is thus isolated, suspended to the body wall. At this point, the laparoscope is transferred to the caudal port and endoscopic grasping forceps are inserted through the larger, sub-umbilical port to grasp and retrieve the ovary. The intra-abdominal pressure is reduced, the trocar is removed and the stay sutures are used to elevate the body wall as the ovary is removed. A slight twisting or rotating motion enhances removal of the ovary. Following inspection, the trocar is then replaced and the procedure is repeated for coagulation and transection of the right ovary.

An ovariohysterectomy can be performed using a similar approach; however, with only one working port it can be difficult to mobilise the ovary and keep it retracted to gain access to the broad ligament. If so, an additional port can be placed to provide caudo-medial retraction while the energy modality is used to coagulate and divide the broad ligament to the level of the uterine arteries and uterine bifurcation. Once both broad ligaments are transected, the uterine body is coagulated and cut or ligated. If the uterine body is small, the LigaSure, ENSEAL or Harmonic Scalpel can be used to coagulate and cut it. If very large, the uterine body may need to be ligated. The caudal midline trocar is removed and the incision enlarged so that the uterine body can be exteriorised. An extracorporeal ligature can then be used to ligate it in the same fashion as in open surgery (technically performing a laparoscopy-assisted ovariohysterectomy). Another alternative is to use pre-tied loop sutures. The pre-tied loop is introduced and the ovaries and uterine horns are passed through it such that the loop can be positioned on the uterine body. The nylon cannula is broken and advanced to tighten the loop, taking care to avoid incorporating other structures into it. When the loop is tight, the suture tail is cut with laparoscopic scissors. The uterus is then transected and removed from the sub-umbilical port.

If the tissue is suspected to be friable, malignant or infected, a specimen-retrieval bag can be utilised to safely remove the tissue while protecting the body wall from contamination. The bag is introduced through one of the ports, tissue is placed in it and the mouth of the bag is closed for withdrawal from the body. Final inspection is performed to ensure haemostasis and the port sites are closed routinely. Complications are rare, and the most common are iatrogenic trauma to the spleen or other abdominal organs during insertion and removal of laparoscopic equipment, electrocautery injury to surrounding tissue, subcutaneous emphysema and inflammation of the port sites. Usually these complications are self-limiting and are treated conservatively with no serious consequence.

Recent studies have evaluated the operative time and potential complications of using one or two ports in laparoscopic ovariectomy procedures. Both methods result in acceptable outcomes; however, the one-port technique may require greater laparoscopic skills or result in longer surgical time (Dupré et al., 2009).

Gastropexy

Prophylactic gastopexy is performed to prevent gastric volvulus in large-breed dogs that may be predisposed to developing gastric dilation and volvulus (or GDV) syndrome. The *laparoscopy-assisted gastropexy* can be performed at the same time as laparoscopic ovariectomy in female dogs. In male dogs, when the procedure is performed at the same time as castration, the surgeon may choose to perform an *endoscopically assisted gastropexy* to avoid placement of an umbilical port. Biomechanical studies of the forces required to disrupt the adhesion site following minimally invasive approaches suggest that the adhesion is as strong as intact stomach and clinical experience indicates that the gastropexy performed with minimally invasive techniques is reliable and strong. Although several techniques have been advocated, the one described by Dr Rawlings and co-workers is technically easiest and most widely used and will be described here (Rawlings et al., 2001, 2002).

Laparoscopy-assisted gastropexy

Ideally, 10 mm laparoscopic Babcock forceps and at least one 10 mm trocar are needed for this procedure. Instruments of 5 mm can be used, but they are not as robust in elevating the stomach to the body wall and can result in more tissue trauma. Following general anaesthesia the animal is positioned in dorsal recumbency. The abdomen is prepared for aseptic surgery and widely draped, especially on the right side, just caudal to the ribs. As with laparoscopic ovariectomy, the procedure begins with open insertion of a 5 or 10 mm trocar cannula approximately 3 cm caudal to the umbilicus on ventral midline. This port serves as the camera port during the procedure. The laparoscope is connected to a camera and the camera is connected to a monitor. Surgeons view the procedure on the monitor placed at the animal's head. The abdomen is distended with carbon dioxide and pressures are kept low to avoid compromising venous return and tidal volume. With the laparoscope inserted in the sub-umbilical port, entry of a second 10 mm trocar is directly visualised. The port is located approximately 3 cm caudal to the last rib just lateral to the rectus abdominis muscle on the right side. Next, the 10 mm Babcock forceps are inserted to elevate the liver lobes and expose the ventral aspect of the stomach. If the stomach is incorrectly positioned the Babcock forceps are used to reposition it in a normal location. A point on the antrum of the stomach, approximately 5 cm cranial to the pylorus, and midway between the greater and lesser curvature, is identified for the gastropexy. The Babcock forceps are used to grasp and elevate the gastric wall and to move it to the base of the trocar cannula (Fig. 5.10A). If there is considerable tension on the stomach, reducing the intra-abdominal pressure may assist in this step. As the Babcock forceps and cannula are withdrawn, the incision in the skin and abdominal fascia is extended to 4–6 cm. A muscle-splitting approach to the

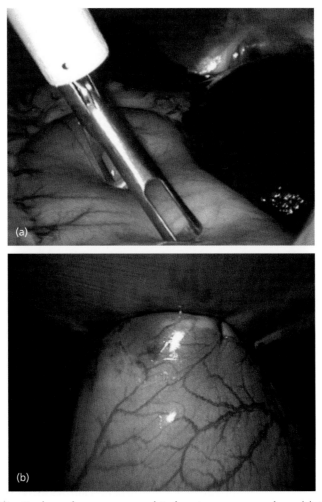

Fig. 5.10   During a laparoscopy-assisted gastropexy procedure, (a) 10 mm Babcock forceps are used to grasp the stomach midway between the greater and lesser curvature about 5 cm proximal to the pylorus. (b) Final laparoscopic photograph showing the sutured gastropexy site.

external and internal abdominal oblique muscles can be utilised. Pneumoperitoneum is lost as the gastric wall is exteriorised. Two stay sutures with size 2-0 monofilament suture are placed to grasp and elevate the gastric wall and the Babcock forceps are then removed. A 4–5 cm seromuscular incision of the gastric wall is made, down to, but excluding, the gastric mucosa. A Gelpi retractor aids in exposure of the layers of the abdominal wall. The seromuscular layer of the stomach is then sutured to the internal fascia and transversus abdominis muscle in a continuous pattern with synthetic absorbable suture. After the stay sutures are removed, the external abdominal fascia is sutured over the defect using a continuous pattern with synthetic absorbable suture. The subcutaneous tissue and the skin are closed routinely. A final inspection with the laparoscope is performed (Fig. 5.10B), the carbon dioxide is allowed to escape and the camera port is removed. The fascia, subcutaneous tissue and skin are closed routinely. A 5% lidocaine patch can then be applied to the skin around the incision.

Totally laparoscopic technique

This technique requires three midline ports, two needle holders and endoscopic suture. The stomach can be sutured to the abdominal wall from inside the abdomen without the need for full-thickness incision in the body wall. Although technically more difficult, this technique appears to result in more rapid return to activity than the laparoscopy-assisted approach (Mayhew and Brown, 2009). The stomach is temporarily anchored to the body wall at the proposed gastropexy site with a single, percutaneously placed stay suture. Adjacent incisions are then made in the abdominal wall and seromuscular layer of the stomach with laparoscopic Metzenbaum scissors. One technique uses a pair of laparoscopic needle holders to suture the stomach to an incision in the transversus abdominis muscle using a simple continuous pattern with 2-0 absorbable suture on a ski-shaped needle. During suturing, and especially during tying of the initial knot, the abdominal pressure is reduced so that the stomach is apposed to the body wall with less tension. The lateral margin is sutured first with one continuous pattern. The suture is then tied and cut and another strand is used to suture the medial margin. The stay suture is then removed. As an alternative to needle holders, the Endo Stitch™ 10mm Suturing Device (Covidien) is available with absorbable, silk, nylon and polyester materials in sizes 0 to 4-0 suture. If this device is used, at least one of the ports must be 10mm in diameter. The Endo Stitch is a suturing device with two jaws and a design that allows a needle (with suture swaged in the centre) to be passed between the jaws by activating a toggle switch on the handle. By closing the jaws on tissue and flipping the toggle switch, the needle is passed from one jaw through the tissue to engage the other jaw of the instrument. Thus, the needle is held securely at all times and orientation is maintained. Once the needle is passed through the stomach and through the body wall it is possible to tie a surgical knot by passing the needle around the free end of suture, creating a loop, and passing the needle through the loop (Fig. 5.11). For complete instructions readers should refer to the manufacturer's website and DVDs. No matter which technique is selected, the surgeon must develop laparoscopic suturing skills in a box trainer and, preferably, on a cadaver prior to attempting these procedures on client-owned animals.

Endoscopically assisted gastropexy

This technique requires a flexible endoscope and a 76mm-long needle with size 2 polypropylene suture (Dujowich and Reimer, 2008). The

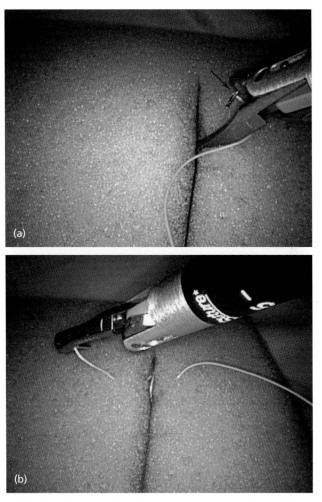

Fig. 5.11   (a) The Endo Stitch device uses a needle with suture swaged in the centre (arrow). The needle is secured in one jaw of the instrument. (b) The jaws are closed around the tissue and the needle is passed to the other jaw by a toggle switch on the handle of the instrument.

animal is positioned in 30° left oblique recumbency and prepared for aseptic surgery. Following insertion of the endoscope, the stomach is inspected and distended with air from the endoscope. The abdominal wall is palpated with forceps while the pyloric antrum is viewed to identify the site for gastropexy. Once the correct orientation of the antrum to the body wall is obtained, two stay sutures are placed. A large needle is passed percutaneously caudal to the thirteenth rib through the body wall and into the antrum of the stomach while viewing with the endoscope. The needle is passed back out through the skin and secured with haemostatic forceps. A second suture is placed in the same manner approximately 4–5 cm aboard to the first. An incision is then made between the two sutures through the skin, subcutaneous tissue and body wall until the gastric surface is seen. A 3–4 cm incision is then made through the gastric serosa and muscularis down to the level of, but excluding, the gastric mucosa. Like the laparoscopy-assisted gastropexy, the seromuscular layer of the stomach is then sutured to the transversus abdominis muscle. The external fascia, subcutaneous tissue and skin are closed routinely. The stay sutures are removed and final endoscopic inspection is performed.

The surgeon occasionally encounters an animal with a pre-existing partial twisting of the stomach. Using the laparoscopic approach this is easily recognised and grasping forceps can be used to reposition the stomach to its normal anatomic location prior to gastropexy. A twist can also be recognised endoscopically and can potentially be repositioned using the endoscope, although this is somewhat difficult. The endoscopic techniques have the potential for unrecognised trapping of omentum or other abdominal contents between the gastric and abdominal walls so careful palpation and repositioning of the animal may be required prior to stay-suture placement.

With each of these procedures, following surgery the animals are given a lidocaine patch and postoperative analgesics, which usually consist of parenteral opiod medication and non-steroidal anti-inflammatory drugs for 3–4 days. Owners are instructed to limit activity for 2–3 weeks while the adhesion forms. In animals that are very active after surgery the most common postoperative complication is seroma formation along the gastropexy incision site, which resolves with conservative therapy.

Laparoscopic cryptorchid castration

If physical examination does not reveal one or both testicles in the scrotum or inguinal area, laparoscopic visualisation of inguinal rings and peritoneal cavity can assist with definitive identification and location of retained testicles. In addition, this technique is associated with less tissue trauma, postoperative pain and wound complications. If the spermatic cord is visualised entering the inguinal ring, the testis is located outside the peritoneal cavity or just inside the inguinal ring (the so-called peeping testicle) (Freeman, 1999). If only the gubernaculums is seen entering the inguinal ring, the testis is located inside the abdominal cavity. It can be found by tracing the gubernaculum from the inguinal ring, the ductus deferens from the prostate, or by identifying and tracing the pampiniform plexus to the testicle.

A laparoscopic or laparoscopy-assisted technique can be performed, depending on available equipment. If an energy modality such as LigaSure, ENSEAL or Harmonic Scalpel is available the laparoscopic approach is performed. If not, the laparoscopy-assisted technique is easiest and quickest.

Both techniques begin with the animal positioned in dorsal recumbency and prepared for aseptic surgery with wide draping. An initial 5 or 10 mm port is placed on the midline just caudal to the umbilicus for insertion of the laparoscope and viewing of the abdominal cavity. Once the location of the testis is identified, a second 5 or 10 mm port is placed on the opposite side, depending on the size of the retained testicle and whether the initial port is 5 or 10 mm. If both testicles are retained they can usually be removed with only two ports, but the surgeon should not hesitate to place a third port, if necessary. During insertion of additional ports, careful palpation of the proposed trocar insertion site should be performed to avoid trauma to the caudal deep epigastric vessels.

When using two ports it is necessary to use a percutaneous suture or the laparoscopic spay hook to suspend the testicle to the abdominal wall to elevate and isolate the ductus deferens and pampiniform plexus from underlying structures. The technique is similar to that for suspending the ovary in an ovariectomy procedure. The grasping forceps hold the testicle next to the body wall while the needle or hook is inserted and rotated to grasp a portion of the testicle and elevate it to the body wall. The grasping forceps are removed and the vessel-sealing device is inserted and placed across the gubernaculum, pampiniform plexus and spermatic cord in succession. The device is activated to coagulate and then cut the tissue (Fig. 5.12). If desired, a double seal can be performed on the pampiniform plexus prior to transection. An alternative to using the vessel-sealing device is to use ligating clips or sutures. Initially, the technique was described using pre-tied ligatures (Gallagher et al., 1992). Once ligation and transection are complete, the testicle is removed from one of the port sites. If a 10 mm port is placed on the midline, as a less traumatic approach, the laparoscope is transferred to the second port and the testicle is removed from the midline location with Babcock grasping forceps, removing the trocar cannula as the testicle is withdrawn. Otherwise, the laparoscope is left in place and the testicle is removed through the parapreputial port. If a laparoscopy-assisted gastropexy is being performed during the same procedure, the second 10 mm trocar is placed in the right cranial quadrant and the testicle can be removed through this port. The port sites are closed routinely in layers.

When using the laparoscopy-assisted technique, the second port is placed *on the same side* as the retained testicle. Babcock forceps are used to grasp and elevate the testicle until it can be exteriorised. The incision may need to be extended slightly for adequate exposure. Ligation of the gubernaculum, pampiniform plexus and spermatic cord is performed with suture outside the abdominal cavity, similar to open surgery. If the testicle is neoplastic, measures to protect the port site from the potential for neoplastic seeding should be taken. If there is evidence of testicular torsion, appropriate exposure may be needed to ensure an easy removal.

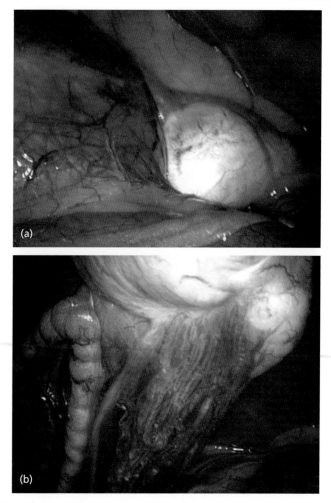

Fig. 5.12 Photographs demonstrating a laparoscopic cryptorchid castration.: (a) the testicle is identified in the inguinal region, just beside the urinary bladder; (b) when the testicle is suspended, the ductus deferens and the pampiniform plexus are identified. The Harmonic Scalpel is then used to coagulate and transect these structures.

Laparoscopy-assisted cystoscopy

Cystoscopy performed with a rigid endoscope may be a procedure that is performed by veterinarians specialised in internal medicine; however, surgeons who perform cystoscopy find application of the technology useful in minimising the approach to management of urinary calculi that are too large or too numerous for other treatment modalities such as laser lithotripsy, urohydropropulsion or traditional cystoscopy with stone retrieval using a basket (Rawlings, 2009). The advantages of laparoscopic cystoscopy are that bladder trauma is limited to a very small incision and there is less likelihood of urine contamination of the abdominal cavity. With a single very large stone, the abdominal incision and incision in the bladder must be large enough to retrieve the stone. Most often, the laparoscopy-assisted cystoscopy is performed in male dogs because females have a larger urethra and are more amenable to retrieval of larger stones with the traditional cystoscope. The *laparoscopy-assisted cystoscopy* approach involves placing a midline trocar for viewing abdominal contents prior to placing a second port for exteriorising a portion of the urinary bladder (Rawlings et al., 2003). Recently, the *keyhole transvesicular cystourethroscopy* procedure has been advocated to avoid the need for the laparoscopic approach (Runge et al., 2008). The bladder is distended and a small laparotomy is made on the midline. The cranial portion of the bladder is grasped and exteriorised. After this, the steps of both procedures are the same and will be described in detail.

Both techniques use a rigid cystoscope, which provides excellent visualisation of the internal surface of the bladder and proximal urethra, ideally ensuring that all stones are removed and that any surface irregularities are seen and biopsy samples taken for further evaluation. The cystoscope comprises a 30° 2.7 mm rigid scope with a 14.5 French sheath for most cases (Fig. 5.13). A smaller cystoscope, which uses a 1.9 mm scope, is available for cats and small dogs. Other equipment needed for the procedure includes a stone basket which fits through the working channel of the cystoscope sheath and a variety of forceps, including alligator forceps, arthroscopy forceps and 5 mm laparoscopic grasping forceps. Irrigation fluids with a pressure cuff are connected to the cystoscope to provide constant irrigation and clearing of the site. When numerous small stones are present, a 5 mm threaded trocar cannula, such as the Thoracoport™ (Covidien), can be inserted into the bladder and

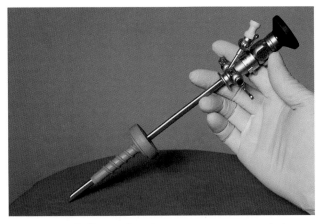

Fig. 5.13 Photograph illustrating the 2.7 mm cystoscope being used with a 5 mm Thoracoport™ cannula.

the cystoscope can then be repeatedly passed through the trocar without traumatising the bladder (Fig. 5.13). Similar to patient management for traditional cystotomy, azotemia and urinary tract infection should be resolved and the animal evaluated for other systemic abnormalities prior to surgery. Radiography documents the number and location of radiopaque stones and ultrasound examination of the kidneys, ureters and bladder is useful in detecting small or radiolucent stones and determining if there are irregularities in the bladder wall or trigone. For animals with recurrent bladder infection, it is wise to obtain a full-thickness biopsy of the bladder wall for culture at the time of surgery. Perioperative antibiotics are administered and the abdomen is prepared for aseptic surgery with wide draping. The prepuce is flushed with antiseptic solution in male dogs and draped into the surgical field.

When performing laparoscopy-assisted cystoscopy the initial 5 mm trocar is placed on the midline at or just caudal to the umbilicus. The laparoscope is inserted and visual inspection of the abdomen is performed. A second 5 or 10 mm trocar is then placed on the midline in female dogs or lateral to the prepuce in male dogs for insertion of the 5 or 10 mm Babcock forceps. The forceps are used to grasp the apex of the bladder and lift it to the trocar site as the cannula is removed (Fig. 5.14). Usually, the 10 mm incision is sufficient for exteriorisation of the bladder, but it can be extended if needed. While holding the bladder apex with the forceps, a minimum of two cruciate stay sutures are placed in the bladder wall and used for retraction. Some surgeons use four quadrate interrupted sutures on the bladder wall and some suture the bladder wall to the skin to prevent abdominal contamination with urine during the procedure (Rawlings et al., 2003). Another option is to insert a threaded trocar cannula, but care must be taken with the reusable ones to ensure that the screw tip does not traumatise the bladder wall. The cystoscope is connected to the camera, light source, irrigation fluids and egress tubing. After scope insertion into the bladder and appropriate fluid distension, visual inspection is performed. The bladder is lavaged and inspected, taking care to ensure that any portion of the bladder that is cranial to the cystotomy site is thoroughly examined. In male dogs one can pass a urethral catheter to occlude the urethral lumen and to serve as an additional means of flushing the urethra.

The wire stone basket is efficient for retrieval of calculi (Fig. 5.15). This device can be passed through the working channel of the cystoscope into the bladder past the calculi and opened. The calculi are then captured with the basket, which is subsequently brought to the end of the cystoscope. The cystoscope is removed and the basket is opened to deliver the calculi. Some calculi are too large to capture in the stone basket. For these, forceps can be inserted alongside the cystoscope and used to grasp the stone. The forceps and cystoscope are removed and reinserted to remove each stone (Fig. 5.16). Smaller calculi may be removed by placing a suction device inside the bladder and flushing through the urethra. The urethral catheter is passed to ensure a smooth

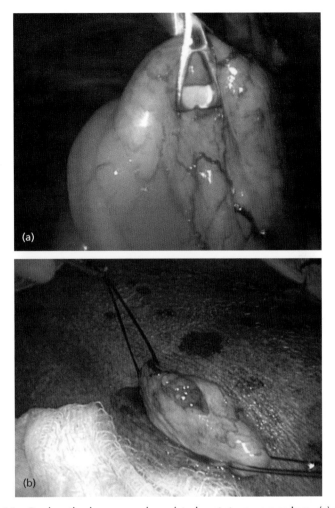

(a)

(b)

Fig. 5.14   During the laparoscopic assisted cystotomy procedure, (a) 10 mm Babcock forceps are used to elevate the urinary bladder to the body wall. (b) The trocar is removed, the abdominal incision extended and the bladder exteriorised and secured with a pair of stay sutures.

passage, flushed, and the proximal portion of the urethra is inspected to ensure removal of all calculi.

If bladder polyps are noted during cystoscopy then a biopsy sample should be obtained to differentiate them from transitional cell carcinoma (Rawlings, 2007) (Figs 5.17 and 5.18). The abdominal incision is extended to exteriorise the bladder and a scalpel blade or laser fibre can be used to resect the bladder wall at the base of the polyp, or a partial cystectomy can be performed if the lesions are diffuse. If the polyp is associated with a single large calculus, one may choose to simply obtain a biopsy by grasping them together with a stone basket or biopsy forceps.

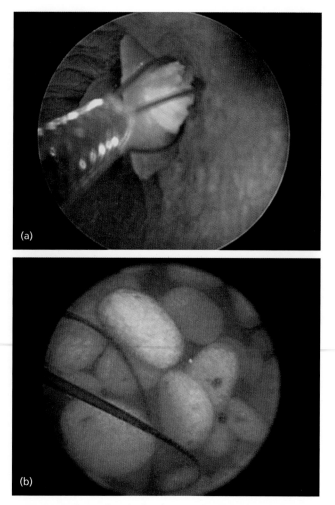

Fig. 5.15 Cystoscopic retrieval of urinary calculi with a stone basket inserted through the working channel of the cystoscope. (a) The basket is used to snare single irregular stones, or (b) multiple stones may be captured in the device.

Inflammatory polyps may then regress if the chronic source of irritation is removed.

The cystotomy is then closed with a single layer of sutures and the bladder is replaced in the abdominal cavity. The second port site is closed in layers (external sheath of rectus abdominis muscle, subcutaneous tissue and skin) and the abdomen is insufflated and finally examined. The camera port is then removed and the site closed routinely. Lidocaine patches are applied to the areas around the skin incisions for local analgesia. Following surgery, radiographs should be taken while the animal remains anaesthetised to ensure that there are no residual calculi. Post-

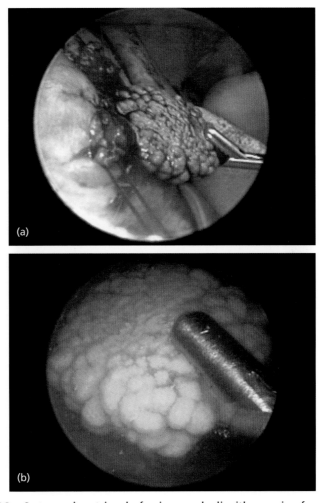

Fig. 5.16 Cystoscopic retrieval of urinary calculi with grasping forceps. (a) Alligator forceps are inserted alongside the cystoscope to grasp a single large calculus. (b) The forceps and cystoscope are removed from the bladder through a very small incision in the bladder.

operative care is similar to that following open surgery, with fluids and postoperative analgesics, antibiotics and dietary modification.

Feeding-tube placement

Animals may be fed enterally through a tube placed in the oesophagus, the stomach or intestine. The choice of tube type depends on the disease state, anticipated length of time the tube will be used and whether the animal will remain hospitalised or will need to be fed at home. The intestinal feeding tubes are best utilised for hospital feeding using a

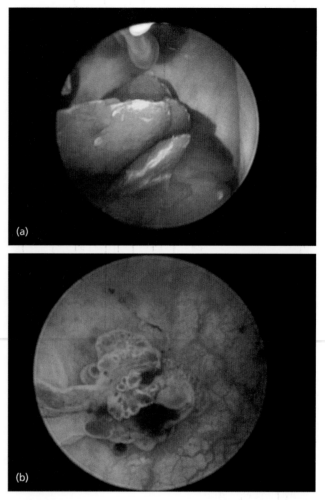

Fig. 5.17   Bladder polyps may be associated with a single large irregular calculus. (a) Cystoscopic view of an irregular calculus and polyp visible at 12 o'clock. (b) Following removal of calculi, a pedunculated polyp is visualised inside the bladder.

constant rate infusion when either postoperative vomiting is anticipated or the stomach needs initial bypass. Gastric and oesophageal feeding tubes are used when the risks of vomiting or regurgitation are minimal; with these, feedings can be performed at home. The gastric feeding tubes can be placed with open, laparoscopic or percutaneous endoscopic gastrostomy (PEG) techniques. One very useful combination is the gastro-jejunal (or G-J) tube wherein a gastric feeding tube is placed using an open technique and the intestinal tube is fed through the gastric tube into the stomach and down into the small bowel. The intestinal feeding is performed while the animal is recovering in the hospital and then the

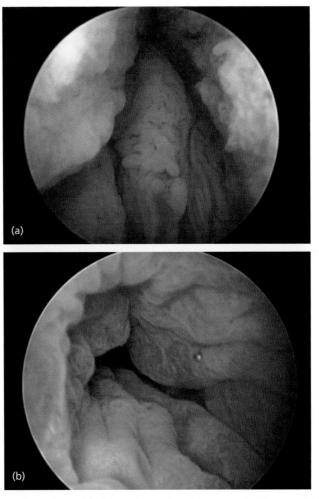

Fig. 5.18 The urinary bladder trigone is a frequent site for transitional cell carcinoma (TCC). (a) Typical appearance of TCC as a fimbriated growth in the region of the trigone. (b) Following urolith removal, the trigone is somewhat oedematous, but otherwise normal in appearance.

jejunal tube is removed and the animal can be continued to be fed through the gastric tube by the owner. Recently, there have been reports of laparoscopy-assisted percutaneous gastrostomy tube placement in children to minimise the complications associated with traditional PEG placement of gastrostomy tube (Takahashi et al., 2008). In these cases, the gastroscope is inserted while the surgeon views the stomach with the laparoscope and the stomach is stabilised it with grasping forceps. A catheter is introduced percutaneously through the body wall and into the stomach under direct vision. In this way, the proper location can be identified by both the surgeon and the endoscopist. The guide wire is

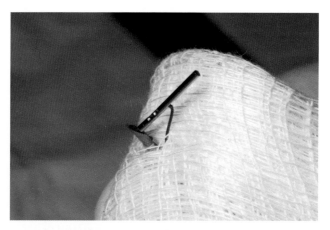

Fig. 5.19 A T-fastener is composed of a size 2-0 nylon suture swaged to the centre of a 1 cm piece of tubing. The device is loaded into an applier that has a beveled tip. The tip penetrates tissue, and the T-fastener is deployed from the applier by a central push rod. The T-fastener toggles in tissue as the applier is removed and traction is applied to the suture, enabling secure fixation of the suture in tissue.

then passed and the PEG tube is inserted in the usual manner. If it is necessary, the stomach can be additionally anchored to the body wall using T-fasteners (Thornton et al., 2002), sutures passed percutaneously or sutures placed laparoscopically. T-fasteners resemble nylon clothing tags, in that suture is swaged to the centre of a 1 cm hollow needle (Fig. 5.19). The needle/suture combination is loaded into a hollow delivery device which can be inserted percutaneously into the stomach. After the needle/suture is deployed into the gastric lumen, tension is applied to the suture such that the needle toggles. The suture is then secured on the surface of the skin.

Although intestinal feeding tubes can be placed using a totally laparoscopic technique, it is easier and faster to place them using a combination of laparoscopic and open techniques. The animal is placed in dorsal recumbency and after sterile preparation and draping the initial camera port is placed on the midline. For duodenal or jejunal feeding a 10 mm trocar is inserted on the right side just lateral to the rectus abdominis muscle. Babcock forceps are then inserted and used to grasp and elevate the duodenum or jejunum to the body wall. The trocar sleeve is removed, and the antimesenteric surface of the bowel is sutured to the body wall. A purse-string suture is sewn in the intestine and, following a small incision, an 8 French tube is threaded into the centre and advanced in an aboral direction for approximately 15 cm. The purse-string suture is tightened and, if necessary, a second one is placed for additional reinforcement. The abdominal fascia is then closed over the defect, the subcutaneous tissue and skin are sutured, and the tube is secured to the surface of the skin with a Chinese finger-trap friction suture. A light dressing and stockinette bandage are placed to support the tube to the abdominal wall. Potential complications of jejunostomy tubes include blockage of the feeding tube, premature dislodgement, self-mutilation, dermatitis around the site, fistula, leakage, and transient diarrhea and vomiting associated with feeding (Freeman, 2009).

Advanced laparoscopic procedures

Laparoscopic cholecystectomy, laparoscopy-assisted cholecystostomy tube placement and laparoscopic adrenalectomy have been performed by veterinary surgeons with advanced laparoscopic skills in carefully selected clinical cases. For additional information, refer to Mayhew's recent description of these techniques (Mayhew, 2009). Murphy et al. (2007) described the technique for cholecystostomy for temporary biliary diversion in cases of extrahepatic biliary tract obstruction. Laparoscopy is used to view and stabilise the gall bladder in a location that corresponds to the right cranial ventral body wall, just caudal to the costal arch. An 8–10 French locking-loop catheter is introduced percutaneously through the body wall to finally reside in the gall bladder. The locking loop is then fixed by pulling the string to hold the catheter in place. If successful, the catheter should remain inserted for 3–4 weeks to prevent leakage. Laparoscopic cholecystectomy could be selected in cases of uncomplicated gall bladder mucocele. Mayhew et al. (2008) reports using a four-port technique to provide adequate exposure and visualisation to enable dissection and ligation of the cystic duct using endoscopic ligating clips or extracorporeally tied sutures. The gall bladder is dissected from the hepatic fossa and placed in a specimen retrieval bag for extraction from the umbilical port. Techniques for both right and left laparoscopic adrenalectomy have been reported in seven dogs (Jiménez Peláez et al., 2008). Visualisation is excellent; however, the location of the adrenal gland adjacent to large vessels makes excellent haemostasis an absolute requirement for successful laparoscopic technique (Fig. 5.20). In the early part of the learning curve, the wise surgeon should be comfortable in having a low threshold for converting to an open procedure when necessary to ensure operative safety.

A few cases of laparoscopic splenectomy and laparoscopic nephrectomy have been performed in carefully selected cases in client-owned animals, enabled by the vessel-sealing devices such as LigaSure, ENSEAL and the Harmonic Scalpel. The camera port is placed at the umbilicus and the animal is rotated to lateral recumbency to expose the kidney. Dissection proceeds with the vessel-sealing device, and final haemostasis of the major blood supply is achieved with a combination of the vessel-sealing device and clips or an endoscopic stapler. The organ may be placed in a specimen-retrieval bag and the umbilical incision is extended along the midline to provide an adequate length for extraction.

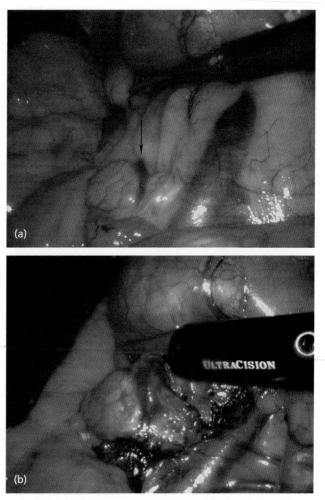

Fig. 5.20 (a) The left adrenal gland is normally situated cranial to the renal vein. It is identified by the large phrenicoabdominal vein (arrow) which courses over the centre of the gland. (b) Precise dissection is achieved with the Harmonic Scalpel. From Freeman, L.J. (ed.) (1999) *Veterinary Endosurgery*. Mosby, St. Louis, MO, Plates 26 and 28. Reproduced with permission from Elsevier.

Notes

Natural-orifice translumenal endoscopic surgery (NOTES) is an emerging area of surgery that began in 2004 when Dr Anthony Kalloo and his colleagues at Johns Hopkins University (Baltimore, MD, USA) reported on the results of using a flexible endoscope to enter the abdominal cavity through the stomach and perform procedures in pigs (Kalloo et al., 2004). We have recently begun experiments on the potential benefits of this approach for animals and our preliminary results indicate that dogs

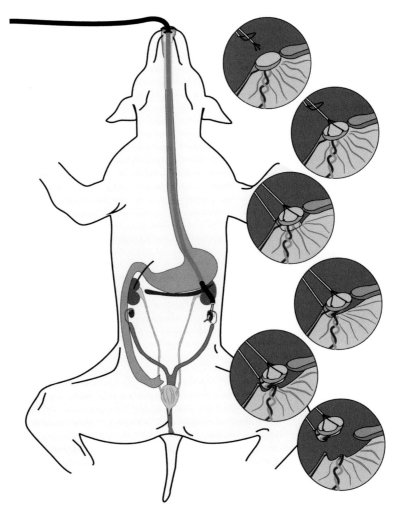

Fig. 5.21 Line drawing simulating the NOTES ovariectomy procedure performed through a transgastric approach. From Freeman et al. (2009). Reproduced with permission from Elsevier.

undergoing transgastric NOTES procedure for bilateral ovariectomy (Fig. 5.21) have less pain than those undergoing open surgery (Freeman et al., 2009, 2010). The technique requires operators skilled in endoscopy and in laparoscopy to work together to perform these procedures, the operative times are prolonged and instrumentation is currently still in development. At present, human NOTES procedures are being performed under Institutional Review Board protocols using both the transgastric and transvaginal approaches for cholecystectomy, but it is not known yet whether these techniques will prove to have a clinical benefit over traditional laparoscopy.

References

Culp, W.T., Mayhew, P.D. and Brown, D.C. (2009) The effect of laparoscopic versus open ovariectomy on postsurgical activity in small dogs. *Veterinary Surgery* 38, 811–817.

Davidson, E.B., Moll, H.D. and Payton, M.E. (2004) Comparison of laparoscopic ovariohysterectomy and ovariohysterectomy in dogs. *Veterinary Surgery* 33, 62–69.

Devitt, C.M., Cox, R.E. and Hailey, J.J. (2005) Duration, complications, stress, and pain of open ovariohysterectomy versus a simple method of laparoscopic-assisted ovariohysterectomy in dogs. *Journal of the American Veterinary Medical Association* 15, 227, 921–927.

Dujowich, M. and Reimer, S.B. (2008) Evaluation of an endoscopically assisted gastropexy technique in dogs. *American Journal of Veterinary Research* 69, 537–541.

Dupré, G., Fiorbianco, V., Skalicky, M., Gültiken, N., Ay, S.S. and Findik, M. (2009) Laparoscopic ovariectomy in dogs: comparison between single portal and two-portal access. *Veterinary Surgery* 38, 818–824.

Freeman, L.J. (1999) Minimally invasive surgery of the reproductive system. In *Veterinary Endosurgery*, Freeman, L.J. (ed.), pp. 205–217. Mosby, St Louis, MO.

Freeman, L.J. (2009) Gastrointestinal laparoscopy in small animals. *Veterinary Clinics of North America, Small Animal Practice* 39, 903–924.

Freeman, L.J., Keller, W., Trenka-Benthin, S. and Gallagher, L. (1992) Canine laparoscopic ovariohysterectomy: surgical model for evaluation of pre-tied ligatures [abstract]. *Veterinary Surgery* 21, 238.

Freeman, L.J., Rahmani, E.Y., Sherman, S., Chiorean, M.V., Selzer, D.J., Constable, P.D. and Snyder, P.W. (2009) Oophorectomy by natural orifice transluminal endoscopic surgery: feasibility study in dogs. *Gastrointestinal Endoscopy* 69, 1321–1332.

Freeman, L.J., Rahmani, E.Y., Al-Haddad, M., Sherman, S., Chiorean, M.V., Selzer, D.J., Snyder, P.W. and Constable, P.D. (2010) Comparison of pain and postoperative stress in dogs undergoing natural orifice translumenal endoscopic surgery, laparoscopic, and open oophorectomy. *Gastrointestinal Endoscopy* 72, 373–380.

Gallagher, L.A., Freeman, L.J., Trenka-Benthin, S. and Stoloff, D.R. (1992) Laparoscopic castration for canine cryptorchidism [abstract]. *Veterinary Surgery* 21, 411–412.

Hancock, R.B., Lanz, O.I., Waldron, D.R., Duncan, R.B., Broadstone, R.V. and Hendrix, P.K. (2005) Comparison of postoperative pain after ovariohysterectomy by harmonic scalpel-assisted laparoscopy compared with median celiotomy and ligation in dogs. *Veterinary Surgery* 34, 273–282.

Jiménez Peláez, M., Bouvy, B.M. and Dupré, G.P. (2008) Laparoscopic adrenalectomy for treatment of unilateral adrenocortical carcinomas: technique, complications, and results in seven dogs. *Veterinary Surgery* 37, 444–453.

Kalloo, A.N., Singh, V.K., Jagannath, S.B., Niiyama, H., Hill, S.L., Vaughn, C.A., Magee, C.A. and Kantsevoy, S.V. (2004) Flexible transgastric peritoneoscopy: a novel approach to diagnostic and therapeutic interventions in the peritoneal cavity. *Gastrointestinal Endoscopy* 60, 114–117.

Mayhew, P.D. (2009) Advanced laparoscopic procedures (hepatobiliary, endocrine) in dogs and cats. *Veterinary Clinics of North America, Small Animal Practice* 39, 925–939.

Mayhew, P.D. and Brown, D.C. (2009) Prospective evaluation of two intracorporeally sutured prophylactic laparoscopic gastropexy techniques compared with laparoscopic-assisted gastropexy in dogs. *Veterinary Surgery* 38, 738–746.

Mayhew, P.D., Mehler, S.J. and Radhakrishnan, A. (2008) Laparoscopic cholecystectomy for management of uncomplicated gall bladder mucocele in six dogs. *Veterinary Surgery* 37, 625–630.

Murphy, S.M., Rodríguez, J.D. and McAnulty, J.F. (2007) Minimally invasive cholecystostomy in the dog: evaluation of placement techniques and use in extrahepatic biliary obstruction. *Veterinary Surgery* 36, 675–683.

Rawlings, C.A. (2007) Resection of inflammatory polyps in dogs using laparoscopic-assisted cystoscopy. *Journal of the American Animal Hospital Association* 43, 342–346.

Rawlings, C.A. (2009) Surgical views: endoscopic removal of urinary calculi. *Compendium on Continuing Education for the Practicing Veterinarian* 31, 476–484.

Rawlings, C.A., Foutz, T.L., Mahaffey, M.B., Howerth, E.W., Bement, S. and Canalis, C. (2001) A rapid and strong laparoscopic-assisted gastropexy in dogs. *American Journal of Veterinary Research* 62, 871–875.

Rawlings, C.A., Mahaffey, M.B., Bement, S. and Canalis, C. (2002) Prospective evaluation of laparoscopic-assisted gastropexy in dogs susceptible to gastric dilatation. *Journal of the American Veterinary Medical Association* 221, 1576–1581.

Rawlings, C.A., Mahaffey, M.B., Barsanti, J.A. and Canalis, C. (2003) Use of laparoscopic-assisted cystoscopy for removal of urinary calculi in dogs. *Journal of the American Veterinary Medical Association* 222, 759–761, 737.

Rudd, R.G. and Hendrickson, D.A. (1999) Minimally invasive surgery of the urinary system. In *Veterinary Endosurgery*, Freeman, L. (ed.), pp. 226–236. Mosby, St Louis, MO.

Runge, J.J., Mayhew, P., Berent, A. and Weisse, C. (2008) Keyhole transvesicular cystourethroscopy for the retrieval of cystic and urethral calculi in dogs and cats, *Proceedings of the 43rd Annual Meeting American College of Veterinary Surgeons*, 23–25 October, San Diego, CA, p. 29.

Takahashi, T., Okazaki, T., Kato, Y., Watayo, H., Lane, G.J., Kobayashi, H., Segawa, O., Kameoka, S. and Yamataka, A. (2008) Laparoscopy-assisted percutaneous endoscopic gastrostomy. *Asian Journal of Surgery* 31, 204–206.

Thompson, S.E. and Potter, L. (1999) Electrosurgery, lasers, and ultrasonic energy. In *Veterinary Endosurgery*, Freeman, L.J. (ed.), pp. 61–72. Mosby, St Louis, MO.

Thornton, F.J., Fotheringham, T., Haslam, P.J., McGrath, F.P., Keeling, F. and Lee, M.J. (2002) Percutaneous radiologic gastrostomy with and without T-fastener gastropexy: a randomized comparison study. *Cardiovascular and Interventional Radiology* 25, 467–471.

van Goethem, B., Schaefers-Okkens, A. and Kirpensteijn, J. (2006) Making a rational choice between ovariectomy and ovariohysterectomy in the dog: a discussion of the benefits of either technique. *Veterinary Surgery* 35, 136–143.

Weil, A.B. (2009) Anesthesia for endoscopy in small animals. *Veterinary Clinics of North America, Small Animal Practice* 39, 839–848.

Wildt, D.E. and Lawler, D.F. (1985) Laparoscopic sterilization of the bitch and queen by uterine horn occlusion. *American Journal of Veterinary Research* 46, 864–869.

Chapter 6
Thoracoscopy
Romain Pizzi

Introduction

Many surgeons who work on humans prefer to refer to video-assisted thoracic surgery (or VATS) instead of using the term thoracoscopic surgery. This highlights one of the main benefits that endosurgery brings to thoracic surgery: visualisation. The use of the term also recognises that some procedures cannot be completed solely via thoracoscopy. Enhanced visualisation can however help reduce wounds to a mini-thoracotomy, without the need for rib retraction and the subsequent associated postoperative pain. Even if still performing an intra-thoracic procedure in a standard open technique, use of an endoscope can help improve this with excellent illumination and magnified visualisation. The ultimate aim of thoracoscopy should be safe, visual surgery, with the secondary benefit of smaller wounds and resultant lower postoperative morbidity. Small open thoracotomy incisions on their own just lead to poor visualisation, and resultant unsafe surgery.

While minimally invasive thoracic surgery has benefits for the patient in terms of reduced postoperative morbidity, there is notably also the benefit for the veterinarian of reduced postoperative care. There is often no need to maintain an indwelling chest drain postoperatively.

It should be obvious, as regards personal professional ethics as well as veterinary jurisprudence, that one should not attempt to perform thoracoscopic procedures unless already familiar with standard open thoracotomy techniques. Thoracoscopy is not an alternative to standard thoracic surgery, but a refinement. It still requires the same preoperative assessment, diagnostics and decision making. Conversion to a standard

Clinical Manual of Small Animal Endosurgery, First Edition. Edited by Alasdair Hotston Moore and Rosa Angela Ragni.
© 2012 Blackwell Publishing Ltd. Published 2012 by Blackwell Publishing Ltd.

open thoracotomy may be needed for a number of reasons (Radlinsky, 2009), and an emergency situation, such as major intra-thoracic haemorrhage, is certainly not the time to learn how to perform a thoracotomy. Wide clipping, preparation and draping are advisable for even what is presumed to be a brief and simple procedure such as lung biopsy, in case of the need for emergency conversion, or a change in procedure or approach. Human surgical studies have demonstrated that early elective conversion to open surgery carries a much better postoperative prognosis that later emergency conversion.

General principles and techniques

While the majority of a procedure such as a lung lobectomy may be completed thoracoscopically, a mini-thoracotomy is usually still needed for tissue extraction. Extraction-site metastasis of neoplasia is a real risk, and efforts to limit the size of an extraction-site wound by pulling tissue directly through the site should be avoided when possible. Brisson et al. (2006) reported port-site metastasis of a mesothelioma after just a diagnostic thoracoscopy, and this risk needs to be conveyed to owners. Even if the aetiology of a lesion is infectious rather than neoplastic, this carries a risk of a wound-site infection.

Instrumentation

A sterile thoracotomy instrument set and rib retractors should always be available in case of the need for conversion to open surgery. Shorter, 20 cm-long, instruments are very useful for the majority of thoracoscopic procedures, as the ergonomics of using the longer 30 cm instruments commonly used in laparoscopy can be very awkward. Standard 30 cm instruments are rarely truly needed in any but the occasional giant breed. In small and medium-sized dogs, puppies and cats, as well as for fine dissection procedures such as vascular ring anomalies, 3 mm diameter paediatric instruments are ideal. Almost as wide a range of different instruments are available as in the 5 mm diameter size (Fig. 6.1).

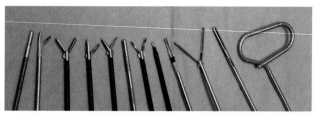

Fig. 6.1 A wide range of 3 mm-diameter paediatric instruments, including retractors and needle holders, are ideal for thoracoscopy in small patients or where fine, precise dissection is needed.

Endoscope selection

Although a range of different rigid endoscopes can be used for thoracoscopy, the most useful with the widest range of application is a 5 mm, 30 cm-long endoscope with a 30° viewing angle, often also favoured for small animal laparoscopy. Although some find the slightly offset view initially disorientating when placing instruments, this rapidly resolves after a small amount of use. By rotating the endoscope a wider area can be examined. The offset view can be used to look around the side of structures to a degree, as well as allowing visualisation of port placement and instrument entry in the same side of the chest wall as the optical port. This limits the risk of levering the endoscope against the adjacent ribs with resultant risk of injury to the patient and damage to the endoscope. The offset angle also allows a more ergonomic horizontal positioning of the endoscope during procedures.

In small patients, the length of this endoscope can interfere with instrumentation use and prove awkward. If still using a 5 mm port, the author finds that a 4 mm, 30°, 18 cm-long arthroscope proves an excellent alternative, with almost as good visualisation and light transmission as a 5 mm endoscope. This size endoscope, commonly used for human arthroscopy, is also relatively sturdy. In small patients, use of a dedicated 3 mm, 30°, 18 cm-long endoscope allows the use of only 3 mm ports, and enables interchange of the endoscope and instruments between the different ports. Alternatively, some prefer the use of a 2.7 mm, 30°, 18 cm-long endoscope (the so-called universal veterinary endoscope) via a 3 mm port, as this may already be owned by a practice and used for rhinoscopy and cystoscopy. This diameter of endoscope is quite delicate and will not withstand leverage or rough handling, and so is most commonly used with a protective sheath. Visualisation and light transmission, even with a 300 W xenon light source, are notably inferior, with at most 20–25% the illumination of a comparable 5 mm endoscope.

For those surgeons preferring perixiphoid transdiaphragmatic placement of the primary optical threaded cannula in dorsal recumbency thoracoscopy, a 0° endoscope is needed for safe visual placement of the port. Good alternative techniques that do not require this specific port placement for procedures are available (see below).

Reuse of single-use disposable instruments

Some instruments are only available as single-use disposable items. These are frequently reused by veterinarians to save costs. While not endorsed by the manufacturers, re-processing (re-sterilisation) of some of these single-use items is now allowed in human surgery in many countries according to strict criteria. Items such stapler handpieces are well suited to reuse, while other items such as haemostatic clip applicators tend to easily become contaminated with blood internally, and as such are relatively poor candidates for reuse. If reusing single-use items then careful cleaning as well as a pre-sterilisation examination are essential if infection or patient injury are to be avoided.

Thoracoscopy ports

Ports for thoracoscopic surgery do not need valves, as in the majority of cases no insufflation is performed. The most suitable ports are soft and pliable, with a blunt atraumatic trocar that is unlikely to damage structures during insertion. These soft ports protect the intercostal vessels and nerves from trauma, and reduce the risk of leverage injuries. Threaded ports are useful as they are not easily dislodged, and also can be fixed with minimal shaft length protruding into the chest cavity. This is helpful as the available operating space in some locations in the chest can be quite small. Disposable Thoracoports (Covidien) are well suited to veterinary companion animal thoracoscopy, and can be resterilised with ethylene oxide or liquid solutions and reused a reasonable number of times. The numbering system is slightly confusing, with the 5.5 mm Thoracoport accommodating instruments up to 6 mm in diameter, and the 11.5 mm Thoracoport accommodating instruments up to 12 mm in diameter (suitable for stapler insertion) (see Fig. 6.2). The 5.5 mm port is suitable for extraction of small endoloop lung biopsies, and the 11.5 mm port is suitable for extraction of pericardium (partial or subtotal pericardiectomy) in most cases.

While reusable steel laparoscopy cannulae can also be used for thoracoscopy there are a number of disadvantages to their use. These can-

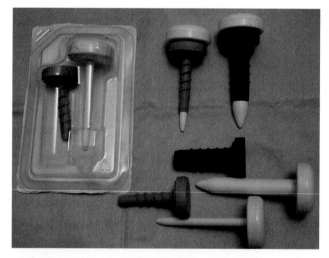

Fig. 6.2 Soft Thoracoports are threaded but atraumatic and well suited to thoracoscopy with 5 mm instruments. The 5.5 mm Thoracoport accommodates instruments up to 6 mm in diameter, and the 11.5 mm Thoracoport accommodates instruments such as endoscopic staplers up to 12 mm in diameter.

nulae are often too long to be ideally suited to thoracoscopy. Valves should be removed to prevent the risk of a tension pneumothorax developing during anaesthesia, interfering with adequate lung ventilation. These rigid cannulae, particularly if threaded, also carry a risk of traumatising the intercostal vessels and nerves in medium-sized and smaller animals. If care is not taken when angulating instruments there is a risk of the applied leverage through the larger 10–15 mm cannulae causing inadvertent rib fractures. Sharp-tipped trocars used for blind (Veress needle) laparoscopic access are unsuitable for inserting cannulae into the chest, as these carry a high risk of causing lung laceration or other injury.

Ports of 3 mm are useful in small paediatric patients, or for fine dissections. These are currently only available from a small number of manufacturers. The author has a particular preference for YelloPort+ cannulae (Surgical Innovations). These are reusable, but are plastic and light weight. Instead of being threaded, they have a finely grooved shaft that is both atraumatic and provides good retention in port sites (see Fig. 6.3). Ports of 3 mm are similar in diameter to many small-gauge chest drains, and so there is minimal risk of developing pneumothorax postoperatively, eliminating the need for postoperative chest drain insertion. Perpendicular cannula ends are preferable to angled ends, which result in a longer portion of cannula protruding into the chest cavity. Even though this may make a difference of only 3–5 mm, this can be sufficient to interfere with the jaw movements of instruments when operating in a very small space, such as when performing a vascular ring anomaly in a 2 kg puppy.

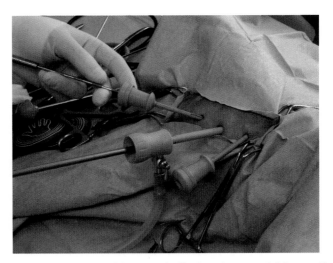

Fig. 6.3 These 3 mm reusable ports (YelloPort+) are useful in small patients or for fine dissection. These plastic ports are light weight, and instead of being threaded they have a finely grooved shaft that is both atraumatic as well as providing good retention in port sites.

Haemostatic clip applicators

Reusable and disposable minimally invasive surgery haemostatic clip applicators are available, most commonly in 10 mm diameter, but also more recently in 5 mm diameter. Right-angled applicators are also available in 10 mm diameter. Whereas single-use disposable applicators are easier to use (being double action), are less likely to drop clips and allow application of multiple clips without needing to reload, they are not good candidates for reuse as they tend to accumulate blood internally, and even with prolonged cold-water soaking in an upright position there is no method of ensuring this has been completely removed. Single- and double-action reusable applicators are available depending on preference. Reusable applicators need to be removed and reloaded for each clip. One needs to check whether these are for Weck, Ethicon, Covidien or Helka clips, as well as the specified clip size (10 mm are most commonly medium or medium-large), as applicator makes and clip sizes are not interchangeable. The 5 mm reusable clip applicators are most suitable for thoracoscopic procedures.

Extraction bags

A multitude of different extraction bags are commercially available. The most commonly encountered types are single-use clear plastic bags. The best, however, are those made of impervious leakage- and rip-proof 'parachute' material such as the E-sac (Espiner Medical), which cannot break or leak even if some considerable force is applied during extraction (see Fig. 6.4). The only real risk of leakage with this type of extraction bag comes from inadvertent damage from a scalpel or scissors if trying to enlarge the extraction site while the bag is in it, or if using these

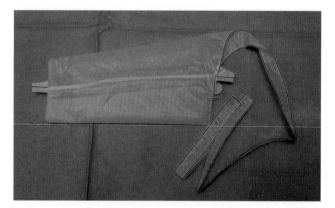

Fig. 6.4 An impervious leakage- and rip-proof endoscopic extraction sac made from 'parachute' material (E-sac), well suited to removal of lung tissue through a mini-thoracotomy site, and prevention of port-site metastasis when removing tumours.

instruments to morcellate tissue inside the bag. The neck of the bag is brought through the extraction site, and any samples for histology or microbiology taken. In the absence of a dedicated endosurgical extraction bag, the finger cut off a silicon glove can be used for extraction of samples such as small endoloop lung biopsies. These are not as easy to manipulate and use. Fingers of latex gloves are less suitable, as they are weaker and more easily broken, and also have a tendency to stick closed with moisture when trying to insert a sample.

The extraction-site wound can also be limited when using a rip-proof bag. The neck of the bag is exteriorised and samples taken for histology and culture as needed (this may be aided by inserting the endoscope into the bag; however, the endoscope should not then be re-inserted into the chest without adequate cleaning; an alternative is to use a different smaller endoscope for this purpose). After this, sponge-holding forceps are inserted into the neck of the bag and used to mash the tissue, which can then be removed piecemeal via the bag's neck, or alternatively it will simply allow removal via a smaller wound as the tissue is less rigid. This procedure unfortunately is not as effective with lungs, especially if fibrosis is present, as it is with liver. Scissors should not be inserted into the bag in an effort to cut the tissue, as this could result in cutting the bag with subsequent leakage of contents into the chest.

Staplers

Endosurgical stapling equipment is among the most expensive single-use consumable items that a veterinary surgeon may consider purchasing. Less costly extracorporeal ligatures are more suited to some veterinary thoracoscopic procedures. Endosurgical staplers produce two to three lines of staples on either side of tissue, as well as cutting between these staple lines. Different staple cartridge lengths (30, 45 and 60 mm) and different staple sizes (2.0–4.8 mm) are suited to different tissue thicknesses and procedures. As a rough guide, a 2.0 or 2.5 mm staple leg length is generally suitable for most peripheral lung, while partial or complete lobectomies in medium and larger dogs usually require a 3.5 mm staple leg length. Endosurgical staplers with 2.0–3.5 mm staples suited to thoracoscopy need a 12 mm port for insertion.

Of current endosurgical staplers the Endo GIA universal stapler (Covidien) is the best suited to veterinary thoracoscopic surgical use. The universal handpiece can be reused with care a reasonable number of times and re-sterilised with ethylene oxide. Straight and articulated (called Roticulator) cartridges of differing length and different staple sizes can all be used with the same universal handpiece. Each individual staple cartridge contains its own anvil and blade. While Ethicon endosurgery ETS staplers provide a better-quality sturdy steel anvil as part of the handpiece, and are hence favoured by many colorectal surgeons working with humans, they are not as suitable for veterinary thoracoscopic use. The main disadvantage for veterinary surgeons is that despite reloads being available the cutting blade and anvil are actually in the handpiece. The blade will become blunt after a few firings, meaning that the handpiece is not suitable for reuse, and notably increasing a procedure's cost. Reloads are also limited to the same cartridge length as the handpiece (30, 45 or 60 mm), requiring increased stocking expense, although different staple-length reloads for different tissue thicknesses can be used with the same handpiece.

Articulated-staple cartridges (Endo GIA Roticulator, Covidien) are marginally more costly than straight-staple cartridges, but much better suited to thoracic surgery, where limited space and limited manipulation, for example of a lung hilus, is possible. Occasionally tissue sectioning is not complete, or staple cartridge misfiring may occur.

For this reason at least two staple cartridges should be available when planning their use in a procedure.

Knot pushers

A knot pusher is highly recommended for placing extracorporeal knot ligatures, such as for peripheral lung biopsies, or for vascular ligations. A closed-end knot pusher (i.e. with a hole at the distal end) is preferable to the open or grooved knot pusher most commonly offered by veterinary suppliers, which is more difficult to manipulate, and doesn't allow as precise knot positioning. Knot pushers are available in 5 mm and paediatric 3 mm diameters.

Retractors

Lung retraction is more difficult and limited in comparison to open thoracic surgery, where one can pack the lungs away with the use of large moist swabs, or simply 'grab something and shove it to the side'. Fan retractors are the most commonly available retractors, but are 10 mm in diameter, needing a large port for insertion. These also risk traumatising the lung or other delicate structures when closing the blades, or on the edges of the fan blades, which in reusable retractors may become sharp over time. Disposable fan retractors (Endo Retract, Covidien) also add to procedure costs. Although reusable flexible 5 mm retractors such as those made by Snowden Pencer and Surgical Innovations are relatively expensive instruments for veterinary surgeons, they are much less traumatic, and easier to use once formed, to hold lung out of the way. Smaller, circle-shaped retractors or standard liver-retractor shapes are available. Their main disadvantage aside from cost is the relatively long lead-in length of the unformed retractor head, which makes them unsuitable for insertion into small chests, or small spaces.

A simple blunt palpation probe may be sufficient for lung retraction in some procedures, such as vascular ring resections, if combined with suitable ventilator settings (Fig. 6.5). To a degree some retraction can also be attained via positioning and gravity, just as for laparoscopy. Ventilation of a single lung, or low-pressure carbon dioxide insufflation

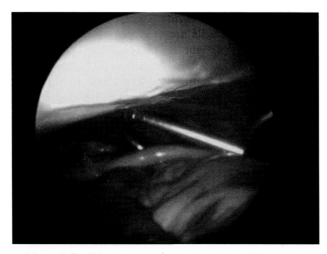

Fig. 6.5 Although flexible lung retractors can be useful in dorsal recumbency thoracoscopy, there is often insufficient space for their use in lateral recumbency, where a simple palpation probe is better suited to retraction of lung in the limited operating space.

of the pleural space, have also been used to increase the operating space available during thoracoscopy, but carry disadvantages (see below).

Electrosurgery and related modalities

Monopolar surgery

Monopolar electrosurgery holds the advantage over bipolar electrosurgery of allowing cautery as well as cutting dissection, but has limited application in thoracoscopic surgery as its use in proximity to the heart is best avoided. It carries a higher risk of causing inadvertent injury than bipolar surgery, or an ultrasonic scalpel. Care is especially needed in small veterinary patients with thick coats, which can prevent good contact with the return electrode (ground plate) and result in burn injuries. The safety of monopolar surgery can be increased by using higher-frequency current, referred to as radiosurgery (Surgitron, Ellman), in the order of 3.8–4.0 MHz, which has less reliance on good contact with the return electrode. The cutting and dissecting function of monopolar electrosurgery is increasingly being replaced in human surgery by ultrasonic scalpels (see below), which coagulate and cut tissues via ultrasound, with little collateral heat generation, and no risk of contact plate burns.

Bipolar electrosurgery

Bipolar electrosurgery is more suitable to thoracoscopic surgery than monopolar surgery and provides precise controlled electrocautery with the current path confined to tissue grasped between the instrument tips. This modality also works well in irrigated environments or when haemorrhaging has occurred. A small gap needs to be maintained between the instrument tips for cautery to function. If bipolar forceps fail to function during a procedure it is often the tips that have bent and are touching each other directly, resulting in a short circuit and no cautery. Opening the tips slightly usually results in a return of function.

Tissue feedback controlled bipolar surgery

Handpieces are available in 5 and 10 mm diameters, with an integrated blade, allowing one to seal and cut tissue without having to change instruments, hence shortening surgery time. Examples are LigaSure, made by Valleylab, and Enseal, by Ethicon. The tool can be used to seal blood vessels up to 7 mm in diameter, and it may be suitable for taking peripheral lung biopsies (see below). The control unit measures tissue impedance and gives an audible signal once tissue has been sealed. This also prevents overlong application with char formation leading to an increased inflammatory response. The main disadvantage of this system is that the instruments are single-use, disposable and relatively expensive, adding to the costs of veterinary thoracoscopic procedures. Whereas handpieces are commonly reused and re-sterilised by liquid or ethylene oxide sterilisation, they can be difficult to clean, and only suitable for very limited reuse. Some surgeons do not favour them, as the jaws can become sticky with coagulum during surgery, and laparoscopic clip applicators are generally favoured for haemostasis of important vascular structures in human surgery.

Ultrasonic scalpel

Unlike electrosurgery, this modality uses an ultrasound transducer in the handpiece to transmit vibrations down the shaft of the instruments to the tip. This generates heat, which coagulates vessels in a similar way to electrosurgery, but with none of the electrosurgical risk. Examples include Harmonic ACE (Ethicon), AutoSonix (Covidien) and Sonosurg (Olympus). Ultrasonic scalpels are regarded as effectively sealing vessels up to 3 mm in diameter. They generate less heat than standard electrosurgery, with minimal collateral heat propagation, and are useful for dissection around delicate structures. Unfortunately, as with tissue feedback controlled bipolar surgery, they also utilise expensive single-use handpieces that add to veterinary procedure costs (with the exception of the Olympus Sonosurg system, which has reusable handpieces). They are similarly difficult to clean, and have a limited lifespan if reused and re-sterilised by liquid immersion or ethylene oxide gas.

Endosurgical suturing and ligation

Extracorporeal suturing

Tying endosurgical locking slip knots or extracorporeal sutures, also referred to as endoloops, formed outside the body, and then positioned and tightened internally with a knot pusher, is an extremely useful technique to master in veterinary endosurgery. While commercially prepared loops are available (Surgitie, Covidien; Endoloop, Ethicon) they cannot be passed around fixed structures such as the ligamentum arteriosum, plus it is more economical to prepare them oneself. Carpenter et al. (2006) found hand-tied extracorporeal knots in both monofilament polydioxanone and braided multifilament polyglactin 910 to be as secure and reliable as commercially available endoloop ligatures for use in veterinary endosurgery. They can be used to ligate vessels, including arteries up to 3 mm in diameter, as well as for taking biopsies of lung and other structures.

There are numerous different knots described that are suitable. The initial endosurgical extracorporeal knot used was the Roeder knot (Hage, 2008). Originally implemented for tonsillectomies, its locking is unreliable unless used with catgut suture which swells on absorbing moisture, 'locking' the knot, and so it has fallen out of favour. There are several modifications of the Roeder knot that are still useful, however. One modification, the Meltzer knot (Fig. 6.6), is the basis of commercial

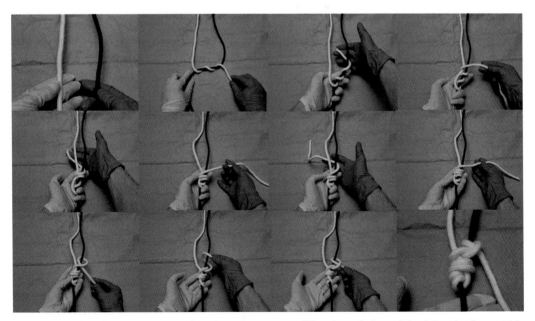

Fig. 6.6 Tying the extracorporeal Meltzer knot, a modification of the original Roeder knot. This knot is also the knot used in commercially available pre-tied endoloops.

prepared loops, and is reliable for lung biopsies and ligations with both monofilament and braided synthetic suture materials. The Weston knot is another popular extracorporeally tied endosurgical slip knot, but although less bulky and relatively easier to tie it has a much lower knot strength than the Meltzer knot (Sharp et al., 1996).

It does take some practice to become familiar with forming and utilising the Meltzer knot. While this knot can be formed and reliably used with monofilament sutures, it is easiest to prepare and use when made with braided suture materials such as polyglactin 910 (Vicryl, Ethicon; Polysorb, Tyco), which have less memory. It is also possible to pre-prepare several loops and sterilise them so they are ready for use in surgery. Trostle et al. (2002) demonstrated that ethylene oxide sterilisation of pre-tied monofilament polydioxanone suture loops did not have any adverse effect on suture failure strength. Small peripheral lung biopsies provide an ideal situation for becoming proficient with their use (see below), and it is markedly less costly than using an endoscopic stapler.

The standard open-ended or notched knot pushers most commonly offered by veterinary endosurgical suppliers are poorly suited to precise knot placement, loop manipulation and adequate tightening. A closed-ended knot pusher (with a hole at the distal end) is preferable, allowing precise knot positioning as well as application of a tight-locked knot under tension.

Intracorporeal suturing and ligation

Internal suturing and knot tying are more difficult than extracorporeal knot tying, and currently of limited application in veterinary thoracic endosurgery. Application for the thoracoscopic repair of some diaphragmatic hernias, as in humans, does currently warrant further investigation, and may be aided by the use of disposable suturing devices such as the Endo Stitch applicator (Covidien), rather than endosurgical needle holders and J-shaped endoski needles. Intracorporeal tying of ligatures is seldom indicated in thoracoscopy. Not only is the increased technical difficulty and limited space disadvantageous, but more importantly it is difficult to apply adequate tension to ligate any but the smallest vascular structures (Fig. 6.7). While dedicated 5mm and even 3mm paediatric needle holders are available, grasping forceps with locking handles are equally suitable for simply tying intracorporeal ligatures. Andrews and Lewis (1994) investigated the use of endoscopic haemostatic clips as an alternative to knotting, for securing untied suture ends, but found this to be significantly weaker than knots, and their use for this purpose is hence not recommended.

Anaesthesia

General anaesthesia is required for thoracoscopic procedures. Preoperative assessment, anaesthetic preparation and monitoring requirements are essentially the same as for traditional open-chest surgical procedures.

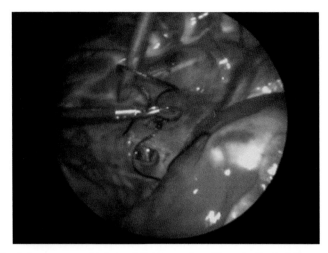

Fig. 6.7 Intracorporeal tying of ligatures is seldom indicated in thoracoscopy. Not only is the increased technical difficulty and limited space disadvantageous, but it is also difficult to apply adequate tension to ligate any but the smallest vascular structures. In this case 3 mm instruments, including a needle holder, are being used to ligate the ligamentum arteriosum. The application of an extracorporeal knot with a 3 mm knot pusher is quicker, easier, requires less operating space and can also be applied under tension, making this a better method of thoracoscopic ligation.

While ventilation by means of bagging the patient by hand is possible, mechanical ventilation is highly recommended. This allows adjustment of the ventilator settings such as tidal volume, to prevent inflated lungs completely obscuring the chest cavity during a procedure. A degree of lung atelectasis will always occur, and usually results in an increase in the partial pressure of carbon dioxide (P_aCO_2), and decrease in the partial pressure of oxygen (P_aO_2), that is normally not particularly clinically significant. Multiparameter monitoring that includes capnography is recommended. An electrocardiographic (ECG) trace during cardiac procedures such as pericardiectomy is useful. Contact with the epicardium by instruments can result in ventricular premature contractions (or VPCs), or may cause a more clinically important ventricular tachycardia.

Insufflation of the chest with low-pressure carbon dioxide (4 mmHg) has been performed to increase the working space of a hemithorax for procedures in lateral recumbency; or occasionally as an adjunct to single-lung ventilation to initially evacuate the lung in the operated hemithorax. As for laparoscopy, valved cannulae are required. Insufflation of the chest may cause significant haemodynamic compromise, and the moving partially ventilated lung is still prone to instrument trauma (Potter and Hendrickson, 1999). In the author's limited initial experiences with the technique it did not yield a notable improvement in operating space or any other benefits, and is not recommended.

Single-lung ventilation by means of endobronchial blockers or selective bronchial intubation directed by preoperative bronchoscopy has been reported in a number of studies. While some have regarded this as essential for safe lateral recumbent thoracoscopic procedures (Potter and Hendrickson, 1999), many others have performed the same procedures with no more difficulty without this technique. Single-lung ventilation notably increases the anaesthetic time, as well as having effects on anaesthesia and requiring attentive monitoring throughout. There is a learning curve to these techniques, and single-lung ventilation should be established in the operating theatre immediately before thoracoscopy. Dislodgement can occur with moving or positioning of the patient. Incorrect placement can result in the lung in the operative hemithorax remaining inflated. Depending on the initial placement, inflation of the balloon can also result in displacement into the carina or trachea. Initial placement or confirmation of both techniques requires bronchoscopy.

Kudnig et al. (2006) found single-lung ventilation in thoracoscopy comparable with clinical parameters encountered in bilaterally ventilated lungs in dogs undergoing open thoracotomy. This was believed to be due to hypoxaemic vasoconstriction in the atelectic lung and shunting of blood flow to ventilated regions of lung, reducing ventilation/perfusion mismatching. Radlinsky (2008), however, highlights that single-lung ventilation in ill patients may be more difficult, and recommends the addition of $5\,cmH_2O$ positive end expiratory pressure (PEEP), in an effort to recruit more alveoli in the ventilated lung and reduce ventilation/perfusion mismatching. Potter and Hendrickson (1999) recommend that initially during one lung ventilation half the tidal volume is used (4–5 ml/kg for a medium-sized dog) with double the respiratory rate (20 breaths/min), and that this is gradually changed during the first 30 min to a more normal tidal volume (10 ml/kg) and respiratory rate (10–12 breaths/min), while maintaining an airway pressure of $20\,cmH_2O$.

At the end of the thoracoscopy procedure, the bronchial endotrachial tube is withdrawn into the trachea, and the re-ventilation of the atelectatic lung observed with the endoscope. Levionnois et al. (2006) reported the accidental entrapment of an endobronchial blocker tip by staples during a lung lobectomy (see below). The author rarely uses single-lung ventilation, even in lateral recumbency procedures, instead preferring atraumatic lung retraction if needed.

Safe thoracoscopic access

As for laparoscopy, the optical and instrument ports should not be inserted over a lesion or target organ, but a reasonable distance away from and directed towards them to allow good, wide-angle visualisation, and a suitable operating space. Similarly, instruments should ideally always be inserted into the chest under visualisation. With limited space and lung movements this is even more important than in laparoscopy in preventing inadvertent entry injuries.

The most suitable ports for intercostal primary (optical) port placement are soft, flexible ports with a blunt atraumatic trocar (see above). After a skin incision over the selected intercostal site, the port can be bluntly pushed through the intercostal muscles. Alternatively the chest may be entered with blunt dissection with curved artery forceps to initiate a pneumothorax before insertion of the port. The primary ports should not be inserted at or ventral to the costochondral junction. The endoscope is then inserted, and the underlying lung and other structures examined for any injury. The locations of the other ports can then be selected based on the individual's specific anatomy and the procedure to be performed. These ports can be safely placed under endoscopic visualisation. Sharp trocars should not be used for primary access due to the high risk of lung trauma, even if a prior pneumothorax is established.

The Veress needle was originally used for inducing a pneumothorax prior to surgical treatments of tuberculosis and pleural adhesions in humans, before it was later adopted for insufflation prior to laparoscopy. While this double-lumen, guarded needle could still be used before primary port placement, it holds no benefit over simply using a blunt trocar, and can still traumatise underlying lung.

Some favour the use of a paraxiphoid transdiaphragmatic placement of the primary optical port for procedures in dorsal recumbency, such as subtotal pericardiectomy. A threaded cannula is recommended. A 0° endoscope is used for intraluminal visualisation during placement. Insertion of the cannula is directed dorsally, and towards the opposite shoulder. In chronic disease cases with notably thickened pleura insertion can be difficult if not directed adequately dorsally during placement (Radlinsky, 2008).

Exploratory thoracoscopy

Exploratory or diagnostic thoracoscopy is an extremely useful technique, and notably less invasive than an exploratory thoracotomy. Even with advanced diagnostic imaging such as computed tomography scanning, which may localise a specific lesion, sampling is needed for a definitive aetiological diagnosis, such as in the case pictured in Fig. 6.8. In many cases it is not possible to achieve this safely blindly, or under ultrasound guidance. In human surgery, thoracoscopy and excisional biopsy are usually the diagnostic modalities of choice for single isolated pulmonary nodules less than 2 cm in diameter.

The diagnostic yield at histology and microbiological culture of thoracoscopic lung biopsies has been demonstrated to be comparable to open surgical biopsy (Faunt et al., 1998). Thoracoscopy also allows the opportunity to proactively address any haemorrhage or air leakage that may occur at the time of biopsy, rather than as a later unexpected emergency after performing ultrasound-guided needle or Trucut biopsy.

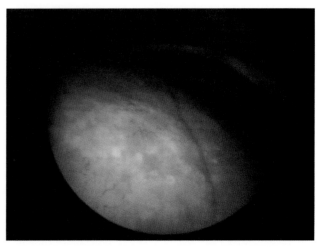

Fig. 6.8   Multiple small pulmonary metastases, demonstrating a rosette appearance, on lateral thoracoscopy in a flat-coated retriever.

Exploratory thoracoscopy and biopsy have also been found diagnostic in all canine and feline pleural effusion cases in which it was performed (Kovak et al., 2002), and thus extremely useful in determining the prognosis and suitable treatment protocol in cases of pleural effusion.

Exploratory thoracoscopy can also be used with lavage for the diagnosis and treatment of pyothorax. Johnson and Martin (2007), however, demonstrated that even chronic cases of pyothorax with adhesions respond extremely well to conservative medical treatment with a single pleurocentesis, no lavage and 6 weeks broad-spectrum antibiosis. Enthusiasm for endosurgery should not encourage one to perform thoracoscopy unnecessarily in these cases, and it should be directed only to those chronic cases that are not responsive to medical treatment, and the ones demonstrating pulmonary masses or consolidation. In these cases the surgeon should be prepared to perform a partial or complete lung lobectomy should this be necessary, if a foreign-body granuloma, abscess or neoplasia is found. Adhesiolysis of multiple strong fibrous adhesions can be time-consuming and care needs to be taken not to injure the lungs and other tissues. The ultrasonic scalpel, in the form of either a dissecting hook or shears, is better suited to pleural adhesiolysis than the monopolar hook or scissors.

Exploratory thoracoscopy is useful in cases of recurrent spontaneous pneumothorax. Emphysematous bullae (Brisson et al., 2003) or isolated lung lesions can be treated by ligation with extracorporeal loop ligatures or other means. Cases with no obvious bullae or other gross abnormalities are more difficult, and saline instillation may help in locating an air leak, by visualisation of bubbles during ventilation.

In cases with no obvious gross pathology, biopsies should be taken of pleura, lung, lymph nodes, pericardium and mediastinum. Biopsies of the pleura can be performed using cup biopsy forceps, or with incision and dissection with curved Metzenbaum scissors. The intercostal vessels and nerves must be avoided. When biopsing lymph nodes, simply grasping and pulling with cup biopsy forceps may result in tearing of the mediastinum and associated vessels, with resultant haemorrhage. The lymph node should be stabilised or grasped with atraumatic forceps for biopsy. The overlying mediastinum and capsule can be incised with Metzenbaum scissors; this will lead to a better sample, with reduced histological crush artefacts.

During exploratory thoracoscopy the surgeon should not forget to examine the thoracic surface of the diaphragm for any unusual conformation. A primary undiagnosed liver tumour can sometimes be recognised by its abnormally shaped impression on the diaphragm (Fig. 6.9).

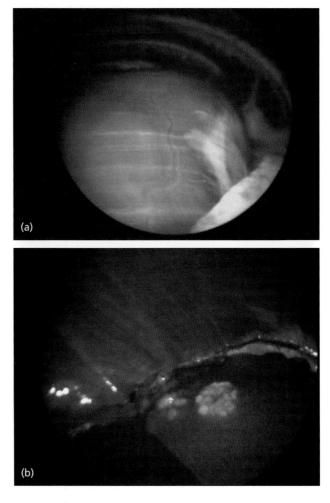

Fig. 6.9 (a) An abnormal nodular surface to the diaphragm visualised during thoracoscopy. (b) A brief exploratory laparoscopy after lung biopsy revealed the presence of an undetected primary hepatic adenocarcinoma.

As for other thoracoscopic procedures, patient positioning and port-site selection are dependent on the anticipated pathology and its location, guided by the results of preoperative imaging. In cases of diffuse pathology, or uncertainty as to which hemithorax is affected, a dorsal recumbency approach is recommended to allow examination of both sides of the chest.

Pericardiectomy

Thoracoscopic pericardiectomy is arguably the best-established and -evaluated of veterinary thoracoscopic procedures (Jackson et al., 1999; Walsh et al., 1999; Dupre et al., 2001; Radlinsky, 2008; Mayhew et al., 2009). The decrease in postoperative pain and stress is well established (Walsh et al., 1999), and the procedure is regarded as the standard of care for pericardiectomy (Radlinsky, 2008). A partial or pericardial window procedure may be performed in either lateral or dorsal recumbency, while a subtotal (sub-phrenic) pericardiectomy requires dorsal recumbency. Dorsal recumbency has the further advantage of not necessitating single-lung ventilation (see below).

While a lateral approach from either side is possible if performing a pericardial window, the left lateral approach gives access to the right atrial appendage and base of the aorta for evaluation of possible neoplasia. Several different lateral recumbency port placements have been described, including the third, fourth and fifth intercostal spaces; second, fifth and ninth intercostal spaces; fourth, sixth and eighth intercostal spaces; or the fourth, sixth and tenth intercostal spaces (Radlinsky, 2008).

Dorsal recumbency is the position of preference in the majority of cases. This allows an examination of both sides of the chest, and allows a subtotal pericardiectomy to be performed. While many veterinary texts advise a technique using a paraxiphoid transdiaphragmatic approach to placement of the primary optical trocar, the author favours an alternative technique. A soft cannula with a blunt trocar is inserted in the left mid chest (typically sixth or seventh intercostal space) dorsal to the costochondral junction. After a brief initial examination of the chest, the next two ports are inserted under visual guidance, as far caudally and ventrally as feasible on either side of the chest. There is marked anatomical variation between different large dog breeds, and this visually directed variable placement is more helpful than identical placement in differing patients. The endoscope is then transferred to the left caudal port, but instruments and endoscope can be alternated between the different ports if needed. In performing a subtotal pericardiectomy, a fourth port placed in the ventral mid right chest is useful and, in conjunction with a second pair of grasping forceps and alternating the endoscope between ports, can aid more rapid completion of the procedure. In dorsal recumbency the heart flops dorsally, which inexperienced surgeons may find disorientating.

If the pericardial effusion has not been at least partially drained preoperatively then a thoracoscopic guided pericardiocentesis is usually needed to allow the pericardium to be grasped and incised. This may be performed with a spinal needle inserted percutaneously, or via a port with a dedicated endoscopic needle. The pericardium is often notably thicker than normal: this should be borne in mind if practising the procedure on cadavers. The sternopericardial ligament and ventral mediastinum may also be thickened, with tortuous vessels that require bipolar cautery before sectioning. If only a pericardium window is performed, the ligament does not need to be sectioned, and a small fenestration is simply made for instrument insertion. For subtotal pericardiectomy, the sternopericardial ligament should be resected ventrally and close to the sternum, otherwise a curtain of mediastinum interferes with instruments and tends to splatter the endoscope end, which then needs to be repeatedly cleaned (Fig. 6.10).

When performing a partial (window) pericardiectomy, a window is cut in the ventral/lateral pericardium, avoiding the right atrial appendage cranially (Fig. 6.11), which could be inadvertently cut with potentially catastrophic results. Potter and Hendrickson (1999) describe the successful use of extracorporeal suture loops to repair accidental trauma to the right atrial appendage during thoracoscopic pericardiectomies in dogs. Suture loops have also been used to perform a palliative resection of a pedunculated atrial haemangiosarcoma in a similar manner (Crumbaker et al., 2010) (Fig. 6.12). Care also needs to be taken not to inadvertently cut lung tissue during ventilation, which may need to be periodically stopped for brief periods during parts of the pericardiectomy (Fig. 6.13). The window needs to be a sufficient size not to simply adhere closed, but not so large that the heart can herniate. Adhesions may be present between the pericardium and epicardium in some areas, and these should be sectioned with care if possible, or another region of pericardium removed. Once an initial incision in the pericardium has been made, a palpation probe may be inserted to investigate the presence of adhesions. If only a pericardial window is performed this may be expanded by making two or three longitudinal incisions or fenestrations just ventral to the phrenic nerves (Radlinsky, 2008). The removed section of pericardium should always be submitted for histopathology, as well as microbiology if indicated.

Subtotal (subphrenic) pericardiectomy (Fig. 6.14) is more time-consuming and technically slightly more difficult, but is indicated in conditions such as restrictive (fibrous) pericarditis (Fig. 6.15) and infectious pericarditis. Anecdotally it also appears to result in better palliation in cases of neoplasia. Subtotal pericardiectomy is started the same as for a partial (window) pericardiectomy in dorsal recumbency, but a fourth port may be required, as described above. The ventral mediastinum is completely resected at the ventral aspect, with the aid of bipolar cautery or an ultrasonic scalpel.

After the initial incision, it is advisable to briefly explore the pericardial space with a blunt palpation probe for adhesions. Large significant

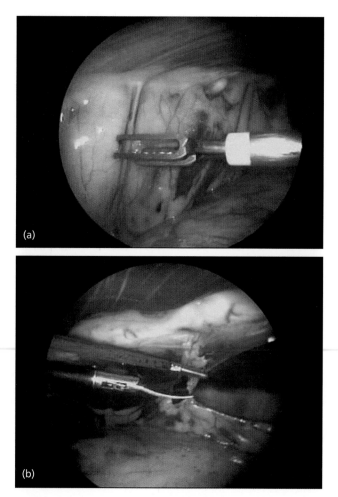

Fig. 6.10   After larger vessels are sealed with bipolar electrocautery (a), the ventral mediastinum is cut close to the sternum (b). While haemorrhage from these vessels is likely to be clinically insignificant, dripping blood tends to soil the endoscope's distal lens and hamper good visualisation.

adhesions may complicate a thoracoscopic subtotal pericardiectomy, and a partial pericardiectomy may instead need to be pursued. The pericardium is then incised laterally towards the heart base, paying attention to avoid the phrenic nerves and vagus. The incision is subsequently extended cranially, taking great care to avoid inadvertent incision into the atrial appendage or edges of the right cranial lung, and then extended on the contralateral side. Lastly the caudal portion of the pericardium is incised, ventral to the vena cava (Fig. 6.16). Adequate visualisation can be achieved by alternating the endoscope and instruments between the different ports, depending on the section of pericardium being incised. A second pair of grasping forceps is useful in manipulating and tensioning

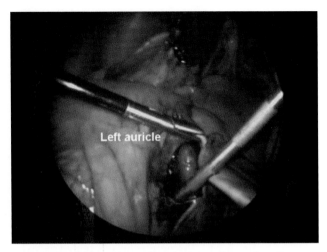

Fig. 6.11 Care should be taken when incising the pericardium to avoid incising the auricles. The initial incision when performing a pericardiectomy is best made further caudally over the ventricles.

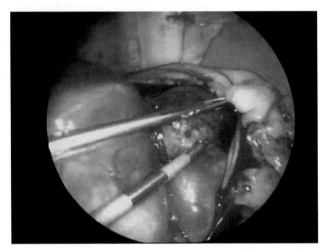

Fig. 6.12 A haemangiosarcoma on the right atrium apparent after a subtotal pericardiectomy. Small pedunculated atrial masses could be considered for palliative extracorporeal knot ligation.

the flaccid cut section of pericardium to make incising easier. Depending on the thickness of the pericardium and amount of associated adipose tissue, a larger 10 mm port is often needed for extraction. The pericardium should be removed through a port, or in an extraction bag, and not pulled through the unprotected incision, to limit risk of port-site metastasis in cases of neoplasia. Port-site metastasis of an invasive mesothelioma has been described after simple exploratory thoracoscopy in

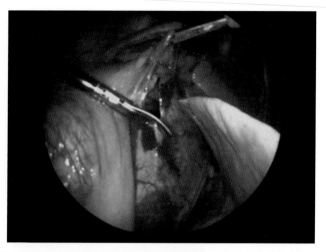

Fig. 6.13 The pericardium is tented away from the underlying heart during incision and care taken to avoid the lung edges during ventilation.

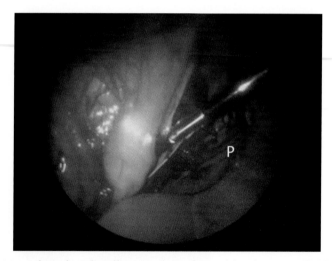

Fig. 6.14 Subtotal pericardiectomy is performed leaving a small fringe of pericardium ventral to the phrenic nerve (P).

a dog (Brisson et al., 2006), and mesothelioma is not an uncommon cause of undiagnosed pericardial effusion.

Aside from cautery of the ventral mediastinum vessels, partly to prevent blood dripping onto the endoscope lens and obscuring visualisation, cautery of even a markedly thickened pericardium is generally not necessary. Use of an ultrasonic scalpel is a good alternative to bipolar electrosurgery for both cautery and incision of the ventral mediastinum, as well as the pericardium, if this is believed necessary.

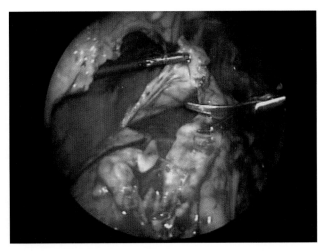

Fig. 6.15 Restrictive pericarditis (fibrosis) requires a subtotal pericardiectomy.

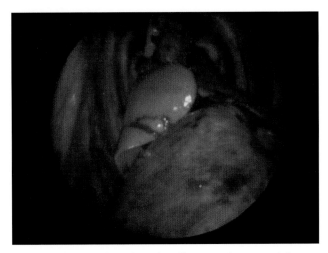

Fig. 6.16 View after a subtotal pericardiectomy from caudal to cranial. Note the small haemorrhagic areas on the epicardium, where adhesions to the pericardium were resected.

Suction of effusion from the pericardial sac in the case of partial pericardiectomy, and from the chest cavity at the end of the procedure in cases of subtotal pericardiectomy, helps in preventing port-site 'seromas' that may occur in the first 12–24 h postoperatively (Fig. 6.17).

While a thoracoscopic partial (window) pericardiectomy is a relatively simple procedure to perform, postoperative outcomes can sometimes be disappointing. It is advisable to be cautious in prognostication for

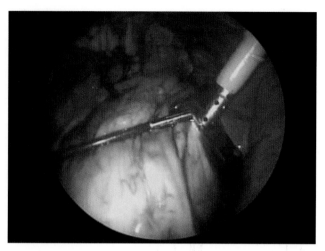

Fig. 6.17   Suction of pericardial effusion after the initial incision reduces soiling of the endoscope's distal lens and improves visualisation during pericardiectomy.

pericardiectomy as a treatment for presumptive idiopathic pericardial effusion. Many cases are not idiopathic; it is just that the underlying pathology has not been diagnosed preoperatively. Owners should be made aware of this fact before agreeing to surgery.

A small number of cases may go on to develop a recurring idiopathic pleural effusion resulting in clinical signs. Good preoperative echocardiography is also recommended to ensure that there are no small 2–3 mm undetected atrial masses before surgery, and the effusion is in fact atrial haemorrhage. Pericardiectomy in these cases risks the animal suffering a large fatal haemorrhage into the chest postoperatively. Comparison of pericardial effusion haematocrit with that of a venous sample preoperatively can be useful. The excised pericardium should always be submitted for histopathology.

Chylothorax: thoracic duct ligation and pericardiectomy

Thoracoscopy for ligation of the thoracic duct combined with pericardiectomy appears to be an acceptable surgical technique for the treatment of cases of idiopathic chylothorax, comparable with the success rates of open thoracic surgery. Surgical outcome is reliant on good preoperative diagnostic assessments, including echocardiography, in an attempt to determine non-idiopathic causes. Thoracoscopy provides an opportunity not only for treatment, but also for exploratory visualisation of the chest and biopsy of lesions. It should be remembered that chylothorax cases arising from a traumatic origin may resolve on their own. Cases associated with congestive heart failure generally have a poor prognosis, and are usually not candidates for surgery. Clients should, however, be made aware preoperatively that despite all this a significant number of idiopathic cases will fail to respond to surgical intervention.

Initial thoracoscopy is performed in sternal recumbency, with three portals placed in the right caudal hemithorax to perform the thoracic duct ligation. Ports are commonly inserted in the eighth, ninth and tenth intercostal spaces, in the dorsal third. They may be placed more caudally in large, deep-chested dogs. The endoscope is placed in the central port, with instruments either side. Placing the central port slightly more ventral than the other ports has the ergonomic benefit when using a 30° endoscope of allowing the scope to be held below the instrument handles, and so results in less 'sword fighting'. While radiographs can help with deciding intercostal-space port placement, the alternative is to place the first port in the eighth or ninth intercostal space, and then place the remaining ports under visualisation in the caudal most accessible intercostal spaces.

The mediastinal pleura is carefully incised over the aorta longitudinally, avoiding the costal arteries. Maryland forceps are used to dissect the mediastinum bluntly; alternatively blunt dissection with curved Metzenbaum scissors is performed. Dissection is first performed ventral to the thoracic duct, with ventral traction of the aorta, until through the mediastinum, then dorsal to the thoracic duct. This is then ligated together with all its visualised branches, either by use of clip applicators (disposable 10 mm or reusable 5 mm) or by placement of an extracorporeal Meltzer knot using non-absorbable braided synthetic suture material (Ethibond Excel, Ethicon), applied with a closed-end knot pusher. A pre-tied endoloop cannot be used, as this is not a loose pedicle.

The patient is then repositioned in either dorsal or lateral recumbency for a pericardiectomy as described above. It is preferable to perform a subtotal pericardiectomy, and hence position the patient in dorsal recumbency. If only a pericardial window is performed, this should be expanded by making two or three longitudinal fenestrations to just ventral to the phrenic nerves.

It must be recognised that although the thoracic duct is generally described as a single structure, there is a very wide variation in anatomy encountered. Methylene blue can be injected into either the popliteal or mesenteric lymph nodes to enhance the identification of the thoracic duct (Enwiller et al., 2003). Coloration of the duct occurs within 10 min and lasts up to 60 min. The technique is useful to visualise whether lymphatic flow into the chest has ceased after ligation, and to detect the presence of other branches. The technique is also useful for identification of the duct before ligation in chronic chylothorax cases where pleural thickening makes visualisation difficult. While less invasive to access, the popliteal lymph node only results in coloration in 60% of cases, and is also poorer. Mesenteric lymph node injection is hence preferable, and may be approached via a small right paracostal laparotomy, or via concurrent right lateral laparoscopy, with the dog positioned in sternal recumbency for the thoracic duct ligation. Two 5 mm laparoscopy ports are inserted: one for insufflation and insertion of the laparoscope/thoracoscope, the other for insertion of a pair of atraumatic grasping forceps. These are used to isolate and grasp a mesenteric lymph node for Methylene blue injection via a percutaneous spinal needle. The technique is advantageous to the injection of aqueous radiographic contrast agents (lymphangiography). In fact, these clear more rapidly, are not visible on thoracoscopy, and need operating-room fluoroscopy via a c-arm, or radiography.

With an alternative technique, demonstrated by MacDonald et al. (2008) in a canine cadaver study, all the tissue dorsal to the aorta and ventral to the vertebrae, including the azygous vein, is ligated *en masse* by means of an extracorporeal Meltzer knot, using non-absorbable braided synthetic suture material. The ligation is performed as far caudally in the chest as possible. The port placement and approach are as for the thoracoscopic thoracic duct ligation technique. The advantages to this method are that it is less time-consuming and also less invasive than dissection and ligation combined with laparotomy/laparoscopy for mesenteric lymph node injection or lymphangiography. A concurrent subtotal pericardiectomy is still advised. True efficacy of this technique in a series of chylothorax dogs has yet to be reported.

Vascular ring anomalies

Vascular ring anomalies causing a megaoesophagus are ideally suited to a minimally invasive endosurgical approach. It must be borne in mind that while a persistent right aortic arch (PRAA) is the most common form of vascular ring anomaly, it is not the only one. In the author's experience it is not uncommon to find a PRAA accompanied by an aberrant left subclavian artery that, if not also sectioned, will not result in resolution of the oesophageal constriction.

As these patients are often very small due to their young age, adequate operating space is a real limitation. While patients may be managed medically to allow them to grow before surgery, this carries the risks of developing megaoesophagus, oesophagitis and aspiration pneumonia, and this should be considered in when making the decision. It is the author's preference to operate early in patients over 3 kg in body weight. While a 5 mm endoscope can still be used in many cases, 3 mm instruments really are preferable, and are absolutely essential in small patients. If attempting to use larger 5 mm instruments there is sometimes not sufficient space to even open the jaws. Longer instruments are also awkward to handle, and not precise enough for accurate careful dissection and so short 20 cm-shafted instruments are required.

Not all puppies with regurgitation after weaning and a dilated cranial oesophagus on barium contrast studies have a PRAA. The base of the heart forms a natural elevation to an idiopathic dilated megaoesophagus and this can appear identical to a vascular ring anomaly on lateral radio-

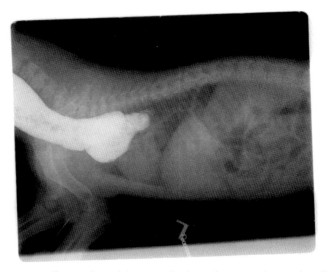

Fig. 6.18   Not all puppies with regurgitation after weaning and a dilated cranial oesophagus on barium contrast studies have a vascular ring anomaly such as a PRAA. The base of the heart forms a natural elevation to an idiopathic dilated megaoesophagus and this can appear similar on lateral radiographs.

graphs (Fig. 6.18). Barium/contrast radiographs should always be taken in a conscious puppy, as anaesthesia can also result in artefactual dilation. Ventrodorsal radiographs may also demonstrate a right-sided aorta and deviation of the trachea. One of the easiest and most reliable diagnostic methods is flexible oesophagoscopy, using a small-diameter gastroscope or bronchoscope, with insufflation of the oesophagus. The aorta can then clearly be seen pulsing through the oesophagus wall in its abnormal right-sided location at the restriction, and can be differentiated from some other anomalies, such as a right ligamentum arteriosum. The lung fields must be carefully evaluated on radiography for signs of aspiration pneumonia which carries a guarded prognosis. The duration of clinical signs is also important for prognosis. There is some evidence that early dilation is partially reversible after surgery, and cases that are operated on when first detected, and also without chronic oesophagitis, hold the best prognosis.

Different approaches and techniques are possible (Radlinsky, 2008). Isakow et al. (2000) described a thoracoscopy-assisted approach, and MacPhail et al. (2001) a thoracoscopic approach, both using 10 mm endoscopic clip applicators. The author prefers a technique completed solely with 3 mm diameter instrumentation and 3.5 mm ports, similar to that used in human paediatric endosurgery. This results in minimal postoperative pain and morbidity. Ligation of the ligamentum arteriosum before sectioning has also been satisfactorily accomplished with extracorporeal sutures, intracorporeal tied sutures and bipolar radiosurgery.

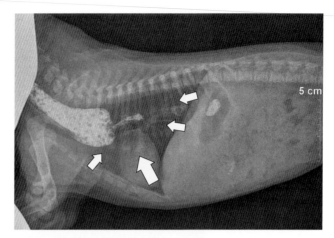

Fig. 6.19 Port-insertion sites for thoracoscopic ligation and transection of ligamentum arteriosum in puppies with vascular ring anomalies causing megaoesophagus. The large arrow indicates the placement of the optical port, in the seventh intercostal space. As space is always limited in these small puppies, the author's preference is to place ports as far apart as possible under visualisation once the first port is placed.

While the literature always emphasises the need for careful dissection and ligation of the ligamentum arteriosum in case of possible patency (patent ductus arteriosus, PDA) in combination with the vascular ring, this is rare. Patency can almost be ruled out entirely with preoperative echocardiography, and attentive auscultation for a typical machinery murmur high on the chest wall.

The patient is positioned in right lateral recumbency. Techniques working from either three caudal ports, viewing caudal to cranial, as well as from ports placed at the third, fifth and seventh intercostal spaces, have been described (Radlinsky, 2008). As space is always limited in these small puppies, the author's preference is to place ports as far apart as possible under visualisation once the first port is placed (Fig. 6.19).

The left cranial lung lobe is retracted dorsally and caudally, and held in place by a 3 mm blunt palpation probe (Fig. 6.20) or flexible retractor (Diamond flex, Surgical Innovations) inserted in the most caudal and dorsal port. The constricting band of the ligamentum arteriosum is not normally visually apparent or palpable (Fig. 6.21), so a wide-bore stomach tube is inserted under thoracoscopic visualisation and the restricting ring can usually then be palpated with the tips of 3 mm laparoscopic Kelly or Maryland dissecting forceps or a palpation probe, and carefully dissected free. If the restriction cannot be found, a 30 ml Foley balloon catheter is inserted into the distal oesophagus, then inflated and gradually retracted orally until the restricting ring is evident.

The author has found 3 mm paediatric Rothenburg double-action bowel forceps extremely useful for initial careful blunt dissection of the

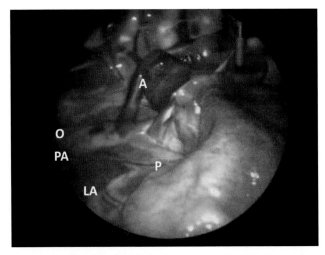

Fig. 6.20 View of the left heart base in a case of PRAA in a puppy. The left cranial lung has been retracted with a 3 mm palpation probe. Labels show the azygous vein (A), oesophagus (O), pulmonary artery (PA), left atrium (LA) and phrenic nerve (P).

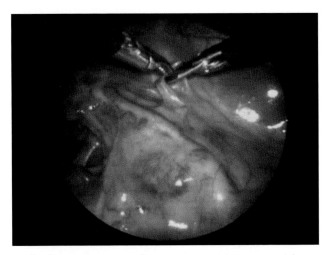

Fig. 6.21 The ligamentum arteriosum may not be apparent in cases of vascular ring anomalies. Careful palpation with a 3 mm dissection forceps once a stomach tube has been placed into the oesophagus will allow one to detect the restricting band.

mediastinum after this is initially incised. In some cases this has allowed completion of the procedure without the need for any electrosurgery. While a PRAA is most common and this is the anatomical position to examine first, other vascular rings are occasionally encountered, and sometimes more than one anomalous vascular ring is encountered. Small tortuous overlying vessels may also commonly be encountered. Even very

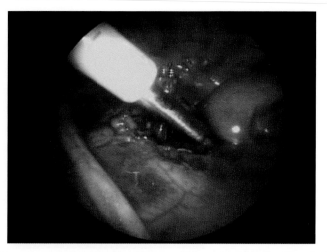

Fig. 6.22   Even minimal haemorrhage will hamper visualisation during dissection of the ligamentum arteriosum in small puppies. A 3 mm suction probe is being used to clear the area in this 3 kg puppy. Note the limited operating space.

small amounts of haemorrhage collect in the dissected space and make visualisation difficult during dissection, and should be removed with a 3 mm suction tube (Fig. 6.22), or pledget if using 5 mm instruments. Once the ligamentum arteriosum or other vessel has been dissected free, it is ligated before sectioning carefully. The author has found application of extracorporeal Meltzer knot ligatures with silk the most reliable method, but has also previously successfully used intracorporeally tied ligatures in larger patients, and careful bipolar radiosurgical cautery with 3 mm forceps (Fig. 6.23). A 30 ml Foley balloon catheter is then inserted into the distal oesophagus, inflated and retracted cranially to check for further fibrous strictures or concurrent vascular constrictions (such as a left subclavian artery) that may have been missed, and to help dilate the oesophagus, which may have other fibrous bands. These may be broken down by sharp or blunt dissection (Fig. 6.24). Finally the retracted cranial lung is replaced, ensuring that the lobe is not in torsion while visualised as the ventilation volume is gradually increased and the atelectatic region is ventilated again. Closure is standard (see below), and no indwelling postoperative chest drain is needed in these cases.

PDA

While thoracoscopically assisted ligation of PDA has been reported in dogs (Borenstein et al., 2004), surgical ligation of PDAs has largely been surpassed by interventional cardiology techniques such as the implantable canine Amplatzer device, which have been shown to be suitable even

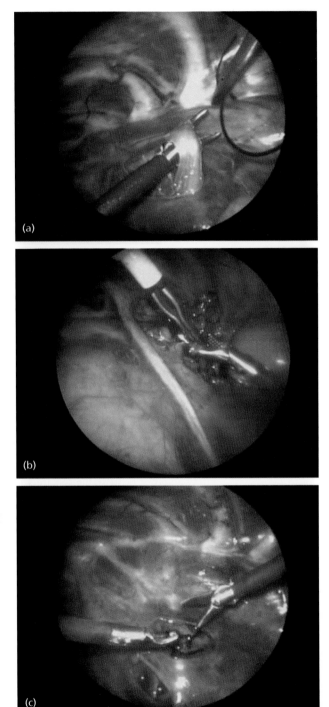

Fig. 6.23 (a) Passing suture behind the ligamentum arteriosum for ligation in a case of PRAA. Extracorporeal knot application with a 3 mm knot pusher is the method of choice. (b) Sealing of the ligamentum arteriosum with 3 mm bipolar forceps before sectioning in a small, 5-week-old puppy with a PRAA. Note the proximity of the phrenic nerve. (c) Sectioning of the ligamentum arteriosum after ligation in PRAA.

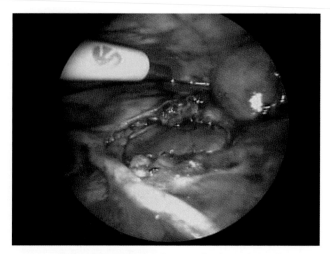

Fig. 6.24   View of the oesophagus after sectioning of the ligamentum arteriosum, ballooning and dissection of remaining fibrous restrictions.

in patients under 3 kg body weight, with a periprocedural mortality rate of less than 2% when performed by experienced cardiologists (Smith and Martin, 2007; Blossom et al., 2010). This is truly minimally invasive in nature, performed via vascular access under fluoroscopic guidance. Surgical ligation of PDAs has not been shown to have a lower perioperative mortality, or better outcome than interventional cardiology techniques. Cadaver studies demonstrate that adequate access to, and safe dissection around, the medial aspect of the ductus arteriosum may not be possible in many cases. It is extremely difficult to safely dissect around the ductus with the limited angulation afforded by thoracoscopic instruments. It may also not be possible to safely pass sutures for extracorporeal ligation with a knot pusher.

Currently vascular access interventional cardiology techniques remain the technique of choice and recognised standard of care for PDAs.

Lung biopsy

Thoracoscopic visualisation and lung biopsy are valuable modalities in numerous pulmonary conditions where less invasive modalities such as bronchoscopic directed bronchoalveolar lavage (BAL) has been unsuccessful in yielding a diagnosis. One of the most common applications for thoracoscopy in humans at present is the diagnostic excision of solitary peripheral lung masses 2 cm or less in diameter. While smoking-related primary neoplasia is common in humans, veterinary patients often have diffuse pulmonary disease on diagnostic imaging, well suited to small peripheral lung biopsies. Thoracoscopic lung biopsy diagnostic histology and microbiology yields are comparable with those from open surgical biopsy (Faunt et al., 1998). A number of different potential methods have been described, all with differing advantages and disadvantages. These include endoloop ligatures (Meltzer knot), endoscopic staplers, bipolar tissue feedback sealing devices (LigaSure) and ultrasonic scalpels (Autosonix, Covidien; Ultracision, Ethicon Endosurgery).

Port placement and patient positioning are dependent on the localisation of lesions, with both dorsal and lateral recumbency suitable. As for all minimally invasive surgery, the optical and instrument ports should not be placed over a lesion, but away from and directed towards a lesion to allow suitable operating space.

Pre-tied loop ligatures, either commercially available (Surgitie, Covidien), or hand-tied Meltzer knot loops applied with a knot pusher, are ideal for 1–2 cm peripheral lung biopsies. They have the advantage of being markedly less costly than endoscopic staplers, and also do not require the larger 12 mm-diameter ports that staplers require. This makes them well suited to small patients, as well as regions difficult or impossible to access with staplers. They can even be applied through 3 mm diameter ports in small patients, although they generally need at least a 5 mm port for retrieval. Lung biopsies also provide an ideal opportunity for the surgeon to become more proficient with hand tying and placing extracorporeal sutures, useful for more advanced procedures such as vascular ring anomalies where a commercial pre-tied loop ligature cannot be placed. Loop ligatures can also be used for the treatment of bullous emphysema (Brisson et al., 2003).

While Adamiak et al. (2008) described the use of Roeder knot loop biopsies of lung tumours in dogs, this knot, if unmodified, is no longer recommended for use in endosurgery. The unmodified Roeder knot has poor security unless used with catgut suture, which swells when wet. Catgut is not recommended in thoracoscopic surgery due to intense inflammatory reaction, occasional sensitivity reactions and high associated incidence of postoperative adhesion formation (Boothe, 2003). A modification of the Roeder knot, the Meltzer knot, is used in commercial endoloops and can be used securely with both multifilament and monofilament synthetic suture materials (see above and Fig. 6.6). Other suitable knots for use include the Weston and Tayside knots, and are detailed on the veterinary laparoscopy website (see Further resources at the end of this chapter).

Loop-ligature lung biopsies (Fig. 6.25), are performed through two instrument ports. Atraumatic grasping forceps are inserted through the loop of the ligature, and then used to gently grasp the edge of the lung region to be biopsied. The loop is then advanced over the tissue and the loop tightened before the suture ends are trimmed and the distal tissue is cut with Metzenbaum scissors. At first use the technique may feel unwieldy. The secrets are to use a small loop, and to place the tip of the knot pusher precisely where the knot is desired, then pull the long arm of the ligature tight, rather than using the instrument to try and push the knot down to the lung surface. Rotation of the knot-pusher shaft

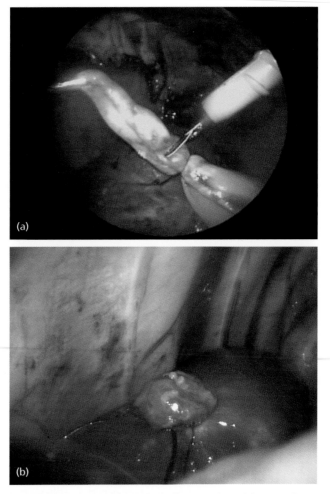

Fig. 6.25   (a) Extracorporeal knot loop-ligature lung biopsy using 3 mm instruments. The 5.5 mm soft Thoracoport allows extraction through the port of the 2 cm biopsy sample. (b) View of a peripheral loop-ligature (extracorporeal knot) lung biopsy site.

will also rotate the loop should this be twisted or lie incorrectly. A closed-end knot pusher (i.e. with a hole at the distal end) is preferable to the open or grooved knot pusher most commonly offered by veterinary suppliers, which is more difficult to manipulate, and doesn't allow for as precise knot positioning. Knot pushers are available in 5 and 3 mm paediatric diameters.

Removal of larger lesions, wedge excisional biopsies and partial or complete lobectomies require the use of endoscopic staplers. As a rough guide, a 2.0 or 2.5 mm staple leg length is generally suitable for most peripheral lung, while partial or complete lobectomy in medium and larger dogs usually requires a 3.5 mm staple leg length. The short 30 mm-long articulated (Endo GIA Roticulator) staple cartridge is often the most suitable in limited operating space, and where one is unable to adequately retract structures such as the lung hilus. A spare cartridge should always be available in the eventuality of a misfire. Endosurgical staplers require placement of a 12 mm port for their insertion, which also allows easy insertion of an endosurgical specimen-retrieval bag.

There has been recent interest in human surgery in the use of bipolar tissue-sealing devices and ultrasonic scalpels as an alternative to endoscopic staplers. This holds both cost advantages as well as only requiring a 5 mm port for insertion, rather than the 12 mm port needed for staplers. Bipolar tissue feedback pulmonary wedge resections of solitary small peripheral pulmonary nodules in humans have been performed using LigaSure, which was found to be comparable in safety and efficacy of air-tight sealing to endoscopic stapling in 22 human patients (Kovacs et al., 2009). Use of a 5 mm ultrasonic scalpel (Ultracision or Autosonix) was also found to yield results comparable to use of an endoscopic stapler for taking peripheral lung biopsies in an experimental animal model study (Molnar et al., 2004).

While current knowledge appears to suggest that the use of the 5 mm LigaSure bipolar tissue sealing device or ultrasonic scalpel may be suitable for peripheral lung biopsies, there is no published work evaluating its safety, efficacy or predictability when used in abnormal or diseased small-animal lung tissue. The use of extracorporeal loop ligatures currently appears to remain the most cost-effective, evidence-based technique for peripheral lung biopsy in veterinary companion animals.

Partial and complete lung lobectomy and pneumolobectomy

Thoracoscopy-assisted lobectomy techniques have been described in canines in a number of reports (Lansdown et al., 2005; Levionnois et al., 2006; Radlinsky, 2008; Laksito et al., 2010). Even if the procedure is completed entirely thoracoscopically in a suitably sized patient, a conversion of one of the port sites to a mini-thoracotomy is still needed for tissue removal. This should ideally be performed via a rip-proof, leak-proof retrieval bag to prevent pleural and extraction-site contamination, infection or metastasis. By avoiding rib retraction, postoperative pain and morbidity are still reduced in comparison to a standard intercostal thoracotomy. Thoracoscopy-assisted lung lobectomy is complicated by the wide variation in canine chest anatomy. Ironically, breeds with laterally compressed chests such as Irish setters and Weimaraners appear in most cases to be easier to perform lateral thoracoscopy on, and to access the hilar region, than round-chested breeds such as Labradors, contrary to what one may expect. Conversion to a standard thoracotomy is more likely to be necessary due to poor visibility or access when performing a cranial lung lobectomy in a small patient, or when performing lobectomy of the right middle or accessory lobes.

In some cases of partial lobectomy it is possible to exteriorise the affected portion of the lung lobe by conversion to a mini-thoracotomy of one of closest port sites, with no rib retraction to reduce postoperative pain. After the affected region and a margin of normal lung have been exteriorised, standard stapling or suture techniques are used before resection just as in open thoracic surgery, and the remaining lung then replaced in the chest at the end. Using this technique it is possible to utilise recently available hydrolysable lung sealants (PleuraSeal, Covidien) to help prevent air leakage postoperatively, should this be judged a risk.

Port-site selection is based on preoperative radiographs of the specific patient's anatomy, as well as the lobe to be removed. Patients are positioned in lateral recumbency. For lobectomy of the caudal lobes, a ventral and two dorsally placed ports, in a triangle, allow the best visualisation, manipulation and dorsal access to the hilus, although the ergonomics may be awkward. For the other lobes, ports are best placed some distance caudo-ventral to the intended hilus or resection site, to allow an adequate operating space and visualisation, ergonomic triangulation of instruments and sufficient lead-in distance for the insertion of the endoscopic stapler, if the procedure is to be performed thoracoscopically. When performing partial or complete lobectomy, hilar lymph node biopsy is highly recommended and should always be performed in cases of suspected neoplasia. Cup biopsy forceps can sometimes result in tearing loose of the lymph node and associated haemorrhage, and, if access allows, biopsy is best performed with stabilisation of the lymph node with atraumatic grasping forceps. Incision of the overlying mediastinum or capsule also results in fewer histological artefacts.

Whereas some authors favour single-lung ventilation for lung lobectomy (Lansdown et al., 2005; Laksito et al., 2010), this increases anaesthetic time as well as having effects on anaesthesia (see above), and requires attentive monitoring throughout. Single-lung ventilation requires bronchial intubation or endobronchial blockers inserted in the operated lung side. Levionnois et al. (2006) reported the accidental entrapment of an endobronchial blocker tip by staples during a lobectomy, and recommended the removal of the guidewire before staple placement, if this mode of single-lung ventilation is used. However, there is a learning curve to both techniques.

The use of a pericardial fat pedicle to reinforce the bronchial stump in humans undergoing a video-assisted lobectomy to reduce the risk of the postoperative development of a bronchial fistula has been reported. This perhaps merits further evaluation, as does endosurgical application of lung sealants such as PleuraSeal, to help prevent air leakage, in selected veterinary patients such as those undergoing pneumolobectomy.

Thymoma resection

Mayhew and Friedberg (2008) described the thoracoscopic resection of modestly sized, non-invasive thymomas in two dogs in which preoperative computed tomography scans had revealed a maximum size of 4.5 cm, with no evidence of vascular invasion. Thoracoscopy was performed using one-lung ventilation via a bronchoscopically placed double-lumen endobronchial tube. A harmonic scalpel was used for dissection with the capsule intact, and the thymomas were placed in endoscopic retrieval bags for removal. One dog was free of recurrence 18 months later, while the other was euthanased 5 days postoperatively due to aspiration pneumonia. This dog had myasthenia gravis, megaoesophagus and aspiration pneumonia diagnosed preoperatively. While thoracoscopic resection of modest-sized thymomas is feasible, the postoperative outcome is dependent on preoperative assessment and careful patient selection.

Port-site closure and postoperative care

Before closure the surgeon should check for adequate reventilation of atelectatic lung lobes that were retracted or collapsed during single-lung ventilation. If a lung lobe was retracted or pulled back, as for vascular ring anomaly surgery, it should be checked that there is no lobe torsion. Instrument port sites can be visualised after the cannulae are removed for any haemorrhage, although this is uncommon. A two-layer suture closure is generally sufficient for port sites, with a rapidly absorbable monofilament (Monocryl, Ethicon; Caprosyn, Covidien) for muscular and intradermal layers.

A narrow-gauge chest drain is inserted percutaneously at the end of a thoracoscopic procedure, under visualisation with the endoscope. It should not be inserted through a port site, but through its own site. It is left in place while all the ports are closed, and then the pneumothorax is drained (Fig. 6.26). The drain is then removed. Indwelling postoperative chest drains are not needed in most procedures, but port-site seromas can occasionally occur in the 12–24 h postoperatively in cases of pleural effusion, chylothorax and pericardiectomy. These may be best prevented by suctioning of effusions from the chest cavity at the end of the procedure and application of a light chest bandage for the first 12 h postoperatively.

Postoperative morbidity is low in most cases that do not require a mini-thoracotomy, and the majority of cases can be given a small amount of food and taken for a brief walk for a few minutes outside within 2 h of recovery from anaesthesia. However, cases are normally best hospitalised overnight for observation. Analgesic requirements are usually similar to those for minor abdominal surgical procedures. Cases requiring a mini-thoracotomy will need additional analgesia, as for open thoracic surgery cases.

Further resources

www.vetlapsurg.com or www.veterinarylaparoscopy.com   The internet portal for all aspects of minimally invasive surgery in all veterinary

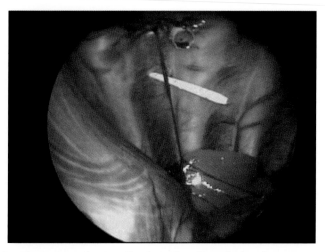

Fig. 6.26 Thoracoscopic visualisation of a chest-drain placement at the end of thoracoscopy. Note that this is not inserted via a port site. The small-gauge drain is simply used to drain the pneumothorax, and an indwelling drain is not needed for most procedures.

species. This website has numerous videos and pictures, and useful handouts and documents that can be downloaded, including the veterinary endosurgery safety checklist.

www.websurg.com   This is a human endosurgery website. There are a large number of surgery videos which are useful in demonstrating techniques, although unfortunately the majority of common human procedures are very different to those commonly performed in companion animal veterinary practice.

Further reading

Cantwell, S.L., Duke, T., Walsh, P.J., Remedios, A.M., Walker, D. and Ferguson, J.G. (2000) One-lung versus two-lung ventilation in the closed-chest anesthetized dog: a comparison of cardiopulmonary parameters. *Veterinary Surgery* 29, 365–373.

McCarthy, T.C. and Monnet, E. (2005) Diagnostic and operative thoracoscopy. In *Veterinary Endoscopy for the Small Animal Practitioner*, McCarthy, T.C. (ed.), pp. 229–278. Elsevier Saunders, St Louis, MO.

Radlinsky, M.G. (2009) Complications and need for conversion from thoracoscopy to thoracotomy in small animals. *Veterinary Clinics of North America, Small Animal Practice* 39, 977–984.

References

Adamiak, Z., Holak, P. and Piórek, A. (2008) Thoracoscopic biopsy of lung tumors using a Roeder's loop in dogs. *Polish Journal of Veterinary Sciences* 11, 75–77.

Andrews, S.M. and Lewis, J.L. (1994) Laparoscopic knot substitutes. An assessment of techniques of securing sutures through the laparoscope. *Endoscopic Surgery and Allied Technologies* 2, 62–65.

Blossom, J.E., Bright, J.M. and Griffiths, L.G. (2010) Transvenous occlusion of patent ductus arteriosus in 56 consecutive dogs. *Journal of Veterinary Cardiology* 12(2), 75–84.

Boothe, H.W. (2003) Suture materials, tissue adhesives, staplers, and ligating clips. In *Textbook of Small Animal Surgery*, Slatter, D. (ed.), 3rd edn, pp. 235–244. Elsevier, Philadelphia, PA.

Borenstein, N., Behr, L., Chetboul, V., Tessier, D., Nicole, A., Jacquet, J., Carlos, C., Daniel, P. and Laborde, F. (2004) Minimally invasive patent ductus arteriosus occlusion in 5 dogs. *Veterinary Surgery* 33, 309–313.

Brisson, B.A., Geggiti, F. and Bienzle, D. (2006) Portal site metastasis of invasive mesothelioma after diagnostic thoracoscopy in a dog. *Journal of the American Veterinary Medical Association* 229, 980–983.

Brisson, H.N., Dupre, G.P., Bouvy, B.M. and Paquet, L. (2003) Thoracoscopic treatment of bullous emphysema in 3 dogs. *Veterinary Surgery* 32, 524–529.

Carpenter, E.M., Hendrickson, D.A., James, S., Franke, C., Frisbie, D., Trostle, S. and Wilson, D. (2006) A mechanical study of ligature security of commercially available pre-tied ligatures versus hand tied ligatures for use in equine laparoscopy. *Veterinary Surgery* 35, 55–59.

Crumbaker, D.M., Rooney, M.B., Case, J.B. (2010) Thoracoscopic subtotal pericardiectomy and right atrial mass resection in a dog. *Journal of the American Veterinary Medical Association* 237, 551–554.

Dupre, G.P., Corlouer, J.P. and Bouvy, B. (2001) Thoracoscopic pericardectomy performed without pulmonary exclusion in 9 dogs. *Veterinary Surgery* 30, 21–27.

Enwiller, T.M., Radlinsky, M.G., Mason, D.E. and Roush, J.K. (2003) Popliteal and mesenteric lymph node injection with methylene blue for coloration of the thoracic duct in dogs. *Veterinary Surgery* 32, 359–364.

Faunt, K.K., Jones, B.D., Turk, J.R., Cohn, L.A. and Dodam, J.R. (1998) Evaluation of biopsy specimens obtained during thoracoscopy from lungs of clinically normal dogs. *American Journal of Veterinary Research* 59, 1499–1502.

Hage, J.J. (2008) On the origin and evolution of the Roeder knot and loop–a geometrical review. *Surgical Laparoscopy Endoscopy & Percutaneous Techniques* 18, 1–7.

Isakow, K., Fowler, D. and Walsh, P. (2000) Video-assisted thoracoscopic division of the ligamentum arteriosum in two dogs with persistent right aortic arch. *Journal of the American Veterinary Medical Association* 217, 1333–1366.

Jackson, J., Richter, K.P. and Launer, D.P. (1999) Thoracoscopic partial pericardiectomy in 13 dogs. *Journal of Veterinary Internal Medicine* 13, 529–533.

Johnson, M.S. and Martin, M.W. (2007) Successful medical treatment of 15 dogs with pyothorax. *Journal of Small Animal Practice* 48, 12–16.

Kovács, O., Szántó, Z., Krasznai, G. and Herr, G. (2009) Comparing bipolar electrothermal device and endostapler in endoscopic lung wedge resection. *Interactive Cardiovascular and Thoracic Surgery* 9, 11–14.

Kovak, J.R., Ludwig, L.L., Bergman, P.J., Baer, K.E. and Noone, K.E. (2002) Use of thoracoscopy to determine the etiology of pleural effusion in dogs and cats: 18 cases (1998–2001). *Journal of the American Veterinary Medical Association* 221, 990–994.

Kudnig, S.T., Monnet, E., Riquelme, M., Gaynor, J.S., Corliss, D. and Salman, M.D. (2006) Effect of positive end-expiratory pressure on oxygen delivery during 1-lung ventilation for thoracoscopy in normal dogs. *Veterinary Surgery* 35, 534–542.

Laksito, M.A, Chambers, B.A. and Yates, G.D. (2010) Thoracoscopic-assisted lung lobectomy in the dog: report of two cases. *Australian Veterinary Journal* 88, 263–267.

Lansdown, J.L., Monnet, E., Twedt, D.C. and Dernell, W.S. (2005) Thoracoscopic lung lobectomy for treatment of lung tumors in dogs. *Veterinary Surgery* 34, 530–535.

Levionnois, O.L., Bergadano, A. and Schatzmann, U. (2006) Accidental entrapment of an endo-bronchial blocker tip by a surgical stapler during selective ventilation for lung lobectomy in a dog. *Veterinary Surgery* 35, 82–85.

MacDonald, N.J., Noble, P.J. and Burrow, R.D. (2008) Efficacy of en bloc ligation of the thoracic duct: descriptive study in 14 dogs. *Veterinary Surgery* 37, 696–701.

MacPhail, D.M., Monnet, E. and Twedt, D.C. (2001) Thoracoscopic correction of persistent right aortic arch in a dog. *Journal of the American Animal Hospital Association* 37, 577–581.

Mayhew, P.D. and Friedberg, J.S. (2008) Video-assisted thoracoscopic resection of noninvasive thymomas using one-lung ventilation in two dogs. *Veterinary Surgery* 37, 756–762.

Mayhew, K.N., Mayhew, P.D., Sorrell-Raschi, L. and Brown, D.C. (2009) Thoracoscopic subphrenic pericardectomy using double-lumen endobronchial intubation for alternating one-lung ventilation. *Veterinary Surgery* 38, 961–966.

Molnar, T.F., Szantó, Z., László, T., Lukacs, L. and Horvath, O.P. (2004) Cutting lung parenchyma using the harmonic scalpel–an animal experiment. *European Journal of Cardiothoracic Surgery* 26, 1192–1195.

Potter, L. and Hendrickson, D.A. (1998) Therapeutic video-assisted thoracic surgery. In *Veterinary Endosurgery*, Freeman, L.J. (ed.), pp. 169–191. Mosby, St Louis, MO.

Radlinsky, M.G. (2008) Rigid endoscopy: thoracoscopy. In *BSAVA Manual of Canine and Feline Endoscopy and Endosurgery*, Lhermette, P. and Sobel, D. (eds), pp. 175–187. British Small Animal Veterinary Association, Gloucester.

Sharp, H.T., Dorsey, J.H., Chovan, J.D. and Holtz, P.M. (1996) The effect of knot geometry on the strength of laparoscopic slip knots. *Obstetrics and Gynecology* 88, 408–411.

Smith, P.J. and Martin, M.W. (2007) Transcatheter embolisation of patent ductus arteriosus using an Amplatzer vascular plug in six dogs. *Journal of Small Animal Practice* 48, 80–86.

Trostle, S.S., Hendrickson, D.A. and Franke, C. (2002) The effects of ethylene oxide and gas-plasma sterilization on failure strength and failure mode of pre-tied monofilament ligature loops. *Veterinary Surgery* 31, 281–284.

Walsh, P.J., Remedios, A.M., Ferguson, J.F., Walker, D.D., Cantwell, S. and Duke, T. (1999) Thoracoscopic versus open partial pericardiectomy in dogs: comparison of postoperative pain and morbidity. *Veterinary Surgery* 28, 472.

Chapter 7
Urethrocystoscopy and the Female Reproductive Tract
Philip J. Lhermette

Introduction

Urethrocystoscopy has been widely used by doctors and gynaecologists in the human field for many years. Indeed, this was the most common and earliest application of endoscopy in the late nineteenth and twentieth centuries.

The female urinary and reproductive tracts are difficult to image in their entirety, being partly encased within the bony girdle of the pelvis. Radiography, ultrasonography, computed tomography or magnetic resonance imaging may all be used, with or without contrast media, to provide information on pathology and morphology and each has its own merits and disadvantages. Radiography and ultrasonography are widely used in conjunction with endoscopy as they are widely available and provide vital information on those parts of the urinary tract not visible from the lumen. Endoscopy provides a means to directly visualise the female urinary and reproductive tracts, identify abnormal structures and take biopsy samples for histological analysis. Many abnormalities can also be treated during the examination. In veterinary medicine, this modality has been greatly underused and provides minimally invasive access to the whole of the lower urinary tract in the bitch for obtaining biopsies for culture and histology and the diagnosis and treatment of many conditions.

Clinical Manual of Small Animal Endosurgery, First Edition. Edited by Alasdair Hotston Moore and Rosa Angela Ragni.
© 2012 Blackwell Publishing Ltd. Published 2012 by Blackwell Publishing Ltd.

Indications for urethrocystoscopy

Urethrocystoscopy may be employed for investigation of a wide range of conditions affecting the lower urinary and reproductive tracts. Persistent cystitis, stranguria, pollakiuria, vaginal discharge, urinary incontinence, reproductive problems, trauma and neoplasia are all indications for direct examination.

Equipment

Although flexible endoscopes are commonly used for urethrocystoscopy in the male dog, where the length of the urethra precludes other choices, the female urinary tract lends itself to the superior optics and versatility of the rigid endoscope. A 2.7 mm-diameter, 18 cm endoscope with a 30° angle of view and a matching cystoscopy sheath will be adequate for the vast majority of bitches and may even be used in many queens. The limiting factor in large breeds is the length of the instrument, and it may be necessary or preferable to use a 4 mm-diameter telescope with a length of around 33 cm and a viewing angle of 30° for these patients as the extra length facilitates examination of the bladder. This will require a matching cystoscopy sheath and instrumentation at additional cost. However, even in large breeds it is often possible to carry out a full examination with the shorter endoscope by careful external abdominal manipulation of the bladder during the procedure. In cats and small breeds of dogs an arthroscopy sheath may be used with the 2.7 mm endoscope as it has a smaller cross section than the cystoscope. However the lack of an instrument channel limits the usefulness of this approach. Biopsies can be taken blind by pointing the instrument at the site of interest and carefully removing the endoscope from the sheath, to allow insertion of biopsy forceps directly down it. The endoscope is then replaced in the arthroscope sheath and the biopsy site inspected. Smaller endoscopes of 1.9 or 2.4 mm diameter may also be used but are usually too short to reach the bladder except in very small kittens.

The cystoscopy sheath has two taps with Luer fitting, one on either side, for instilling and removing fluid respectively. A further tap on the top of the sheath controls the opening to the instrument channel that runs along the top of the telescope and accommodates semi-flexible biopsy forceps, grasping forceps or scissors. Other instruments such as laser fibres or injection needles can also be passed through this channel. Typically, this channel on the sheath of a 2.7 mm endoscope accommodates 7 French (2.3 mm diameter) instruments.

A light guide cable and light source, ideally xenon or metal halide, are also required.

Finally a camera system and monitor are essential, not only to carry out the procedure hygienically, but also because the vastly improved magnification and image quality will make diagnosis and treatment much easier.

Urethrocystoscopy procedure

Urethrocystoscopy is performed under general anaesthesia, usually on a tub table or on a wire grid over a suitable tray for collecting fluid. Urine samples for bacterial culture are indicated in most candidates for urethrocystoscopy and are best obtained by cystocentesis prior to the procedure. The room is arranged so that the monitor is at the head of the patient, which makes orientation during the examination more straightforward. The patient may be positioned in ventral, lateral or dorsal recumbency according to personal preference. For routine urethrocystoscopy this author prefers to position the patient in ventral recumbency with a rolled up towel under the caudal abdomen to elevate the pelvis a little. The tail is held or taped out of the way. In this position anatomical structures are in their normal orientation and a full examination can be carried out following a set routine.

The endoscope is mounted into the cystoscope sheath and the camera and light guide cable attached. The light source is switched on and the camera white-balanced. A litre bag of sterile saline is attached via a giving set to one of the Luer taps on the cystoscope sheath and the clamps on the giving set are opened so that flow can be controlled with the forefinger operating the Luer tap on the cystoscope sheath.

It is not usually necessary to clip the peri-vulvar hair unless it is very long or is soiled and matted. The cystoscope sheath is lubricated with a little sterile water-soluble lubricating gel and the tip is introduced into the dorsal commisure of the vulva in a cranio-dorsal direction to avoid the clitoral fossa. With the tip of the cystoscope just inside the vulvar lips, firm pressure is applied with the thumb and forefinger to form a watertight seal around the sheath. The saline flow is turned on and the vestibule observed on the monitor as it distends with saline. Once sufficiently distended, saline flow can be turned off. The vaginal os is observed dorsally with the urethral opening below (Fig. 7.1), and the

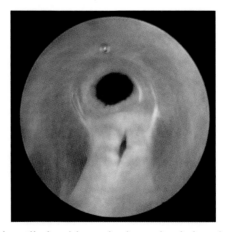

Fig. 7.1   Normal vestibule with urethral opening below the vaginal os (dog in ventral recumbency).

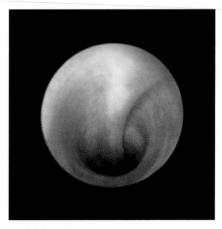

Fig. 7.2   The dorsal vaginal fold.

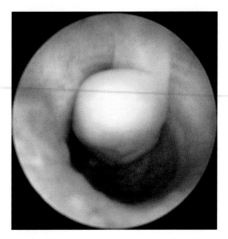

Fig. 7.3   Normal cervical opening on the ventral surface of the cranial end of the dorsal vaginal fold.

cystoscope is advanced cranio-dorsally to it. At this point the vagina extends cranially and the angle of insertion of the cystoscope is altered to follow its lumen to the cervix, which appears as a small slit on the ventral surface of the prominent dorsal fold at the cranial end of the vagina (Figs 7.2 and 7.3). In the entire bitch the vaginal wall may have extensive linear folds but in most neutered bitches this structure is relatively smooth with just a dorsal fold which extends from about mid vagina and increases in size as it approaches the cervix. The endoscopist will often encounter an air bubble in the caudal vagina near the vaginal os. The cranial vaginal lumen is often reflected here and it is important not to mistake this for the lumen itself. The endoscope must be redirected cranially in order to follow the vagina to the cervix. In entire bitches the appearance of the vaginal wall will vary according to the stage of the oestrus cycle. The walls become thickened and more folded during oestrus, becoming thinner and less prominent during anoestrus.

Having examined the vagina, the cystoscope is withdrawn as far as the vestibule and redirected ventrally into the urethral opening. Saline flow is turned on again to distend the urethra as the cystoscope passes down. Once in the urethra, the surgeon may relax the grip on the vulva as a watertight seal is no longer required. Great care must be taken when passing a 30° endoscope down a narrow lumen such as the urethra. The natural instinct is to keep the lumen central in the field of view. However, with a 30° endoscope this would result in the tip of the endoscope running along the mucosa at an angle of 30° which could result in damage or even perforation. Viewing the image as you pass a bare endoscope into the cystoscopy sheath will demonstrate that the lumen of the sheath is right at the bottom of the image on the monitor. This is the orientation that must be maintained in the urethral lumen. It is standard for the angle of view of rigid endoscopes to be directed away from the light post, and the endoscopist can use this to maintain orientation during the procedure.

The walls of the relaxed urethra comprise many longitudinal folds which gradually disappear as the lumen expands. In the queen there is a prominent dorsal fold which usually remains visible throughout the procedure. The mucosa should look pink and smooth (Fig. 7.4) and should be observed for abnormalities as the cystoscope passes down the urethra. Erythema, petechial haemorrhages, transitional cell carcinoma (TCC) or the openings of ectopic ureters are easily seen (see later).

The entrance of the bladder at the trigone is indicated by the presence of yellow, often turbid, urine (turbidity is a regular feature of normal urine during rigid endoscopy). Once the tip of the cystoscope is in the bladder, saline flow is turned off and a brief examination of the bladder

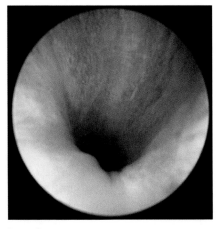

Fig. 7.4 A normal urethra.

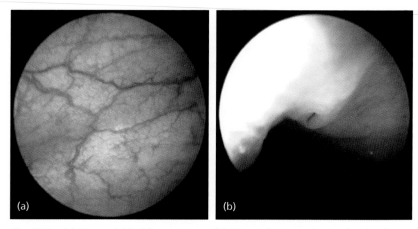

Fig. 7.5   (a) Normal bladder mucosa. (b) Normal ureteral opening in the trigone.

and trigone is carried out to detect gross abnormalities such as masses or uroliths. Urine is then drained from the bladder by opening the tap opposite the saline inflow tap on the cystoscope. A 60 ml syringe can be attached to this tap or alternatively a second giving set may be used to drain urine by gravity into a suitable container. Once the bladder has been emptied, saline flow is re-started to refill the bladder. Sometimes several flushes are required to completely clear the bladder of urine or particulate material. The whole of the bladder mucosa should be examined (Fig. 7.5a). Care must be taken not to over-distend the bladder as this can lead to mucosal damage and bleeding, especially if the mucosa is already inflamed through cystitis. The aim should be to maintain a crinkly, undulating surface that is not under tension. This also facilitates the taking of biopsies if these are required. To avoid over-filling, the flow of saline is turned off once the bladder is sufficiently full to allow examination of the surface. Over-distension also moves the apex of the bladder further away from the endoscope at the trigone, making visualisation of the bladder wall difficult or impossible. In large breeds it is necessary to keep the bladder quite flaccid in order to examine the whole of the bladder mucosa, and it is sometimes helpful to have an assistant gently manipulate the bladder through the abdominal wall to bring all areas of the mucosa into view.

Haemorrhage from the bladder mucosa may present a problem since quite small amounts of blood will impair the view. In the rare cases that this interferes with the examination it may be preferable to insufflate the bladder with air or carbon dioxide to enable a complete examination. Carbon dioxide is preferred as air embolism may be a potential complication of insufflation with room air.

Once the bladder is partially filled with clear saline the image is improved and detailed examination is carried out. The openings of both ureters should be examined (Fig. 7.5b) and urine observed entering the bladder (see Fig. 7.13c, below). With the bitch in ventral recumbency the openings are positioned at roughly 10 and 2 o'clock near the trigone. They appear fairly prominent in the flaccid bladder but may be reduced to flattened slits as the bladder becomes more distended. The endoscope is withdrawn almost back to the urethral opening and rotated around its long axis by rotating the light guide post. This enables the surgeon to utilise the 30° angle of view to visualise the entire trigone. The rest of the bladder mucosa is then examined for polyps, masses or other abnormalities.

Once the examination is complete and any biopsies have been taken the bladder is drained and the endoscope gently removed. If biopsies of the vestibule or vagina are required, these are taken at the end of the procedure as haemorrhage may otherwise hamper the view.

Postoperative care

Antibiotics are not usually required following this procedure unless indicated by underlying pathology. Analgesia is advisable and is provided by opiates pre- and immediately postoperatively and continued with non-steroidal anti-inflammatories if renal function is not compromised.

Careful observation for 24–48 h postoperatively is advisable following more invasive procedures such as laser resection of TCC. Urethral spasm or occlusion of the urethra by adhesions or seroma can occur and may require catheterisation.

Complications

The use of cold saline for irrigation, especially in a small patient, can act as an appreciable heat sink and lead to hypothermia. Careful monitoring of core body temperature throughout the procedure is recommended. The use of saline at body temperature is advisable, especially in patients of small size.

Complications of diagnostic cystoscopy are rare and are almost always the result of iatrogenic trauma or over distension of the bladder with saline. Bruising and trauma to the urethra may lead to urethral spasm and swelling. In rare cases urethral perforation can occur, especially if the angle of view of the endoscope is not taken into account when advancing down the urethra in small patients. Perforations will usually respond to the placement of an indwelling Foley catheter for 48–72 h to allow healing to take place. Surgical repair is rarely required.

Over-distension of the bladder may result in haemorrhage from the mucosa which interferes with the examination but is rarely a major cause for concern for the patient. Severe over-distension could result in rupture of the bladder wall where it has been weakened by pathological processes and this will require surgical repair. However, this is extremely unlikely where saline irrigation is supplied under gravity feed.

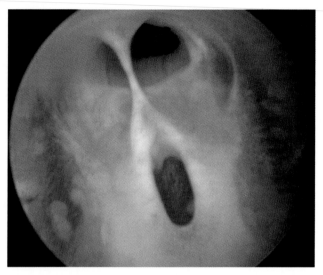

Fig. 7.6   A paramesonephric remnant. Note the presence of lymphoid follicles in the vestibule.

Pathological conditions

Paramesonephric remnant

A paramesonephric remnant (vaginal septum, persistent hymen, vaginal web) is a fairly common finding in bitches (Fig. 7.6). It is typically seen as a dorsoventral band of tissue at the vaginal os immediately cranial to the urethral orifice and may be a thin band of mucosa or more substantial. Paramesonephric remnants are often asymptomatic; however, in the author's experience they can be associated with persistent cystitis and/or vaginitis. They are also commonly found in association with other anatomical anomalies such as ectopic ureters. Where vaginitis is present it is common to see multiple small pale swellings throughout the mucosa of the vestibule. These are lymphoid follicles and are a normal reaction to inflammation (Fig. 7.6).

Resection of a paramesonophrenic remnant is performed with Metzenbaum scissors passed alongside the cystoscope or using a diode laser fibre via the instrument channel (Figs 7.7 and 7.8). Passing surgical scissors alongside the cystoscope often causes loss of a watertight seal, thus impairing direct visualisation during resection. A pair of 5 mm laparoscopic scissors may be used instead of the surgical scissors and this improves the chances of maintaining the watertight seal. 7 French scissors designed for the instrument channel of the cystoscope are not substantial enough to cut this tissue. Resection with a diode laser, if available, is quick and efficient and prevents any haemorrhage.

Occasionally a completely bipartite vagina may be seen where a septum completely separates the vagina into two parts, each of which

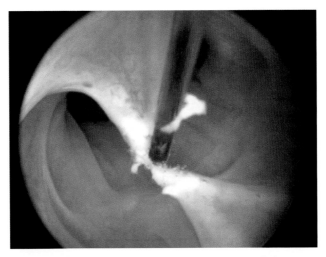

Fig. 7.7   Using a diode laser to resect the paramesonephric remnant.

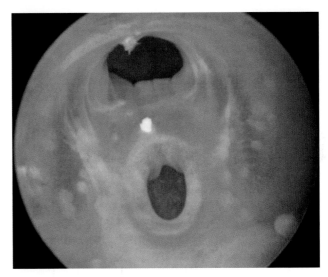

Fig. 7.8   Following resection of the paramesonephric remnant. Note the reduced upward traction on the urethral opening.

can be explored down to a separate cervix at the cranial end. Treatment is not necessary but breeding from affected bitches is not possible or recommended.

Canine herpes virus

Canine herpes virus is a fairly common problem in kennels throughout Europe and the USA. The virus remains latent after primary infection and recrudesces at times of stress, particularly at parturition and pro-oestrus. At these times vesicles may form in the vagina and vestibule. Ruptured vesicles appear as raised red swellings in the mucosa and must be differentiated from lymphoid follicles seen as a result of chronic irritation or infection.

Vaginal polyps

Vaginal polyps may be a cause of persistent vaginal discharge. These may be pedunculated leiomyomas or mucosal fibrovascular polyps. Larger polyps may be extruded and appear as a large pale or red swelling at the vulvar lips. Pedunculated polyps are removed using a radiosurgical polypectomy snare passed through the instrument channel of the cystoscope. Alternatively a diode laser may be used. If the polyp is near the vulva then it may be possible to exteriorise the pedicle through manual traction and then ligate and excise the mass using an open technique.

Vaginal tumours

Leiomyomas may be found either in the vaginal or vestibular lumen or distorting the normal shape of the vagina or vestibule from an extraluminal origin. These tumours are encapsulated, sessile and not easily removed cystoscopically. An episiotomy is usually required.

Transmissible venereal tumours are found in many tropical and subtropical areas of the USA, Africa and Europe and present as irregular, ulcerated masses in the vagina, vestibule and vulva. Chemotherapy is the treatment of choice.

Ectopic ureters

Ectopic ureters are a cause of incontinence in young bitches. More than 95% of ectopic ureters in the dog are intra-mural (Berent et al., 2008), with ureters passing into the bladder wall at the normal position in the trigone and then passing within the wall to open into the urethra, vestibule or vagina. There may be multiple openings and some may not be patent. It is therefore important to assess each case carefully to ascertain the exact anatomy in each case. Normograde or retrograde contrast urography, ultrasound and computed tomography may be used to help ascertain the path and patency of the ureters, and also to assess the ureters and kidneys for pathology not visible from the bladder lumen, such as hydronephrosis and hydroureter (Samii et al., 2004). Ectopic ureters are commonly associated with other lower urinary tract anomalies such as urethral sphincter mechanism incompetence (USMI), paramesonephric remnants and hydroureter.

Ectopic ureters are easily seen during urethrocystoscopy (Figs 7.9 and 7.10), which provides the gold standard for diagnosis. Many appear as slit-like openings into the urethra but some may be very large, making distinction between the urethra and ureter difficult.

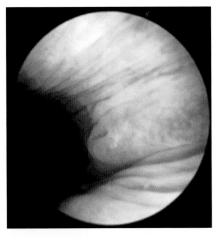

Fig. 7.9 Ectopic ureter opening into the proximal urethra.

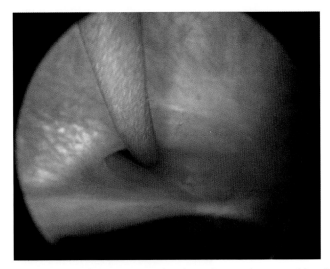

Fig. 7.10 Large ectopic ureter opening into the urethra; a guide wire has been placed into the ureteral opening.

Intra-mural ectopic ureters can be treated using cystoscopic laser ablation (McCarthy, 2006) (Figs 7.11 and 7.12). A 0.89 mm, angled, hydrophilic tip guide wire is advanced up the ureter through the working channel of the cystoscope, which is then removed, leaving the guide wire in place. The cystoscope is then reintroduced and a diode laser fibre is passed through the instrument channel. The laser is used in continuous contact mode at 10–15 W to ablate the common wall between the urethra and ureter as far back into the trigone as possible, using the guide wire to protect the outer wall of the ureter and judge the path and depth of the ureters. Great care must be taken not to resect too far or to penetrate the bladder wall.

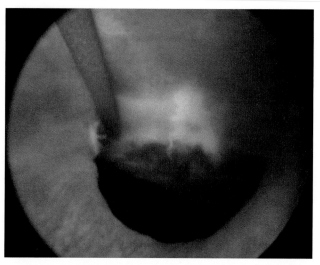

Fig. 7.11   Laser resection of the ureteral opening back into the trigone.

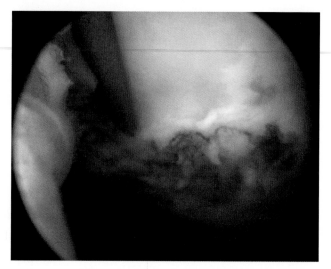

Fig. 7.12   Close-up of laser resection of the ureteral opening back into the trigone.

This procedure provides good improvement in continence in around 65% of cases used alone or around 80% of cases if used in conjunction with oral medication such as phenylpropanolamine or diethystilboestrol. To date, the numbers of animals treated is relatively small, however, and more experience is required to offer a more accurate prognosis. Many of these cases have concurrent USMI and will require additional procedures such as colposuspension or peri-urethral injections of collagen to improve continence further.

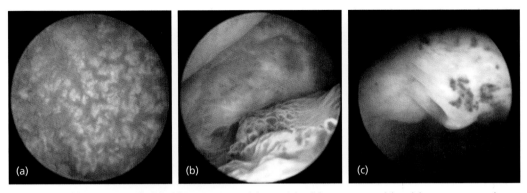

Fig. 7.13 (a) Hyperaemic bladder mucosa with cystitis. (b) Severe cystitis with severe vascular congestion and early polypoid changes. (c) Urine entering the bladder through the ureter. Note petechial haemorrhages on the ureter and bladder mucosa due to severe interstitial cystitis.

Cystitis

Cystitis is a common finding in both dogs and cats (Fig. 7.13). The bladder mucosa may appear thickened, often with petechial haemorrhages, and bleeds easily on distension with fluid. Biopsies should be taken from affected parts, avoiding the ureteral openings. They have to be taken with the bladder in a fairly flaccid state as a taut bladder wall makes obtaining a deep biopsy difficult or impossible. Chronic cystitis may lead to polypoid cystitis (see Fig. 7.15, below), which is a major differential diagnosis for TCC.

Cystic calculi

Cystic calculi are easily diagnosed through urethrocystoscopy (Fig. 7.14) and small stones may be removed using grasping forceps or basket forceps. However, the urethral diameter is the limiting factor and it is only feasible to remove relatively few small stones by this method. They must be removed one by one, removing the cystoscope each time. Larger stones must be removed by laparoscopy-assisted cystoscopy or open cystotomy (Rawlings et al., 2003). Alternatively laser lithotripsy may be used to break down calculi to small pieces that can be removed per urethra (Bevan et al., 2009; Adams et al., 2008). This uses a holmium:YAG (yttrium, aluminum, garnet) laser through a cystoscope to gain direct contact with a stone and break it to small-enough fragments so that the pieces can be withdrawn using a stone basket or by voiding urohydropropulsion.

Cystic polyps

Chronic cystitis may lead to the formation of polypoid cystitis (Fig. 7.15). There is evidence in humans that this may be a precursor of TCC, and polypoid cystitis always warrants aggressive treatment. Small

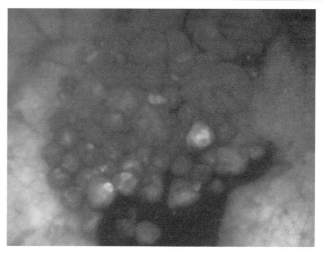

Fig. 7.14   Struvite calculi in the bladder.

pedunculated polyps may be removed using a radiosurgical polypectomy snare passed through the instrument channel of the cystoscope. In most cases the polyps are multiple and sessile and are best removed using a diode laser. The magnification afforded by the cystoscope enables even very small polyps (less than 1 mm) to be removed (Lhermette and Sobel, 2008).

Polypoid cystitis is often both a sequel to and cause of persistence of chronic bacterial urinary tract infection, and this should be managed concurrently.

TCC of the bladder and urethra

TCC is the commonest neoplasm of the urinary tract of the dog. The tumour is slow-growing and slow to metastasise but readily seeds along needle tracts or incisional scars, so percutaneous cystocentesis should be avoided at all costs if TCC is suspected. The tumour has a predilection for the trigone area where the growing mass eventually results in dysuria and tenesmus. Haematuria is a common clinical sign, as well as stranguria and pollakiuria. Typically, the dog is able to pass urine reasonably well when the bladder is distended, but as the bladder emptied and the pressure drops, the urethral diameter reduces and the mass in the trigone and/or urethra blocks the outflow. The harder the dog strains to pass urine the more the mass is forced into the urethra. Although classically described as occurring mainly in the trigone, in the author's experience many of these cases have tumour growing throughout the urethra and often into the vestibule and vagina as well (Figs 7.16 and 7.17). It is also not uncommon to encounter tumours confined almost exclusively to the urethra. The inability to completely empty the bladder usually results in a secondary bacterial

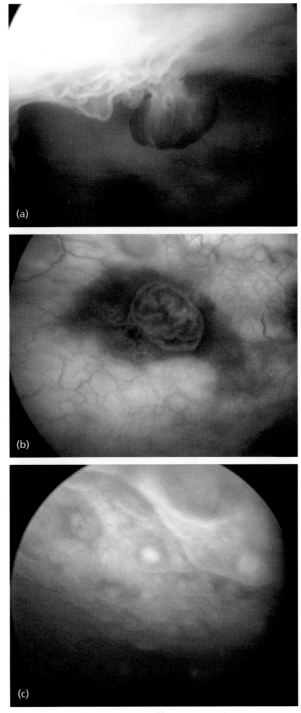

Fig. 7.15   (a) Cystic polyp. (b) Cystic polyp with localised ecchymotic haemorrhage. (c) Polypoid cystitis.

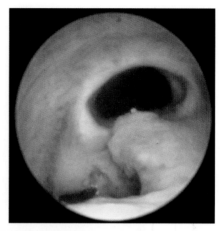

Fig. 7.16   TCC of urethral papilla.

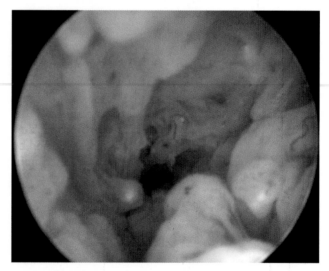

Fig. 7.17   TCC of urethra.

cystitis which is probably why most cases respond initially to antibiotic therapy. In some cases urinary retention may lead to azotaemia, and if tumour affects the ureteral orifice then hydroureter or hydronephrosis may result. Ultrasound examination of these cases is essential to assess areas of the urinary tract not visible from the lumen and also to plan the procedure. Contrast radiography may also be indicated.

TCC is easily visualised at urethrocystoscopy (Lhermette and Sobel, 2008), and may appear in two forms. Most commonly the tumour is seen as a fimbriated, quite friable mass of tissue spread over a wide area of mucosa but without great thickening of the mucosal wall of the urethra or bladder (Fig. 7.18). Alternatively a more solid, singular mass with smooth

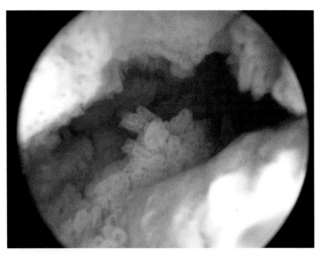

Fig. 7.18   TCC in the trigone showing a classic fimbriated appearance.

surface and forming a solid mass within the wall of the bladder may be seen. This second type may carry a worse prognosis as in the author's experience they are more rapidly growing and refractory to treatment.

Invariably cases are not presented until they are quite advanced and resulting in clinical signs of urinary obstruction: pollakiuria, stranguria, haematuria and tenesmus. Treatment with certain non-steroidal anti-inflammatory agents, especially piroxicam (0.3 mg/kg by mouth every 24 h), is useful and may be combined with other chemotherapeutic agents such as mitoxantrone (5 mg/m2 intravenous every 3 weeks for four treatments) (Upton et al., 2006). However these treatments are most effective if introduced before clinical signs of urethral blockage occur. Laser debulking of the tumour tissue can significantly improve morbidity and relieve clinical signs completely.

A diode laser is passed through the instrument channel of the cystoscope and used to ablate around 90–95% of the tumour tissue. Neoplastic tissue which is not adjacent to the normal margins of the bladder and urethral wall may be ablated in non-contact mode using 10–15 W. This devitalises tissue, which will subsequently slough away. Near the margins of the normal bladder wall and urethral wall contact mode is used at around 9–10 W to give more precise control and a cutting effect. This allows very careful resection of tumour tissues with minimal risk of perforation (Fig. 7.19). If haemorrhage obscures the view the bladder may be drained and filled with carbon dioxide or room air. The former is safer as the risk of air embolism is reduced. Laser ablation carried out in air carries additional risk of perforation since tissue heating and collateral spread are greater without the heat-sink effect of fluid. Great care must be taken not to devitalise deep tissues. Ablation must be done carefully and slowly and can be a time-consuming procedure. Extensive neoplasia may take 2–3 h or longer to ablate.

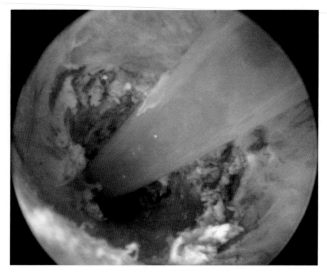

Fig. 7.19 Urethra following laser ablation of TCC with 8 French catheter in place.

Clinical signs usually resolve immediately and tumour regrowth is controlled using chemotherapy (piroxicam and mitoxantrone). In this author's experience a single laser treatment usually gives remission of signs for around 6 months if used alone or 8–12 months if combined with chemotherapy. However, repeat laser debulking at 3–5 month intervals can keep the dog free of clinical signs for considerably longer. Currently the author has three dogs undergoing laser debulking that have been free of clinical signs for over 2 years. Eventually distant metastasis to lungs or lymph nodes is likely to occur.

An alternative to laser debulking is the use of urethral stents placed under fluoroscopic guidance to try and maintain patency. This is also a palliative procedure and does not remove any tumour tissue, which will eventually grow through the stent.

Foreign bodies

Foreign bodies can occasionally be found in the vestibule or vagina. Grass seeds can find their way into the reproductive tract via the vulva and result in a persistent vaginal discharge. These can usually be visualised easily at vaginoscopy and retrieved using grasping forceps. More uncommon foreign bodies are occasionally seen as a result of malicious intent or inquisitive children. The stick in Fig. 7.20 was the result of a penetrating stick injury in the left flank of the dog. The bulk of the stick had been removed following exploratory surgery and laparotomy but the tip of the stick which had penetrated the cranial vagina was missed and resulted in a vaginal discharge a few weeks later. This was retrieved using large grasping forceps alongside the cystoscope.

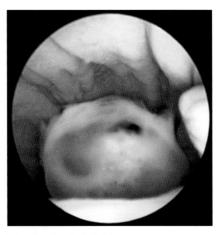

Fig. 7.20 Vaginal foreign body (stick).

USMI

USMI is a common problem in spayed bitches, particularly those with a short urethra and intrapelvic bladder. Many cases respond adequately to medical therapy with phenylpropanolamine or diethyl stilboestrol; however, some cases are refractory to treatment. Surgical correction may be attempted but success rates are often disappointing. Surgery is also rather invasive (although colposuspension can be carried out laparoscopically to minimise the trauma and postoperative discomfort).

An alternative treatment is to use an injection of a bulking agent at three equidistant points submucosally in the proximal urethra to partially occlude the lumen and act as a more effective 'valve'. Several bulking agents have been used, such as silicone, collagen and acellular matrix (Acell™). This does not provide a permanent solution but can provide a good control of continence for 12–18 months in almost 70% of cases (Barth et al., 2005). The procedure can be repeated as necessary. However, not all cases are suitable. In bitches with a very short and very wide-diameter urethra it may prove difficult to provide an adequate occlusion of the lumen and the effects are likely to be much shorter. Urethral diameter varies considerably between individuals, even those of the same size and breed, and careful case selection is vital.

To perform peri-urethral injection of collagen a 2.7 mm endoscope in a cystoscopy sheath is advanced into the urethra as described above. The bladder and urethra are examined for any ectopic ureters and the tip of the cystoscope is withdrawn just inside the proximal urethra. A 23 gauge 25 cm needle is inserted into the instrument channel of the cystoscope. If a sheathed needle is used, as supplied with some of the collagen kits, it generally sits nicely in the centre of the instrument channel. If an unsheathed needle is used it is helpful to place it through a section of thin flexible tubing first. This can be cut to length so it just fits the cystoscope channel. The tubing supplied for transendoscopic

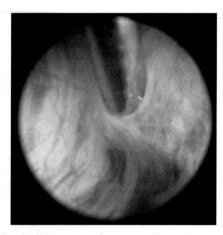

Fig. 7.21   Injecting bulking agent for USMI via a 23 gauge needle in the proximal urethral mucosa.

bronchoalveolar lavage is often suitable. If tubing is not used the needle tends to slip to the side of the telescope making the needle tip difficult to manipulate and visualise. The tubing keeps the needle central above the endoscope and prevents it moving from side to side.

A small flexible connector is attached to the Luer hub of the needle at one end and the syringe holding the bulking agent at the other. The needle tip is advanced into view and the bevel is turned towards the lumen of the urethra. The tip of the needle is advanced into the submucosa (Fig. 7.21) and approximately 1 ml of bulking agent is injected submucosally at three equidistant points around the urethral circumference, keeping the needle *in situ* for 30 s or so after each injection to reduce back flow occurring at removal. It is preferable to have an assistant make the injection since the endoscopist may find it difficult to maintain the tip of the needle in the correct place throughout the procedure. The mucosa will be seen to swell up and partially occlude the lumen after each injection (Fig. 7.22). Dedicated endoscopic equipment is available for this procedure. Although this makes manipulation of the needle more precise for the endoscopist, the diameter of the sheath restricts its application to bitches of approximately 15 kg and larger.

Transcervical catheterisation for artificial insemination

Cervical catheterisation requires considerable practice. The procedure is usually carried out in a conscious bitch and without the benefits of saline infusion to expand the vagina (Lhermette and Sobel, 2008). During oestrus the cervical os is dilated, thus facilitating the procedure. However, sedation may be required in some bitches.

The cystoscope is passed into the vestibule and then through the vaginal os to the cranial end of the vagina. In giant breeds a 4 mm,

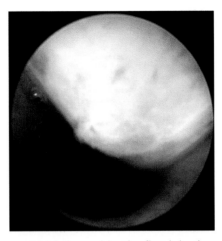

Fig. 7.22 Submucosal bleb formed by the first injection.

30 cm-working-length endoscope may be required due to vaginal length. A catheter deflection device at the tip of the cystoscope is extremely useful to help guide the tip of the catheter into the cervix. This is seen as a small slit on the ventral surface of the dorsal ridge of the vagina at the cranial end. The os is normally surrounded by a fine rosette of grooved mucosa but may be difficult to visualise at all. A 2–2.5 mm semi flexible urinary catheter with a terminal hole is used. A fine guide wire is placed in the catheter to increase rigidity and it is introduced through the instrument channel of the cystoscope and manipulated into the cervical os. The guide wire can then be withdrawn and the catheter gently introduced further into the uterus with a twisting motion.

Further reading

McCarthy, T. (2005) *Veterinary Endoscopy for the Small Animal Practitioner*, pp. 49–135. Elsevier Saunders, St Louis, MO.

Rawlings, C.A. (2007) Resection of inflammatory polyps in dogs using laparoscopic-assisted cystoscopy. *Journal of the American Animal Hospital Association* 43, 342–346.

Tams, T. and Rawlings, C. (2011) *Small Animal Endoscopy*, 3rd edn, pp. 507–561. Mosby, St Louis, MO.

References

Adams, L.G., Berent, A.C., Moore, G.E. and Bagley, D.H. (2008) Use of laser lithotripsy for fragmentation of uroliths in dogs: 73 cases (2005–2006). *Journal of the American Veterinary Medical Association* 232, 1680–1687.

Barth, A., Reichler, I.M., Hubler, M., Hassig, M. and Arnold, S. (2005) Evaluation of long-term effects of endoscopic injection of collagen into the urethral submucosa for treatment of urethral sphincter incompetence in female dogs: 40 cases (1993–2000). *Journal of the American Veterinary Medical Association* 226, 73–76.

Berent, A.C., Mayhew, P.D. and Porat-Mosenco, Y. (2008) Use of cystoscopic-guided laser ablation for treatment of intramural ureteral ectopia in male dogs: four cases (2006–2007). *Journal of the American Veterinary Medical Association* 232, 1026–1034.

Bevan, J.M., Lulich, J.P., Albasan, H. and Osborne, C. (2009) Comparison of laser lithotripsy and cystotomy for the management of dogs with urolithiasis. *Journal of the American Veterinary Medical Association* 234, 1286–1294.

Lhermette, P. and Sobel, D. (2008) Urethrocystoscopy and vaginoscopy. In *BSAVA Manual of Endoscopy and Endosurgery in the Dog and Cat*, Lhermette, P. and Sobel, D. (eds), pp. 142–157. British Small Animal Veterinary Association, Gloucester.

McCarthy, T.C. (2006) Endoscopy brief: transurethral cystoscopy and diode laser incision to correct an ectopic ureter. *Veterinary Medicine Online* 1 September, 2006.

Rawlings, C.A., Mahaffey, M.B., Barsanti, J.A. and Canalis, C. (2003) Use of laparoscopic-assisted cystoscopy for removal of urinary calculi in dogs. *Journal of the American Veterinary Medical Association* 222, 759–761.

Samii, V.F., McLoughlin, M.A., Mattoon, J.S., Drost, W.T., Chew, D.J., DiBartola, S.P. and Hoshaw-Woodard, S. (2004) Digital fluoroscopic excretory urography, digital fluoroscopic urethrography, helical computed tomography, and cystoscopy in 24 dogs with suspected ureteral ectopia. *Journal of Veterinary Internal Medicine* 18, 271–281.

Upton, M.L., Tangner, C.H. and Payton, M.E. (2006) Evaluation of carbon dioxide laser ablation combined with mitoxantrone and piroxicam treatment in dogs with transitional cell carcinoma. *Journal of the American Veterinary Medical Association* 228, 549–552.

Chapter 8

Endoscopy of the Upper Respiratory Tract: Rhinosinusoscopy, Pharyngoscopy and Tracheoscopy

David S. Sobel

Introduction

Endoscopy of the rhinarium, paranasal sinuses, pharynx and trachea comprises a set of procedures quickly and easily mastered by even the most novice endoscopists, providing significant diagnostic information to the clinician. Diagnostic procedures can be easily and confidently carried out in most first-opinion general small animal practices and, with experience, interventional procedures can effectively be performed.

Rhinoscopy is the endoscopic examination of the rhinarium including the nasal conchae and meati. This logically extends to sinusoscopy, in particular the endoscopic examination of the frontal sinuses. Pharyngoscopy can be performed both in a trans-oral fashion as well as via the ventral nasal meatus through the posterior nares. And finally, tracheoscopy is usually performed from a trans-oral approach. Rigid endoscopy is ill-suited for examination or intervention in the distal third of the trachea and more distal portions of the bronchial tree beyond the carina.

Advantages to endoscopic examination of these anatomic locales include the ability to directly visualise structures otherwise inaccessible

Clinical Manual of Small Animal Endosurgery, First Edition. Edited by Alasdair Hotston Moore and Rosa Angela Ragni.
© 2012 Blackwell Publishing Ltd. Published 2012 by Blackwell Publishing Ltd.

without a surgical intervention, significant magnification and very low surgical morbidity. Patients recover from these procedures quickly and are often discharged on the day of the procedure with minimal need for significant aftercare by the owners.

Rhinosinusoscopy, pharyngoscopy and tracheoscopy can be used to diagnose and manage chronic infectious diseases (both bacterial and fungal), foreign bodies of the airways, congenital malformations, and both benign and malignant neoplasms. The use of diode lasers has allowed for expansion of the modalities from simply diagnostic to therapeutic, as laser surgery is often an excellent adjunctive therapy to other therapeutic modalities for a variety of pathological conditions.

Indications

The common presenting clinical signs in most canine and feline patients that should lead the clinician to include upper respiratory endoscopy in their armament of diagnostic modalities include coughing, sneezing and stertorous or stridorous breathing. This can also be accompanied by chronic nasal (or oculonasal) discharge of a serous, mucoid or mucopurulent nature. Epistaxis and/or haemoptysis are often noted. Other common presenting clinical signs include halitosis (unexplained by simple dental disease), facial pruritis or pain, facial deformity, difficulty in prehension and mastication of food, and exophthalmos. Certain of these presentations are easier to appreciate in mesocephalic or dolicocephalic dogs but with careful examination these clinical signs can be appreciated in most canine and feline breeds.

Instrumentation

There is a wide variety of instrumentation available on both the new and used equipment markets. Equipment choices, use, care and maintenance are discussed elsewhere, but a brief overview of clinically relevant equipment is appropriate here.

A high-quality endoscopic video camera is requisite for performing meaningful endoscopic examinations. Less-expensive single-chip camera-coupling device (CCD) cameras, as well as more costly three-chip CCD and high-definition (HD) cameras are available and all perform well. Higher-quality cameras should be paired with appropriate high-quality monitors to maximise the quality of the resultant image. That said, single-chip cameras provide excellent visualisation and resolution. Practitioners collecting images for use in publications or presentations will appreciate the improved image quality with three-chip or HD cameras.

A light source with a flexible fibre-optic light guide cable is also needed. Halogen, xenon and metal halide light sources are available at a variety of cost points. This author prefers the use of a xenon light source, as this provides the brightest and whitest light for the coolest temperature available. Halogen light sources are available and quite inexpensive but the light produced is generally of a lesser intensity with a slight yellow hue.

Irrigation fluid can be delivered via a pressure bag or gravity feed, or via a purpose-built endoscopic irrigation pump.

The majority of rhinosinusoscopy is performed with rigid endoscopes. The most commonly used rhinoscope in my arsenal is the 2.7 mm-diameter, 30° paediatric cystoscope. Manufacturers commonly market this endoscope as a 'multipurpose rigid endoscope'. This designation is appropriate given the multiplicity of procedures that this one endoscope can perform. The scope can be housed in either a cystoscopy sheath or an arthroscopy sheath. The cystoscopy sheath has a beveled, angled distal aperture equal to the 30° angle of the optical end of the endoscope. This allows for a more even laminar flow of irrigant over the lens of the endoscope, providing a cleaner, debris-free image. This sheath also has dual two-way stopcock ports for fluid ingress and egress and an instrument channel port. The downside to this sheath is the slightly larger resultant external diameter relative to the same scope in the arthroscopy sheath. The arthroscopy sheath has a single fluid-irrigation port, but is narrower in diameter, allowing for an easier fit into small-diameter luminal spaces. Operator preference dictates which sheath is used. This author uses the standard paediatric cystoscope sheath for the majority of procedures and will employ the arthroscopy sheath for particularly narrow spaces in smaller dogs and many cats.

Smaller-diameter rigid endoscopes with similar sheaths are also available for use in small canine and feline patients. This author rarely uses these devices, for several reasons. Firstly, the smaller diameter results in a small optical field of view. Secondly, these scopes are quite delicate and susceptible to damage (I have broken more than my fair share of these scopes!). Still, their small diameter gives them great utility in some anatomical situations.

These rigid endoscopes can also be used quite effectively in endoscopy of the frontal sinus, which will be discussed later in this chapter.

While the focus of this chapter is on rigid endoscopy of the upper respiratory tract, a complete rhinoscopic examination does require the use of a small-diameter flexible endoscope. These scopes are usually found as fibreoptiscopes (rather than true video endoscopes) and range in external diameter from 2.9 to 4.1 mm. These scopes generally have two-way deflection and a small-diameter instrument channel with an optional bridge that can allow for simultaneous irrigation and instrumentation placement. These scopes are requisite for 'J manoeuvre' evaluation of the posterior nares and adjacent soft palate.

When rigid tracheoscopy is indicated, the previously mentioned endoscopes can be employed. However, the length of the scope is often the limiting factor. In larger patients the author has employed a 5 mm forward-view laparoscope to achieve a more distal view of the trachea.

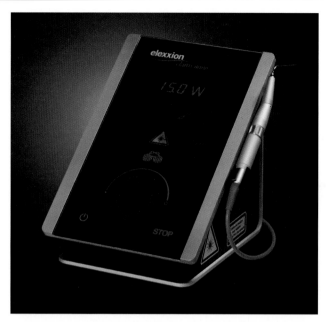

Fig. 8.1   A 810 nm-wavelength digital-pulse diode laser (Elexxion Claros Nano, Elexxion, Germany). Photograph courtesy of Elexxion, Germany.

A variety of hand instrumentation is available for use with this equipment. Biopsy forceps, fluid aspiration catheters and cytology brushes are often used. Flexible equipment can be inserted via the instrument channel of the endoscope sheath. If the arthroscopy sheath is used, the lack of an instrument channel dictates that rigid forceps (for biopsy) be inserted adjacent to the long axis of the endoscope. These forceps are often more robust with a larger biopsy cup than flexible forceps. However, the lack of ability to direct their placement with complete accuracy can make them frustrating to use.

Additionally a variety of accessories for foreign-body retrieval and fibres for laser surgery are available (see Figs 1.2 and 1.13 in Chapter 1 of this volume, and Fig. 8.1).

Anatomy

The limiting factor to the endoscopy of the canine and feline rhinarium and paranasal sinuses is the bony encasement that limits anatomic exploration (Fig. 8.2). The rhinarium is defined by dorsal, middle and ventral meati, each separated by a corresponding concha. The dorsal nasal meatus ends in the cribriform plate at the front of the calvarium and the ventral nasal meatus terminates at the posterior nares, leading into the posterior pharynx. The two sides of the rhinarium are separated by a cartilaginous septum medially, and each side is defined dorsally and

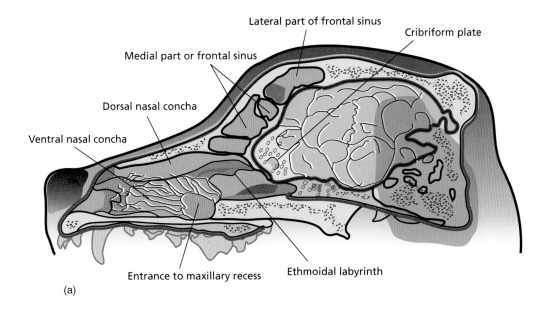

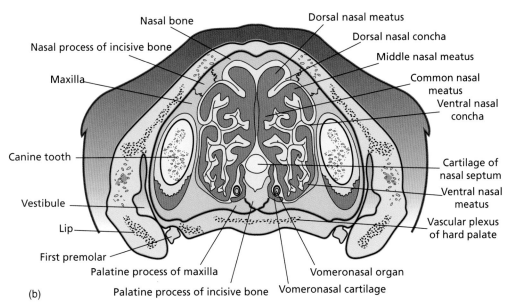

Fig. 8.2 (a) Schematic longitudinal section of the canine nose, showing the local anatomy. (b) Schematic transverse section of the canine nose, showing the local anatomy. Both images reproduced from Lhermette and Sobel (2008). Illustration drawn by Samantha J. Elmhurst, BA Hons, www.livingart.org.uk, and printed with her permission.

laterally by the nasal and frontal bones, laterally and ventrally by the maxillary and palatine bones and rostrally by the nasal planum. The nostrils serve as the aperture into the nasal vestibule. The puncta of the nasolacrimal duct are located in the nasal vestibule along the most ventral aspect of the alar cartilage.

The paranasal sinuses are a series of bilateral, somewhat interconnected, air-filled spaces lined with a highly secretory mucous membrane. As a practical matter, the most clinically significant of the paranasal sinuses is the frontal sinus, which can be accessed endoscopically.

The mucous membrane of the rhinarium extending to the proximal pharynx comprises a ciliated columnar epithelium. These highly vascular membranes, draped over the tremendous surface area of the nasal conchae, serve to warm, humidify and filter the inspired air.

The pharynx is contiguous with the posterior aspects of the rhinarium and the oral cavity, extending caudally to the glottis. Significant structures include the glottis and epiglottis, soft palate, arytenoid cartilages and vocal folds. Bilaterally paired lymphoid tonsils are found in the caudolateral aspects of the pharynx, usually tucked into their tonsillar crypts (Fig. 8.3).

Beyond the arytenoid cartilages is the cervical trachea, the most proximal portions of which can be accessed with rigid endoscopes. More distal aspects of the trachea are best examined via flexible tracheobronchoscopy, which has been well covered in other texts (see Further reading at the end of this chapter).

While the gross external appearance of the rhinarium varies between dogs and cats and from breed type to breed type, the anatomic descriptions noted above are quite consistent.

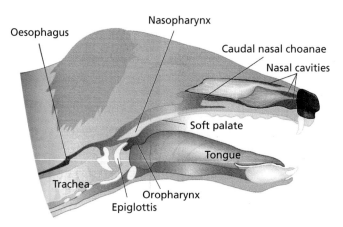

Fig. 8.3 Schematic drawing of the anatomy of the retropharynx. and posterior nasal cavity. Both images reproduced from Lhermette and Sobel (2008). Illustration drawn by Samantha J. Elmhurst, BA Hons, www.livingart.org.uk, and printed with her permission.

Clinical examination and anamnesis

As is often the case, a careful history-taking can help clue the clinician in to the necessity and applicability of endoscopy as part of the diagnostic and therapeutic management of the patient. Understanding the patient's work or recreation history (hunting or herding dogs), home environment (if owners are tobacco smokers) and travel history are very helpful pieces of information. Querying the owner as to the onset and duration of clinical signs, nature of any discharge (colour, character, odour, unilateral versus bilateral) and observation of sneezing, coughing, head shaking and seasonality of clinical signs are all very helpful clues as to the type of disease process.

Examination of the conscious patient in the consultation room will of course focus on the head and respiratory status. The clinician will undertake careful observation of respiratory effort and listening for stertorous or stridorous airflow. Symmetry of the head and face is important. Note should be taken of the nature of any oculonasal discharge; the colour, character, odour and whether it is uni- or bilateral.

Using a paediatric stethoscope, auscultation of the rhinarium with percussion can identify regions of fluid or tissue density. Auscultation of the ventral pharynx and trachea is also important with obvious attention being given to the heart and lungs. Airflow across each nostril should be evaluated. This can be done by blocking one nostril (if the patient is compliant) at a time and sensing airflow with one's hand or cheek. Alternatively, one can use a glass slide to appreciate condensation as an indicator of airflow. With experience, the clinician can learn to appreciate subtleties of turbulence from one side to the other.

If the conscious patient is compliant, an oral exam should be done. Attention should be given to the presence of severe dental disease, oronasal fistulae with notation of abnormalities related to the hard and soft palates, and pharyngeal lesions.

Diagnostic work-up prior to endoscopy

As epistaxis is a common presenting sign for nasal disease, a complete blood count with accurate platelet count is imperative. Buccal mucosal bleeding times and toenail bleeding times can also give a crude measure of platelet function. Coagulation times, including prothrombin time and partial thromboplastin time are also important. Blood pressure measurement should also be performed, as hypertension can be associated with epistaxis. Cats should also be evaluated for hyperthyroidism as a potential cause for hypertension.

Bacterial culture and sensitivity can be performed preoperatively on nasal exudates if samples can be reliably obtained. Serology for fungal disease, in particular aspergillosis, can also be performed prior to endoscopy. Serology may have a high degree of cross-reactivity with other forms of antigenic stimulation (specifically neoplasia); however, even with these limitations there is clinical utility to this test.

In cases where large airway disease is suspected it is advised that cervical and thoracic radiographs be performed. This step is critical in differentiating lower and upper airway disease prior to general anaesthesia. Mass lesions suspected in the cervical neck and thorax may be well visualised with ultrasound imaging.

Diagnostic work-up under general anaesthesia

Once the appropriate pre-anaesthetic workup has been completed and the potential utility of endoscopy has been established, the patient can be placed under general anaesthesia. This presumes that no specific contraindication to general anaesthesia is noted.

With the patient anaesthetised additional imaging studies can be obtained. Where available, computed tomography (CT) and magnetic resonance imaging (MRI) are excellent modalities for examining the rhinarium, paranasal sinuses and brain case. In an ideal situation, these studies can be scheduled concurrently with anticipated endoscopy. More often than not, the need for referral to secondary or tertiary referral practices makes this impossible. However the availability of these advanced imaging modalities is increasing, and access to CT and MRI should be explored.

Radiography of the skull for evaluation of the rhinarium, paranasal sinuses and cervical neck is still standard for this diagnostic work-up in the absence of easy access to CT and MRI. The advent of digital radiography has made doing these studies faster, easier and more reliable. Standard views include the lateral nasal, open-mouth ventrodorsal and the frontal sinus skyline views (Fig. 8.4). The presence of soft-tissue densities in abnormal locales, bony lysis or proliferation, or changes in radiographic symmetry from one side to the other helps the endoscopist plan the procedure(s).

A more detailed oropharyngeal exam can now be done with the patient under anaesthesia. Digital palpation of the upper dental arcade, looking for loose teeth, pockets of subgingival purulent material and soft, pliable maxillary bone are all important observations. If available and clinically indicated, dental radiographs can be taken.

Similarly, digital palpation of the hard and soft palates can detect subtle changes in tissue characteristics from one area to another. An ovariohysterectomy hook can be utilised to reflect the caudal edge of the soft palate cranially to allow for better visualisation of the dorsal pharynx. It is very difficult to visualise the posterior nares using this technique alone.

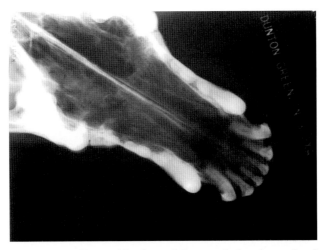

Fig. 8.4   Intraoral radiographic view of the nasal chambers of a dog. A soft-tissue opacity is visible in the right caudal nares. Reproduced from Lhermette and Sobel (2008), with the permission of BSAVA publications. © BSAVA.

Rhinoscopy

Patient positioning

Rhinosinusoscopy should ideally be performed on a wet table or surgical sink to minimise the clutter and fluid spillage from the procedure. This author prefers to perform rhinoscopy with the patient positioned in sternal recumbency with the head slightly elevated with the use of towels, while maintaining a slight ventral pointing of the rhinarium. The endoscopic equipment tower is usually positioned at about the midpoint of the patient's body, with the monitor pointed cranially to allow the operator to visualise the surgical site in an anatomically 'true' position.

Given the large volumes of irrigant solution that is often used in rhinoscopy, care must be taken to ensure that the endotracheal tube is of appropriate size with a functional, well-inflated cuff. Another safeguard against iatrogenic aspiration of irrigant is the use of feminine hygiene napkins or pads to aid in the absorption of fluid. A notch can be cut in the centre of the pad to allow for it to fit around the tube, and several pads can be advanced around the tube and pushed caudally to ensure a good seal to trap fluid and blood.

Effective monitoring of anaesthesia including S_PO_2 and end-tidal CO_2 is of paramount importance. Patients that are morbidly obese or have other cardiorespiratory compromise may require assisted ventilation.

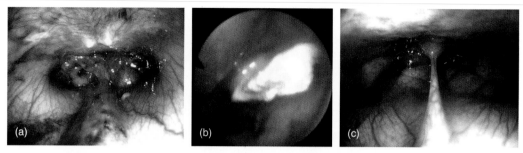

Fig. 8.5 Abnormalities visible on retroflex rhinopharyngoscopy. (a) Neoplastic mass occluding both nasal passages. (b) Foreign body lodged in the posterior nares. (c) Mucous discharge present in the right choana. All images courtesy of Mr P.J. Lhermette.

Retroflexed rhinopharyngoscopy

The first portion of the exam to be performed is examination of the posterior nares and the posterior pharynx. This is usually best performed with the use of a flexible fibreoptiscope. Usually either a bronchoscope or small-diameter flexible urethroscope is used for this purpose. With the patient positioned as previously noted, a mouth gag is inserted to open up the oropharynx and prevent an inadequately anaesthetised patient from biting down on the endoscope. The endoscope is then flexed into a hard 'J' position to form a hook-like appearance. With the point of the 'hook' in the dorsal position, the endoscope is inserted into the mouth and hooked over the caudal edge of the soft palate. With careful manipulation of the tip of the endoscope the operator can now visualise the posterior nares – effectively the caudal terminus of the ventral nasal meatus – looking rostrally. The operator is now in a position to examine the patient for nasopharyngeal stenosis or atresia, masses obscuring one or both posterior nares, or other pathologies (Fig. 8.5). It is not uncommon to see significant lymphoid follicle development on the dorsal floor of the soft palate in front of the posterior nares. Biopsies can be taken of any areas of clinical concern for both histopathology and bacteriological culture and sensitivity. A note of caution is warranted as any biopsy or manipulation of tissue in this region will result in haemorrhage, albeit minimal in most cases. This small amount of haemorrhage will however make subsequent examination of the pharynx and rhinarium more difficult due to blood contamination. With this portion of the examination complete the endoscope can be removed and the mouth gag taken out.

Rostral rhinoscopy

The patient position is maintained as previously described. A bag of saline irrigant solution is hung near the head of the patient to allow for intra-operative irrigation and flushing. In most cases, ongoing irrigation is needed to keep the visual field free of blood and other debris. Some authors have advocated using cool saline and others have suggested the use of dilute adrenaline (epinephrine) or other vasoconstrictive agents in an effort to minimise haemorrhage. This author has not found it necessary to do so.

As previously noted, this author performs the vast majority of rhinoscopy with the 2.7 mm, 30° urethrocystoscope. However, there are some limited circumstances where the small-diameter flexible scope is of value. Small patients or lesions that require odd angulation to visualise adequately may benefit from the two-way deflection afforded by the flexible endoscope.

The rigid endoscope is inserted into the nose via the nostril across the alar cartilage. Generally speaking a slight dorsal deflection of the tip of the endoscope is needed to get over the ventral ridge of the alar cartilage. At this point, fluid irrigation should be begun. It bears noting that even minimal, seemingly innocuous manipulation of the nasal mucosa will cause some haemorrhage. While usually of no clinical significance, the blood can make keeping the field of view clear more difficult. Care should consequently be taken with all intraluminal manipulations.

A systematic examination of the rhinarium should be undertaken. This author usually starts with examination of the dorsal nasal meatus and concha. While it is usually difficult to examine the dorsal meatus to the level of the cribriform plate, significant posterior progress should be made. Ventrally the dorsal aspects of the ethmoid turbinate structures should be quite apparent (Fig. 8.6).

The differentiation between the dorsal (Fig. 8.7) and middle nasal meatus is difficult to appreciate endoscopically and delineation between the two is more academic than clinically important. However, it is still important to document the approximate location of any lesion observed for future reference. It is helpful to note the distance of any significant findings from the nostril, and the approximate location (which meatus, nearby structures, etc.) within the rhinarium. The ability to correlate

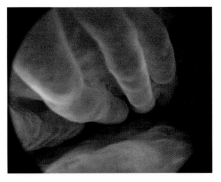

Fig. 8.6 Normal appearance of the turbinates: they are smooth and pink in colour, and seem almost to interdigitate. Photograph courtesy of Mr P.J. Lhermette.

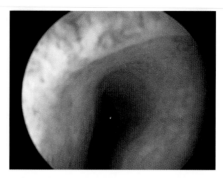

Fig. 8.7 The normal canine dorsal meatus has a vaulted and smooth appearance. Photograph courtesy of Mr P.J. Lhermette.

endoscopic findings in real time with radiographs or CT/MRI images can be very advantageous.

The normal appearance of the nasal mucosa is thin, smooth and very pink. Deviations from this in terms of texture and colour should be noted.

With this portion of the exam complete, the ventral nasal meatus should be explored. The aperture or delineation of the ventral nasal meatus from the middle and dorsal ones can also be very difficult to appreciate endoluminally. Often the ability to enter the ventral meatus is accomplished by feel and experience. This can be one of the more frustrating aspects of rhinoscopy. Sometimes visualising the passage of a nasogastric tube can be helpful. There is a bony shelf that forms a separation between the middle and the ventral nasal meati. The passage to the ventral meatus can be seen ventromedially to the point of insertion of the endoscope at the nostril. A slight ventromedial angulation given to the endoscope should place it in position to fall into the ventral nasal meatus. Alternatively, inserting the endoscope in the middle meatus, and identifying the bony ridge ventromedially, gives a landmark along which to withdraw the endoscope. Once at the rostral edge of this shelf gentle ventromedial pressure should cause the endoscope to drop into the ventral meatus.

The ventral nasal meatus is free of any turbinate or conchal structures and is simply a relatively smooth passage to the posterior nares and pharynx. In most canine patients, even among the smaller breeds, passage into the ventral nasal meatus should encounter limited resistance. Any luminal narrowing or obstruction should be noted. The endoscope can often be advanced to its full length, placing it well into the pharynx. Along the lateral wall, near the edge of the soft palate, it is often possible to see the slit-like opening of the Eustachian tube. Any fluid coming from this slit should be noted as evidence of middle-ear disease.

With the examination of one side complete, the contralateral side can now be examined in the same manner. It has been suggested that in cases of unilateral disease, or where one side is more severely clinically affected, that the most affected side be examined first. The thought behind this approach is to minimise any potential contamination of blood and detritus from one side to the other. If the side of greatest clinical interest should become contaminated with irrigant and other materials from the contralateral side, it may be more difficult for the operator to distinguish contamination artifact from real pathology.

With the examination of both sides complete, the operator can now go back and re-examine any areas of clinical interest for the purposes of taking biopsies for histopathology and culture, removing foreign bodies or resecting mass or inflammatory lesions (see section on laser surgery, below). Multiple biopsy samples should be obtained from any regions with abnormal appearing mucosa, but other representative areas should also be selected for biopsy. Aggressive saline irrigation should continue as even the most gentle technique and small biopsy size will result in haemorrhage that will otherwise limit visibility. Samples should be collected and separated based on anatomical site to aid the pathologist in correctly identifying regions of disease. Wire or foam endoscopic tissue baskets will help preserve the small biopsy specimens for adequate transport in formalin to the laboratory.

This procedure as described is identical for both dogs and cats of all breeds and sizes. It is worth noting, however, that brachycephalic breeds of dog and cat, and smaller individual cats, will provide for a more challenging examination. The reduced space available to the operator will make it more difficult to examine every nook and cranny of the rhinarium. In some cases a smaller-diameter or a flexible fibreoptiscope may be an appropriate choice of equipment. In any event, these patients will often have less-complete examinations by virtue of their unique anatomy.

Sinusoscopy

If, based on radiographs (frontal sinus skyline view), CT or MRI, it is suggested that there is pathology present in the frontal sinus, then endoscopic examination is of tremendous value. Indeed, given the relatively simple structure of the sinus space, and the limited redundancy of the sinus epithelium, the diagnostic yield of the frontal sinus is often greater than the rhinarium.

The landmarks of the frontal sinus should be identified. These are the midline of the skull and the bony prominence that forms the top of the orbit. A 2 cm × 2 cm area should be clipped just medial to this prominence and prepared for aseptic surgery. A hole that is adequate to insert the endoscope is then made into the frontal sinus. A small incision is made into the skin to the level of the periosteum. The size of the incision should be slightly smaller than the diameter of the endoscope and sheath combination. The entry point into the frontal sinus can be made using a small Michele trephine, a Steinmann pin and Jacobs chuck, or a Hall air drill. Slow, careful drilling into the sinus is advised to avoid iatrogeni-cally damaging the far wall of the sinus or delicate deeper structures.

Once the hole is made, it is not unusual for the release of pressure in the sinus to allow for copious discharge to come out of the hole spon-taneously. This discharge, be it fluid or tissue, can be collected for cytol-ogy, culture or histopathology. Once material for culture has been recovered it is advised to give an intra-operative parenteral dose of a broad-spectrum antibiotic. Subsequent antibiotic therapy can be dictated by the clinical presentation and culture results.

The endoscope can now be introduced into the sinus and irrigation should begin. This will allow for clearing of any debris within the sinus and adequate visualisation of the entire cavity. In some cases of severe sinus disease the deep recesses of the sinus and the communication between other recesses of the frontal sinuses and the rhinarium itself can be appreciated.

Biopsies of material present in the sinus can be taken for laboratory evaluation. Residual fluid from irrigation or from underlying disease processes should then be removed. There is little need to try and close the bony defect, but the skin incision can often be closed in a single layer with one or two simple interrupted or cruciate sutures of non-absorbable monofilament suture material.

Review of selected pathologies

Lymphoplasmacytic rhinitis/polyps

The most commonly identified non-infectious, non-neoplastic form of (usually) bilateral nasal disease is lymphocytic or lymphoplasmacytic rhinitis. This can appear as singular or multiple sessile mass-like or polypoid lesions (Fig. 8.8a) or in the form of diffuse thickening and erythema of the nasal mucosa (Fig. 8.8b). It is this author's observation that the ventral and middle nasal meati are most commonly involved, but any portion of the rhinarium and paranasal sinuses can be affected. This disease is thought to have an autoimmune underlying mechanism, but environmental allergens are often implicated as either primary causes or exacerbating factors in this disease.

For discrete masses or polyps surgery is often of benefit (see section on laser rhinoscopic surgery, below) but recurrence is a concern regard-less of the method of management. More diffuse presentations are usually managed medically with corticosteroids being the therapy of choice. On occasion oral antihistamines and/or non-steroidal anti-inflammatory drugs are used with sporadic benefit. Occasionally, where environmental or food allergens are implicated, hyposensitisation therapy can be con-sidered. It is this author's observation that frequently more potent immu-nomodulatory medications (chlorambucil) are needed in conjunction with steroids. Where bacterial infection is a secondary component, appropriate antimicrobial therapy based on culture and sensitivity results is indicated. Images of polyps are shown in Fig. 8.9.

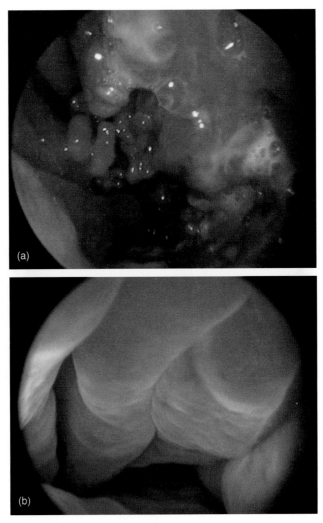

Fig. 8.8 Lymphoplasmacytic rhinitis is the most common nasal disease. It can appear as singular or multiple polypoid lesions (a), or as a diffuse thickening and erythema of the nasal mucosa (b). Both images courtesy of Mr P.J. Lhermette.

Nasal neoplasms

Nasal lymphoma is seen in both cats and dogs and also can present as diffuse thickening and erythema of the nasal mucosa, although focal masses can also be observed. Tissue tends to be markedly friable and will bleed easily with minimal tissue manipulation. While these tissues respond well to resection and ablation with the laser it is critical to treat this disease as a systemic disorder. As such, systematic chemotherapy is indicated. Appropriate protocols are described elsewhere in the veterinary literature.

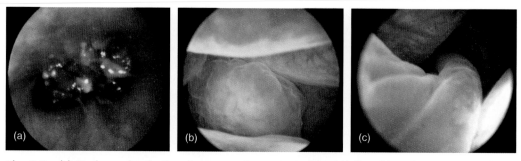

Fig. 8.9 (a) Benign polyp in the choanae as it appears with retroflex rhinopharyngoscopy. (b) Polyp seen at anterior rhinoscopy. In this case there is a solitary polyp, confined to a small area, whereas in (c) the polyp occupies most of the nasal passage. All images reproduced from Lhermette and Sobel (2008), with the permission of BSAVA publications. © BSAVA.

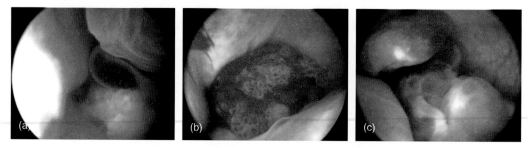

Fig. 8.10 Various images of nasal carcinoma: although the appearance is often pale, the stroma can be markedly vascular. All images courtesy of Mr P.J. Lhermette.

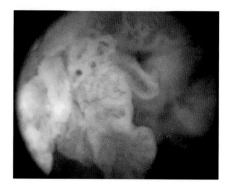

Fig. 8.11 Adenocarcinoma viewed under saline irrigation. Photograph courtesy of Mr P.J. Lhermette.

Nasal carcinoma (Fig. 8.10) and adenocarcinoma (Fig. 8.11) are the most commonly identified nasal cancers and are more frequently noted in older mesocephalic or dolicocephalic breeds of dog, although these tumours can occur in all breeds of dog and cat. These masses can appear as discrete mass foci or diffuse infiltrative lesions. The tissue tends to be relatively pale but the stroma of these masses is often markedly vascular.

It is worth noting that it is often difficult to identify all the margins and anatomic limitations of these lesions at rhinoscopy. As previously discussed, a combination of radiography and/or CT or MRI will help the surgeon delineate the extent of the mass. These tumours are known to be markedly sensitive to radiation therapy and both palliative and curative protocols are described. The diode laser has also been shown to have significant palliative benefit, but should not be regarded as curative or as having a long-term management effect. In patients for whom radiation therapy is not an option, this author often uses a combination of laser ablation and oral piroxicam as a palliative management strategy.

Fungal disease

The most common fungal disease observed in the rhinarium and paranasal sinuses is aspergillosis. *Aspergillus* is a soil-borne environmental pathogen that can cause chronic destructive mycotic rhinitis in the nose and sinuses of, most commonly, sporting dogs, although any breed or lifestyle of patient can be at risk. The fungal plaques are usually identified as fluffy white to grey coalescing colonies with black punctate regions of necrotic debris (Fig. 8.12). The mucosa around these lesions is often markedly distorted and necrotic with dramatic secondary inflammation. Secondary bacterial infection is also often observed with culture. The dorsal nasal meatus and ethmoid turbinates are most commonly affected. The material can be retrieved for biopsy analysis via standard hematoxylin and eosin (HE) staining although special fungal stains and culture methodologies are also available. Therapy often consists of some form of endoscopically guided instillation of an anti-fungal agent (enilconazole, miconazole) often paired with oral therapy (ketoconazole or itraconazole). A complete discussion of the management strategies for this disease can be found elsewhere.

Anterior rhinoscopy is also extremely useful for the retrieval of foreign bodies (Fig. 8.13).

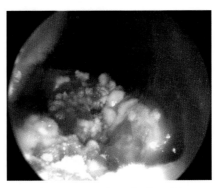

Fig. 8.12 Nasal aspergillosis in the dog: fluffy white to grey coalescing colonies associated with severe turbinates damage. Photograph courtesy of Mr P.J. Lhermette.

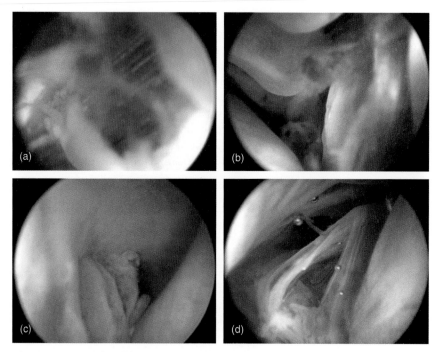

Fig. 8.13 Anterior rhinoscopy is also extremely useful for the retrieval of foreign bodies, which are often surrounded by copious mucopurulent exudate (a, b). Foreign bodies can be sometimes difficult to see, as embedded in the mucosa (c); (d) shows the damage consequent to penetration by a wooden stick. All images courtesy of Mr P.J. Lhermette.

A more exhaustive discussion of the management of nasal pathology can be found in other texts.

Laser endoscopic surgery

This author has adopted relatively routine use of diode lasers in the management of a variety of pathological conditions of the nasal passages over the last 15 years. It is my experience that these devices have significant adjunctive value in the treatment of many different diseases with minimal morbidity.

The lasers of choice for the purposes of endoscopic surgery are surgical diode lasers. While it is beyond the scope of this chapter to discuss the physics behind lasers and their use in surgery, a bit of background is helpful. Diode lasers use diode semiconductors to produce laser light of different wavelengths. The specific wavelength is determined by the characteristics of the particular diode used. The use of diodes (as opposed to some form of gas or metallic lasing medium) makes these devices more reliable, more cost-effective and less prone to mechanical failure than other surgical lasers. More important, however, is the fact that diodes use a slender solid quartz fibre as their delivery system. This makes them ideal for introduction into the operating channel of the endoscope (be it rigid or flexible). In addition, the wavelength of light that is produced by most commercially available surgical diodes ranges from 810 to 980 nm. These wavelengths of light perform particularly well in fluid mediums, such as those encountered in nasal endoscopic surgery. In particular, diodes at the 810 nm wavelength are particularly well absorbed by biological pigments (haemoglobin), thus maximising their thermal effect.

The diodes are used to vapourise and ablate abnormal tissue. This is done by introducing a fibre of appropriate size into the area of interest via the operating channel of the endoscope. A power level is then selected, a pulse interval chosen and the fibre placed in apposition to the affected tissues. The procedure is continued until all grossly identifiable abnormal tissue is removed or until normal anatomical landmarks can no longer be easily identified.

The diode lasers have been used to manage many different types of nasal pathology but their greatest utility is as adjunctive therapy for neoplastic diseases. Often the procedure is performed as part of the initial rhinoscopic examination in the hopes of reducing tumour volume for the benefit of subsequent, more definitive therapy (e.g. radiation therapy). However, we have performed many cases where laser surgery was the sole therapy chosen by the owners, and good success has been noted. It is clear that this procedure does not result in clean surgical margins, but extended periods of control of clinical signs have been observed, often in excess of 6 months. Lack of empirical data makes it difficult to recommend laser surgery as a definitive therapy for nasal neoplasia, but its benefit as an adjunctive or palliative modality is clear.

Currently we are using the 810 nm diode routinely to treat nasal adenocarcinoma and carcinoma, as well as benign inflammatory nasal and nasopharyngeal polyps (Fig. 8.14). Lasers are relatively less

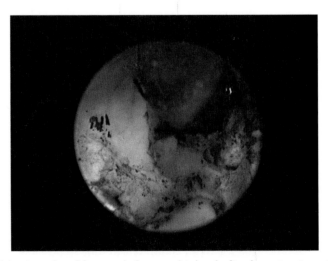

Fig. 8.14 Anterior rhinoscopic image obtained after laser treatment for neoplasia.

effective in the management of nasal chondromas/chondrosarcomas, osteosarcomas/osteomas and lymphomas (note: the latter responds extremely well to the laser but, as lymphoma needs to be managed as a systemic disease, recurrence if very likely with sole laser therapy). A side benefit of laser use is that diodes of this wavelength are haemostatic, neurostatic and lymphostatic, making postoperative complications minimal. The net result is that postoperative oedema, haemorrhage and pain are minimised dramatically.

Postoperative care and complications

The two major complications with any sort of rhinoscopic procedure are haemorrhage and aspiration pneumonia. Life-threatening haemorrhage is rare unless the underlying pathology lends itself to a bleeding diathesis, or there has been an unidentified or incompletely managed coagulopathic tendency. Aspiration pneumonia from irrigant fluid contaminated with blood and other exudate is a preventable complication if patient positioning and proper airway management techniques are adhered to.

Care following rhinoscopy is usually quite minimal. It is usually advised to allow patients to recover from general anaesthesia slowly to minimise rapid spikes in blood pressure. Intra- or perioperative use of acepromazine will help keep the patient's blood pressure on the low normal side, thus minimising hypertension-induced haemorrhage. It is expected that there will be some degree of ongoing epistaxis for a few days following the rhinoscopy. While this is rarely of any clinical concern it can be quite untidy and alarming to owners. Often I will suggest hospitalising the patients for the first postoperative evening in an effort to keep the patient quiet and sedated and to minimise any owner anxiety. Within 3–4 days haemorrhage and discharge as a sole postoperative issue are resolved.

Rigid tracheoscopy

Although a complete examination of the trachea and bronchial tree is best accomplished with a flexible bronchoscope, there is significant value in the use of rigid endoscopes for tracheoscopy. In particular the emergency diagnosis and management of tracheal foreign bodies, as well as procedures such as guided bronchoalveolar lavages and transtracheal aspirates/brushings in smaller patients, are well facilitated by rigid endoscopy.

Patients presenting for rigid tracheoscopy are often in an acute respiratory crisis, so respiratory and ventilatory support is of paramount importance. In most cases the decision to perform rigid tracheoscopy will make the use of an endotracheal tube impossible. Judicious sedation with flow by oxygen support is important in the pre-anaesthetic management. An

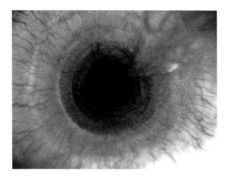

Fig. 8.15   Trachea as seen using a 5 mm, 0° laparoscope. Photograph courtesy of Mr P.J. Lhermette.

intravenous catheter should be placed to allow for the use of intravenous anaesthetics.

For smaller patients presenting for either a diagnostic tracheoscopic exam or emergency foreign body removal, I can sometimes use the 2.7 mm, 30° urethrocystoscope. The obvious advantage to the use of this scope is the ability to introduce operative accessory instrumentation via the instrument channel. However, the short length of this scope limits the distal extent of the exam. In those situations a longer-length, 5 mm, 0° laparoscope (or similar) can be used (Fig. 8.15). Again, without an operating sheath, accessory instrumentation must be slipped alongside the endoscope, allowing for less accuracy in the placement and use of these devices.

With the patient in either sternal or lateral recumbency an induction agent such as propofol is given intravenously. Care must be taken with many of these induction agents, as apnea is a common-dose-related sequela to their use. When the patient is adequately anaesthetised a nasal or oral oxygen catheter is slipped into the trachea to provide supplemental oxygen.

Propofol can be continually administered via continuous-rate infusion or intermittent boluses, but speed and efficiency in these procedures is paramount. With endoscopic guidance, bronchoalveolar lavage can be performed and cytological brushings obtained from the trachea and main stem bronchi.

Foreign bodies can be retrieved from the trachea using standard endoscopic retrieval instrumentation or using long-shafted laparoscopic grasping forceps. Care must be taken to avoid iatrogenic injury to the tracheal mucosa or rings and the surgeon must be prepared to place an emergency tracheostomy tube distal to the point of obstruction (if possible) in the event that the foreign-body retrieval procedure is prolonged.

Other pathologies that can be diagnosed are tracheitis (Fig. 8.16) and tracheal collapse (Fig. 8.17).

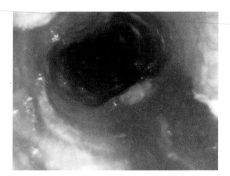

Fig. 8.16   Severe changes associated with tracheitis. Photograph courtesy of Mr P.J. Lhermette.

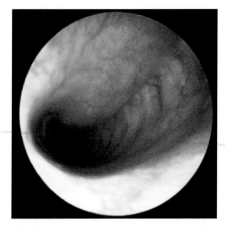

Fig. 8.17   Tracheal collapse; the dorsal tracheal membrane is protruding into the lumen. Photograph courtesy of Mr P.J. Lhermette.

Conclusion

The list of indications for endoscopy of the upper respiratory tract are ever increasing and new and improved techniques and instrumentation will allow veterinary surgeons to address nasal, sinus, pharyngeal and tracheal diseases with minimal morbidity and disruption of normal structures.

Further reading

Beherent, A.C., Kinns, J. and Weisse, C. (2006) Balloon dilatation of the nasopharyngeal stenosis in a dog. *Journal of the American Veterinary Medical Association* 229, 385–388.
Freeman, L.J. (1998) *Veterinary Endosurgery*. Mosby, St Louis, MO.

Johnson, L.R., Clarke, H.E., Bannasch, M.J. and De Cock, H.E.V. (2004) Correlation of rhinoscopic signs of inflammation with histologic findings in nasal biopsy specimens of cats with or without upper respiratory tract disease. *Journal of the American Veterinary Medical Association* 225, 395–400.

Johnson, L.R., Drazenovich, T.L., Herrera, M.A. and Wisner, E.R. (2006) Results of rhinoscopy alone or in conjunction with sinuscopy in dogs with aspergillosis: 46 cases (2001–2004). *Journal of the American Veterinary Medical Association* 228, 738–742.

Lefebvre, J., Kuehn, N.F. and Wortinger, A. (2005) Computed tomography as an aid in the diagnosis of chronic nasal disease in dogs. *Journal of Small Animal Practice* 46, 280–285.

Lhermette, P. and Sobel, D. (eds) (2008) *BSAVA Manual of Canine and Feline Endoscopy and Endosurgery*. British Small Animal Veterinary Association, Gloucester.

McCarthy, T.C. (ed.) (2005) *Veterinary Endoscopy for the Small Animal Practitioner*. Elsevier Saunders, St Louis, MO.

Noone, K.E. (2001) Rhinoscopy pharyngoscopy and laryngoscopy. *Veterinary Clinics of North America Small Animal Practice* 31, 671–689.

Tams, T.R. (1998) *Small Animal Endoscopy*, 2nd edn. Mosby, St Louis, MO.

Willard, M.D. (2002) Respiratory tract endoscopy. In *Small Animal Surgery*, 2nd edn, Fossum, T.W. (ed.), pp. 121–126. Mosby, St Louis, MO.

Windsor, R.C., Johnson, L.R., Herrgesell, E.J. and De Cock, H.E.V. (2004) Idiopathic lymphoplasmacytic rhinitis in dogs: 37 cases (1997–2002). *Journal of the American Veterinary Medical Association* 224, 1952–1957.

Chapter 9

Endoscopy of the Canine and Feline Ear: Otoendoscopy

David S. Sobel

Introduction

Of all of the applications for endoscopy and endoscopic surgery in small animal practice, otoendoscopy is certainly one of the most common and rewarding. Aural disease is a frequent presenting clinical problem to primary care clinicians and represents a common cause of morbidity in canine and feline practice. Otoendoscopy is one of the simplest endoscopic techniques to master and represents a cost-effective use of endoscopic equipment. The equipment used for otoendoscopy is simple and straightforward, and often the endoscopic instrumentation is similar to that for other common endoscopic procedures. For the purposes of this chapter I will presume that the practitioner has a degree of comfort using the standard handheld direct-view otoscope in the awake patient. Our focus will be on the interventions available to the practitioner in using endoscopy to further their diagnostic and therapeutic interventions.

Clinically, otoendoscopy is used to differentiate between otitis externa (aural disease of the pinnae, and vertical and horizontal canals to the level of the tympanic membrane) and otitis media. It is increasingly recognised that otitis media is a common sequela or aetiology of otitis externa. Otoendoscopy is used diagnostically to determine the causes of various aural pathologies (retrieving samples of tissue or exudates for biopsy or cytologic examination, retrieval of materials for bacterial or fungal culture, visualisation of the tympanum). It is also used as an interventional

Clinical Manual of Small Animal Endosurgery, First Edition. Edited by Alasdair Hotston Moore and Rosa Angela Ragni.
© 2012 Blackwell Publishing Ltd. Published 2012 by Blackwell Publishing Ltd.

modality to therapeutically correct underlying pathology (tumour or polyp resection with laser or electrocautery, foreign-body retrieval, deep-ear cleaning and flushing, myringotomy). As such, otoendoscopy is a technique that is valuable for every endoscopist to have in their arsenal.

Indications

The clinical presentations of the patient with aural disease are all too familiar to most veterinary practitioners. Ear shaking or aural pruritis, chronic aural odour and/or discharge, aural pain, hearing loss and peripheral neurological signs consistent with middle-ear disease are all common presenting problems for the patient in need of otoendoscopy. In addition, the clinical progress of patients with confirmed aural pathology can be monitored. Patients with aural disease refractory to therapy can also be evaluated and subsequent treatment plans modified to achieve optimal clinical results.

Instrumentation

Several equipment manufacturers make small animal-specific otoendo-scopes that work extremely well (Fig. 9.1) in most small animal patients. These scopes are 0° or forward-facing endoscopes, with short overall length (approximately 8 cm) and a 5 mm-diameter optical end, and are squat, robust small endoscopes. This makes them ideal for use in the exam room with either a compliant, awake patient or a lightly sedated animal with less risk of damage to the endoscope. A Luer-fitted biopsy channel usually has a diameter of approximately 2 mm and optional bridges with two- and three-way stopcocks can be added to the port to allow for continuous irrigation/flushing as well as the introduction of an instrument via the operative channel.

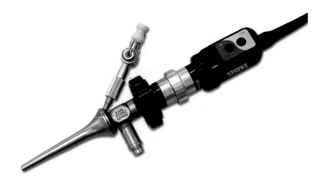

Fig. 9.1 Veterinary otoendoscope with integrated working channel. Reproduced from Lhermette and Sobel (2008), with the permission of BSAVA publications. © BSAVA.

While this author does use 0° otoendoscopes for some diagnostic otoendoscopy, the use of a 2.7 mm, 30° rigid endoscope is preferable for working on larger canine patients and doing most interventional procedures. These endoscopes are often marketed as 'multipurpose rigid endoscopes' but are essentially paediatric urethrocystoscopes in an appropriate sheath (see Fig. 1.2). The advantages to these endoscopes are the increased working length which allows for complete visualisation of the horizontal ear canal in even the largest patients, as well as the increased field of view due to the 30° optical view. This is particularly advantageous in visualising all areas of the ear canal at the level of the junction of its vertical and horizontal portions as well as providing complete visualisation of the tympanum. In addition, these endoscopes have separate ingress and egress channels allowing for adequate fluid irrigation and drainage as well as a separate instrument channel.

A full range of cytology, culture and cleaning brushes as well as curettes, biopsy forceps and graspers are available. The author also uses diode lasers in the endoscopic management of aural disease and the flexible quartz fibres used as a light-delivery system come in diameters that will be accommodated by almost any endoscope (Fig. 9.2). In addition, suction and irrigation devices are also marketed by several manufacturers. These devices allow irrigation of the ear at a controlled, predetermined pressure via the instrument channel of the endoscope through a slender cannula. Similarly the irrigant and collected detritus can be removed via the suction component of these devices (Fig. 9.3). While admittedly lower tech, similar results can be achieved with an irrigation cannula or slender red rubber feeding tube, and a saline-filled syringe.

Standard endosurgery equipment has been discussed elsewhere but high-quality endoscopic video cameras, in both standard and high-definition (HD) resolution, are now available and are quite reasonably priced. Xenon light sources of no less than 150 W are ideal for otoendoscopy, along with the associated flexible fibre-optic light guide cables.

A variety of different accessory instrumentation, including aspiration and irrigation cannulae, biopsy forceps, guarded culturette swabs, ear

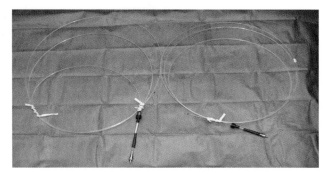

Fig. 9.2 Flexible quartz laser fibres that can be inserted into the otoendoscope and used for illumination.

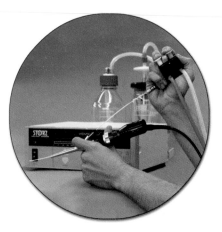

Fig. 9.3   Flushing and suction device (Vetpump 2, Storz, Tuttlingen, Germany). Reproduced from Lhermette and Sobel (2008), with the permission of BSAVA publications. © BSAVA.

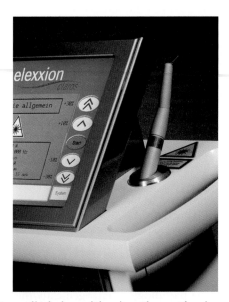

Fig. 9.4   An 810 nm diode laser (Elexxion Claros, Elexxion, Germany).

curettes and many more are available for use in otoendoscopy. Ideally these instruments will be compatible with the operative channel of the particular endoscope chosen, but some operators do choose to utilise instruments that work extraluminal to it.

The advent of low-cost, high-power diode lasers to the veterinary market has greatly enhanced the interventional aspects of otoendoscopy (Fig. 9.4). Lasers of wavelength between 810 and 980 nm will function quite well in the aqueous medium of otoendoscopy. Powers of 8–15 W are usually adequate for most lesions in the ear. A detailed description of lasers, laser physics and laser endosurgery can be found in other texts. Suffice to say that these diode lasers are a great aid in performing myringotomies, ablation of proliferative inflammatory lesions, control of haemorrhage, and resection of polyps and other masses.

Anatomy

The canine and feline outer ear is defined by the external pinna to the vertical canal (Fig. 9.5). The origination of the vertical canal is edged ventrally and laterally by the intertragic notch, a separation between two cartilaginous ridges: cranial and caudal. This can serve as an important landmark for initial insertion of the endoscope. The length and angle of the vertical ear canal varies from breed to breed and between canine to feline. The epithelium of the vertical canal is squamous in nature with variable numbers of hair follicles and progressively more sebaceous and ceruminous glands as the vertical canal progresses deep. The angle forming the demarcation between the vertical and horizontal canals is defined by a firm ridge of cartilage extending caudo-ventrally. Navigating this angle is often times the most challenging portion of otoendoscopy for the novice. The severity of this angle is less in cats and brachycephalic dog breeds, resulting in a more accessible horizontal canal.

The tympanum (Fig. 9.6) is a thin, glistening membrane forming the separation from the external ear and middle ear, at the terminus of the horizontal canal. In the normal ear, the pars flaccida of the tympanum is seen dorsally, occupying approximately one-third of the field of view of the structure. The pars tensa occupies the ventral two-thirds of the visible tympanum and is clinically the more important portion of it (Fig. 9.7). In the normal patient, a bony ridge separating the tympanic cavity from the bulla can be seen ventrally through the pars tensa, while dorso-caudally the manubrium of the malleus in the middle ear is visible (Fig. 9.8). The opacity of the membrane sometimes limits visualisation of these landmarks, although this more often occurs in the diseased intact tympanum (Fig. 9.9). In conditions where the tympanum is ruptured, either via pathology or iatrogenically/therapeutically, with careful cleaning and irrigation, these structures are easily visualised.

Patient preparation

Generally, most patients presenting to have a detailed otoendoscopic exam and/or endoscopic surgery have had a long list of empirical therapies attempted prior to the exam. As such, a careful anamnesis and evaluation of previous clinical pathology studies is indicated. Following the general physical exam a careful neurological exam is also advised.

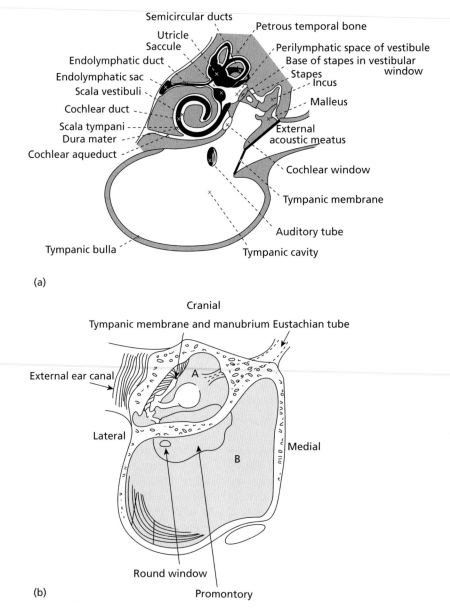

(a)

(b)

Fig. 9.5 Schematic drawings showing the anatomy of the canine (a) and feline (b) ear. In (b), A and B refer to the two compartments of the feline bulla, a smaller dorsal compartment (A) and a larger ventral compartment (B).

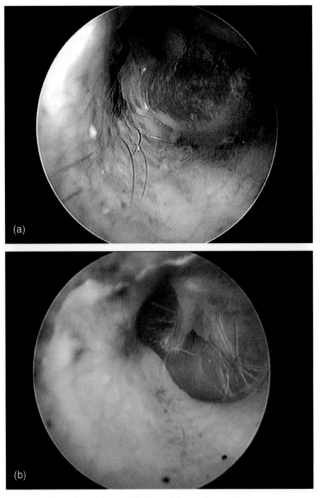

Fig. 9.6 Normal canine (a) and feline (b) eardrum. Images courtesy of Dr G. Ghibaudo.

Particular attention to the cranial nerves and central cortical status is important.

It can also be advisable to coordinate additional imaging studies to be done either prior to otoendoscopy or in conjunction with the procedure. These can include magnetic resonance imaging (MRI) or computed tomography (CT) as well as conventional radiography. MRI is an ideal modality for visualising the middle and inner ear and certainly if there is any concern over central involvement this may be the only way to accurately image the extent of disease.

If there is any indication that a bacterial culture and sensitivity may be required as part of the work-up it is imperative that antibiotics, both oral and topical, be discontinued for at least 3 days, preferably 7 days,

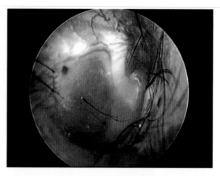

Fig. 9.7 Normal canine tympanum. Apparent is the pars tensa, occupying the ventral two-thirds, through which it is visible the bony ridge separating the tympanic cavity from the bulla. Photograph courtesy of Dr G. Ghibaudo.

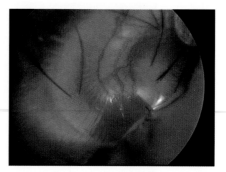

Fig. 9.8 Through this normal canine tympanum the manubrium of the malleus can be seen dorso-caudally in the middle ear, with its associated blood vessels and striations in the pars tensa of the tympanic membrane. Reproduced from Lhermette and Sobel (2008), with the permission of BSAVA publications. © BSAVA.

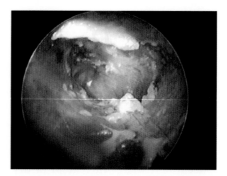

Fig. 9.9 In this case of myringitis in a dog, the opacity of the membrane limits visualisation of the middle ear landmarks. Photograph courtesy of Dr G. Ghibaudo.

prior to the procedure. Some authors advocate the use of glucocorticoids prior to otoendoscopy in the hope of controlling inflammation in the ear canals, a common sequela to otitis externa. This should make passage of the endoscope easier, and should also minimise neurological complications (transient though they usually are) post endoscopy. This author has not found this to be of necessity, and indeed, being able to appreciate the nature of the pathology at its clinically most significant can aid in interpretation of findings and potentially make histopathology more rewarding.

Patients should be starved of food for 12 h prior to the procedure in preparation for general anaesthesia. They should be sedated and induced for anaesthesia in accordance with standard protocols for the particular facility as well as with their general health and cardiovascular status. Given the hyperaesthetic nature of the ears, especially in the diseased state, general inhalation anaesthesia delivered via endotracheal tube is indicated. This also provides an increased measure of safety when using irrigation, to prevent aspiration pneumonia. As otoendoscopy is often done as part of a more extensive upper airway endoscopic work-up, including pharyngoscopy and rhinoscopy, it is prudent to have an anaesthetic and operative protocol to facilitate doing all of these procedures at the same time.

Otoendoscopy operative procedure

Patient positioning is at the preference of the operator and often the design of the operatory room may dictate the patient positioning, location of the surgeon and location of the endoscopic equipment tower. Still, some standardisation is valuable in providing consistent results from case to case. It is advisable the procedure be performed on a wet table or surgical sink table as often copious amounts of irrigant are used. This facilitates keeping the patient warm and dry and minimises flooding the floor of the operating theatre.

The patient is usually positioned in lateral recumbency with the affected side (or the side to be examined first) uppermost. The endoscopy equipment tower is positioned along the dorsal aspect of the patient, at approximately the level of the head, ideally at 11 o'clock to the top of the skull. The surgeon usually stands at approximately 6 o'clock given this orientation. This provides for the most ergonomic positioning of the operator and equipment relative to patient. Occasionally, depending on the specific anatomy of a given patient, it may be beneficial to place a rolled towel under the head to allow the muzzle to point in the downward direction, while slightly elevating the dorsal part of the head. This brings the vertical canal into more linear approximation with the angle of the endoscope and allows for drainage of irrigant out the nose, rather than back into the pharynx.

Once the requisite materials have been laid out and sterilised as per the manufacturer's directions (see Chapter 1) the procedure can commence. Cytological and bacteriological samples are collected before introducing the endoscope into the ear canal. This is done prior to any cleaning or examination of any sort. If needed, deeper samples for the same clinical pathology testing can be obtained from the middle ear later in the procedure.

There is some recent questioning as to the merit of bacterial culture and sensitivity in the ear, citing a wide variability in bacterial species recovered as well as the wide variance of sensitivity patterns among the same species isolates. Still, it seems prudent in cases of resistant, confirmed bacterial infection that samples from both external and middle ear be obtained separately.

Once samples for clinical pathology have been obtained a cursory cleaning of the external ear can be performed. I usually avoid using ceruminolytic cleaners for several reasons. The turbidity obtained with dissolution of the ceruminous wax can be difficult to clear even with subsequent aggressive saline irrigation. Even the mildest ceruminolytic agent can be mildly irritating, causing some degree of oozing of already inflamed aural tissues, further hindering good visualisation. Finally, these agents are generally not sterile preparations, making subsequent culture of the middle ear more difficult. The use of warm sterile saline is in my experience more than adequate to achieve excellent results. This initial cleaning should be done very gently in an effort to avoid causing further iatrogenic damage to the aural tissues and the resultant difficulty in visualisation. Only the most grossly obstructive material should be removed in this initial cleaning. Ideally a suction/irrigation pump apparatus can be used to perform this cleaning, but a red rubber feeding tube of appropriate size with gentle syringe pressure works well.

Fluids used as irrigants in otoendoscopy should be slightly warmer than room temperature to facilitate ceruminolysis and to minimise any transient post-endoscopy temperature-related neurological signs. Irrigation is ideally done with a simple gravity-fed bag of warm saline via a standard administration set. A pressure bag or pump can be used if needed. Again, a suction/irrigation pump can be used via an irrigation cannula that is delivered through the working channel of the endoscope to keep the field of view clear intra-operatively, and to remove any collected blood and debris.

With the endoscope/camera assembly held pistol-style in one hand, the tip of the pinna is held in the other hand and retracted dorsally. This action opens up the vertical canal for easy access of the endoscope. The endoscope is placed in the intertragic notch and angled ventrally into the vertical canal. At the base of the vertical canal the endoscope is deflected medially towards the centre of the head into the horizontal canal. This motion, with continued traction on the pinna and ongoing saline irrigation, should open up visualisation of the tympanum.

The horizontal and vertical canals should each be inspected carefully for masses, excessive ceruminous discharge, polyps, foreign bodies, excessive hair growth, inflammatory changes to the epithelium, etc. Any abnormal lesion can then be biopsied using forceps passed within the operative channel of the endoscope or alongside it. For adequate histological evaluation multiple biopsies should be obtained. If there is still excessive cerumen or other discharges obscuring adequate visualisation, manual removal of debris with biopsy or grasping forceps can be done, or a slightly more aggressive cleaning with an irrigation/suction apparatus may be of value.

A common occurrence is the finding of a sessile mass or polyp lesion of unknown point of origin obscuring visualisation of the horizontal canal and tympanic membrane. Removal or at the very least debulking of the lesion must be done to allow for examination of deeper structures. In these instances the first order of business is to retrieve biopsies for histopathology. Next the diode laser is used to help resect and ablate the mass. Ideally an 810 nm diode laser with a 1000 µm flat-beam fibre is used in contact mode. Powers of 8–15 W are usually needed although very dense, relatively less vascular tissues can require more power. The fibre is inserted into the instrument channel of the endoscope and the laser fired on a continuous cutting mode. The mass is vapourised by progressive cranial-to-caudal, back-and-forth cutting motion in a continuous or short-pulse mode. This usually allows for serial resection of the lesion allowing the operator to identify its point(s) of origin, paying particular attention to surgical margins. With the laser resection complete there may be bits of charred tissue that require removal, usually done with biopsy or rat-tooth-type forceps.

If a laser is not available, manual removal of the mass can be done with grasping of the lesion either with endoscopic forceps or with very small curved haemostatic forceps and gentle traction. While this can be a very effective technique, the subsequent haemorrhage, while not clinically significant, can make the rest of the otoendoscopic exam difficult.

A similar technique using the laser can be employed on proliferative inflammatory lesions or portions of the epithelium that are proliferative to the point of causing an effective stenosis of the canal. These tissues can quite successfully be ablated, allowing for an effective increase in its diameter.

With good visualisation of the vertical and horizontal canals achieved, the tympanum and middle ear can now be evaluated. Any residual tissue or ceruminous material resting against the tympanum can be either gently removed manually or with gentle irrigation to provide an adequate view. Evaluation of the integrity, colour, opacity and vascularity of the tympanum should now be done. The different anatomical portions of this structure should be identified as both surgical landmarks and points of visual reference. The pars flaccida and pars tensa should be clearly identified. If the tympanum is perforated it may be difficult to obtain a truly representative middle-ear sample for cytological and bacteriological evaluation but it certainly can be attempted. A sterile guarded culturette or sterile polypropylene catheter are the preferred tools for this task. If the tympanum is intact, but middle-ear disease is suspected based on the gross appearance of the tympanum (and adjunctive imaging studies), a myringotomy can be performed. The myringotomy has been much maligned in veterinary practice but when used appropriately and judiciously its role in the management of otitis media cannot be underestimated.

A myringotomy can be performed with a variety of instrumentation. Specially designed myringotomy knives are available but are designed for the human patient where navigating the vertical canal towards the horizontal ear canal is not an issue. These can be used in some feline patients. A flexible, small-diameter endoscopic needle can be used via the otoendoscope but frequently the diameter of these needles (25-gauge) limits the effectiveness of the myringotomy. Biopsy or grasping forceps can also be used to make a few punctate holes in the tympanum. Often, if there is increased pressure in the middle ear behind the tympanum, a single puncture will allow a larger tear to result. This author uses the diode laser to perform the myringotomy. In this case, a smaller-diameter fibre, usually 600 μm, is used. With a power setting of 6–10 W, a cruciate-type linear incision is made in the pars tensa of the tympanum, beginning in the craniodorsal aspect and extending caudo-ventrally. The next incision is made caudo-dorsal to cranio-ventral. The advantages of using the laser with this pattern of myringotomy cut involve delayed surgical healing of the tympanum. With good postoperative medical management the canine and feline tympanum can heal very quickly; indeed, in many cases more quickly than one would prefer. In an effort to provide a longer period of middle-ear drainage, the laser myringotomy may prove superior to other methodologies. One of the results of the thermal injury from the laser is the region of cell death that occurs along the margins of the incision. This cell death will produce the effect of delayed healing. While in many clinical scenarios this would be counterproductive, here it achieves the benefit of the desired longer period of middle-ear drainage.

In virtually any event, the tympanic membrane will heal quite adequately with reasonable medical management. With the myringotomy performed and samples obtained for clinical pathology, gentle irrigation of the middle ear will help remove any fluid or more inspissated material from the middle ear.

Selected pathologies of the ear canals and middle ear

While a complete treatise on the pathologies of the ear in dogs and cats is beyond the scope of this chapter, the practitioner must learn to appreciate the most commonly encountered disease conditions seen via an otoendoscopic exam.

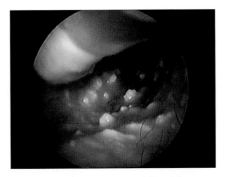

Fig. 9.10 Video-otoscopic image of bacterial otitis externa in a dog. Evident is the exudate along the external ear canal. Photograph courtesy of Dr G. Ghibaudo.

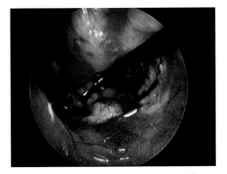

Fig. 9.11 Haemorrhage and ulcerations are commonly associated with *Pseudomonas* otitis externa. Photograph courtesy of Dr G. Ghibaudo.

Otitis externa

Far and away the most common disease seen in clinical practice is otitis externa (or OE). Although many aetiologies are possible, bacterial infection and yeast (*Malassezia* spp.) aural infections are the most frequently encountered. The appearance of the horizontal and vertical ear canals is variable but commonly excessive erythema is noted with variable degrees of oedema depending on whether the presentation is for an acute onset of otitis externa. The glandular epithelium of the canals can become proliferative or in some cases take on a nodular appearance (Fig. 9.10). Secondary ulceration can also be associated with otitis externa, and is commonly associated with *Pseudomonas* infection (Fig. 9.11).

Neoplasms

Benign masses of the aural canals represent the most common type of tumour noted (Fig. 9.12). These lesions can present as multilobulated diffuse lesions or singular sessile and usually obstructive foci.

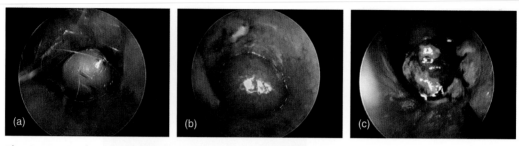

Fig. 9.12 Benign masses of the aural canals represent the most common type of tumour noted. (a) Polyp observed in a canine external ear canal. (b) Polyp visible at video-otoendoscopy in the external ear canal of a cat. (c) Ductal ceruminous adenoma in a dog. Images courtesy of Dr G. Ghibaudo.

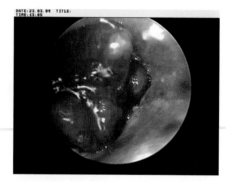

Fig. 9.13 Ceruminous gland adenocarcinoma in the external ear canal of a cat. Reproduced from Lhermette and Sobel (2008), with the permission of BSAVA publications. © BSAVA.

Histopathologically these lesions tend to be either lymphoplasmacytic or plasmacytic. In some cases these lesions can be associated with polyps in other areas of the upper respiratory tract, notably in cats. Depending on the size of the lesions these may be responsive to glucocorticoid treatment, but often this does not obviate the need for surgical resection. In one study of feline patients a recurrence rate of 30% was noted whether sole medical, sole surgical or combination therapy was used.

Masses visible at otoendoscopy may also be malignant in origin (Fig. 9.13) and thus any mass observed in the ear canal should be biopsied (Fig. 9. 14) and submitted for histopathological examination.

Otitis media

Otitis media (or OM) is now understood to be a far more frequent clinical finding than previously thought, and can be found as a separate clinical entity or associated with chronic otitis externa (Fig. 9.15). As a stand-alone finding, often the presenting signs of otitis media may include

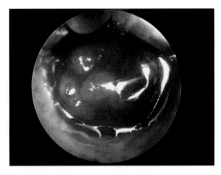

Fig. 9.14 Biopsy of the neoplasm seen in Fig. 9.13, performed with biopsy forceps inserted in the instrument channel of the video-otoscope. The forceps are visible at the top of the image. Reproduced from Lhermette and Sobel (2008), with the permission of BSAVA publications. © BSAVA.

aural pain including head shaking, vocalisation, pawing at the head and ears, and pain on prehension of food with associated dysphagia. These patients can be diagnosed accurately with otoendoscopy. In these cases often the vertical and horizontal ear canals are normal. At the level of the tympanum, however, significant findings are often more obvious. The tympanum, in particular the pars flaccida, is often bulging due the collection of fluid and inflammatory detritus behind the membrane. The tympanum can be thickened and opaque. Often notable hyperaemia can be appreciated. In these cases a myringotomy is often of significant clinical benefit. This can be accomplished in one of several manners. This author finds that the use of a diode laser (810–980 nm) at low levels of power to be of tremendous utility (see above). This is usually done in a cruciate manner with two linear cuts made from rostro-dorsal to caudo-ventral and the second from caudo-dorsal to rostro-ventral. The use of the laser has as a normal sequela to its use delayed tissue healing. This can be of significant benefit in allowing the middle ear to continue to drain for a period of time following the endoscopy. Other methods of myringotomy, including the use of a biopsy instrument, myringotomy knife, curette or loop, work very well but it has been noted that the healing time of the tympanum can be in the order of just a few days, potentially allowing for relapse and recurrence of middle-ear disease.

Once the myringotomy is performed a sterile aspiration catheter should be introduced via the operating channel of the endoscope for collection of material for bacterial culture and sensitivity as well as for fluid analysis and cytology. Gentle but copious irrigation using sterile saline should then be performed. Gravity feed, a pressure bag or a mechanical fluid pump (Fig. 9.3) can be used for irrigation. Irrigation should be done until the effluent runs clean. Following the myringotomy, both topical and systemic antimicrobial therapy, based on culture results from both the middle and external ear, should be undertaken.

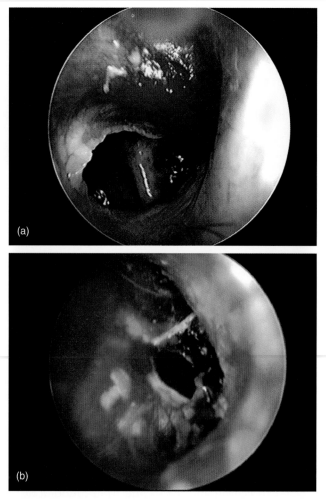

Fig. 9.15   (a) Bacterial otitis media in a dog. (b) Otitis media caused by yeast in a dog. In both cases there is rupture of the tympanic membrane. Photographs courtesy of Dr G. Ghibaudo.

Frequently with severe middle- (and external-) ear disease the patient may present with a tympanum that is already perforated. In these cases the management is similar to that following a myringotomy. However, culture results must be interpreted in light of the potential for contamination from the external ear. Again, copious irrigation should be undertaken. It is worth noting that with appropriate medical management following otoendoscopy the vast majority of ruptured tympanums will heal well.

The clinician must be aware that for middle-ear disease that is refractory to therapy, or is associated with peripheral neurological signs, CT and MRI are excellent adjunctive imaging modalities (Fig. 9.16).

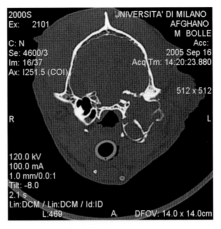

Fig. 9.16 CT scan of a dog with a left cholesteatoma: the middle ear cavity is enlarged, and there are loss of air contrast and lysis of the bulla wall. Reproduced from Lhermette and Sobel (2008), with the permission of BSAVA publications. © BSAVA.

Complications

Complications from otoendoscopy are infrequent and usually self-limiting. Cats seem to be more susceptible to postoperative problems, including head shaking, pain and neurological signs. The caloric and manual trauma from instrumentation and fluid irrigation can result in neurological signs such as enophtalmos, ptosis, miosis and Horner's syndrome. These signs are usually transient and resolve without further therapy, but in rare cases permanent signs such as vestibular anomalies and deafness can ensue. Good technique and the avoidance of ototoxic agents can usually minimise the risk of iatrogenic injury, but owners should be made aware of the risk of these complications.

Conclusion

With the frequency of aural disease in small animal practice it is likely that otoendoscopy will become the standard of care in the management of a vast majority of ear disease in canine and feline practice. The technique is safe, easy to learn and cost-effective. The huge amount of information that can be made available to the clinician via otoendoscopy will prove invaluable and lead to more timely and accurate management of aural disease.

Further reading

Angus, J.C. and Campbell, K.L. (2001) Uses and indications for video-otoscopy in small animal practice. *Veterinary Clinics of North America Small Animal Practice* 31, 809–828.

Cole, L.K. (2004) Otoscopic evaluation of the ear canal. *Veterinary Clinics of North America Small Animal Practice* 34, 392–410.

Cole, L.K., Kwochka, K.W., Podell, M., Hiller, A. and Smeak, D.D. (2002) Evaluation of radiography, otoscopy, pneumatoscopy, impedance audiometry and endoscopy for the diagnosis of otitis media in the dog. *Advances in Veterinary Dermatology* 4, 49–55.

Gotthelf, L.N. (2002) Laser ear surgery. *17th Proceedings of the AVD/ACVD*, pp. 137–138.

Gotthelf, L.N. (2004) Diagnosis and treatment of otitis media in dogs and cats. *Veterinary Clinics of North America Small Animal Practice* 34, 469–487.

Griffen, C.E. (2006) Otitis techniques to improve practice. *Clinical Techniques in Small Animal Practice* 21, 96–106.

Lhermette, P. and Sobel, D. (eds) (2008) *BSAVA Manual of Canine and Feline Endoscopy and Endosurgery*. British Small Animal Veterinary Association, Gloucester.

Morris, D.O. (2004) Medical therapy of otitis externa and otitis media. *Veterinary Clinics of North America Small Animal Practice* 34, 541–555.

Chapter 10
Small Exotic Animal Endosurgery
Romain Pizzi

Introduction

Rigid endoscopy has been well established in avian medicine since the 1970s when it was first used for surgical sexing. It is only more recently that endoscopy has become increasingly utilised in general exotic animal practice in reptiles and small pet mammals. While some endosurgical procedures are well described in the laboratory animal literature, these are often more of use as models for human diseases, than in the types of condition encountered in small pet mammals. The author has yet to see a clinical indication for a Nissen fundoplication in a pet rabbit. Much emphasis is placed on the minimally invasive nature of endosurgery, but the enhanced visualisation, the access to parts of the body and structures difficult to visualise in open surgery, and provision of excellent illumination are also of great benefit to the surgeon working with small exotic species.

In these patients it is possible to perform not only techniques and applications identical to those used in canines and felines, but also other specific procedures, thanks to differing anatomy and the unique disease conditions encountered. Diagnostic endosurgery is particularly useful in species where other imaging modalities are limited due to the species anatomy. Ultrasonographic examination of the rabbit, guinea pig and chinchilla abdomen, for instance, is limited by the voluminous gas-containing caecum, while in birds the air sacs prove a similar limitation. Radiography may similarly not demonstrate small liver metastasis from a primary uterine adenocarcinoma in a rabbit, or small *Aspergillus* fungal air-sac plaques in a parrot; and the osteoderms in the scales of a

Clinical Manual of Small Animal Endosurgery, First Edition. Edited by Alasdair Hotston Moore and Rosa Angela Ragni.
© 2012 Blackwell Publishing Ltd. Published 2012 by Blackwell Publishing Ltd.

plated lizard may overlie and obscure underlying coelomic pathology on radiographs. All these lesions are readily evident with the aid of laparoscopy (Fig. 10.1). Furthermore, although speculums can be used to visualise the oral cavities of rodents and rabbits to evaluate the extent of dental disease, rigid endoscopy provides ease of access, and a well-illuminated and magnified view even at the back of the mouth (Fig. 10.2). Images may also later be shown to owners, in a bid to help them understand the disease process.

This chapter will attempt to give a very broad overview of some of the most common applications for conditions encountered in exotic pet species in general practice, but clearly there are many more applications for rigid-endoscopic techniques not covered here. Endoscopes can be used to visualise any anatomical space, or any potential space that can be created via distention with fluid, air or carbon dioxide, and can also be used in surgically created spaces. While outside the scope of this chapter, endosurgery has been described in amphibians such as frogs (Cook, 1999), fish endosurgery is surprisingly well developed thanks to recent research (Divers, 2010), and endoscopy has even been used for examination of the pulmonary cavity in giant African land snails (Pizzi, 2010).

Although minimally invasive in nature, the majority of endoscopic procedures in exotic pet animals do need anaesthesia for safe restraint, as well as analgesia in surgical applications, just as for all surgical procedures.

Equipment

A 2.7mm-diameter, 30° endoscope and associated operating sheath, originating as a human paediatric cystoscope, has traditionally been the mainstay of exotic pet endoscopy, and is commonly referred to as the 'universal' endoscope. This endoscope may also be used in other applications such as canine rhinoscopy. When choosing endoscopes, one will always be forced to compromise between the diameter of the endoscope and the light-transmission capability and related image size and quality.

While the minimally invasive nature of endosurgery is always emphasised as the main benefit in veterinary patients, the other notable advantage is the excellent visualisation that is possible, as well as illumination, and access to the regions of the body such as the cranial and caudal abdomen not easily visualised by open surgery. Unfortunately emphasis on incision size and number has led to some veterinarians believing that the smallest number of smallest ports is always best. A reduction in 2mm port-site wound size is likely to have minimal effects on postoperative pain and healing, yet the reduction in endoscope size may cause a notable decrease in illumination from the same light source and yields a smaller, poorer-quality image. The ultimate aim of minimally invasive surgery is safer, more physiological surgery, and this is best accomplished with good visualisation. It is up to the individual clinician to decide the best

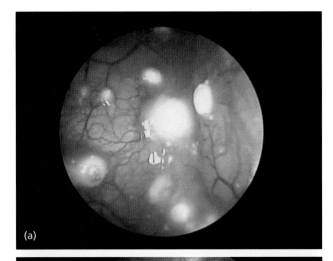

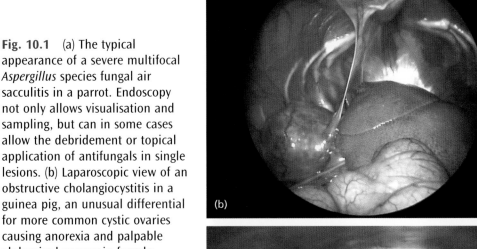

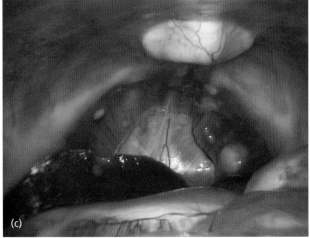

Fig. 10.1 (a) The typical appearance of a severe multifocal *Aspergillus* species fungal air sacculitis in a parrot. Endoscopy not only allows visualisation and sampling, but can in some cases allow the debridement or topical application of antifungals in single lesions. (b) Laparoscopic view of an obstructive cholangiocystitis in a guinea pig, an unusual differential for more common cystic ovaries causing anorexia and palpable abdominal masses in female guinea pigs. Despites the patient's small size, at 1.1 kg, laparoscopy results in excellent visualisation. Care is needed, however, in avoiding trauma to the large, thin-walled caecum and large intestine during entry. (c) Uterine adenocarcinoma metastasis to the peritoneum, diaphragm and liver are evident in this rabbit. Brief laparoscopy provides a useful staging tool for prognostication in these cases.

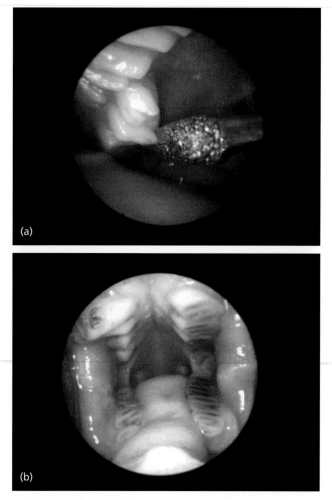

Fig. 10.2   (a) Use of a 4 mm endoscope to visualise filing of dental spurs in a rabbit. (b) Endoscopic visualisation of the small oral cavity of a chinchilla. The first right maxillary premolar is notably overgrown and forming a painful buccal spur, and both upper and lower right dental arcades show uneven dental wear. The oral cavity in small animals is narrow and difficult to illuminate and visualise well without an endoscope.

compromise between endoscope diameter (and hence wound size), and image quality and light transmission.

In contrast, there are clear advantages to the use of instrumentation with small diameter and short shaft length in small exotic animal patients. While the reduction in 'invasiveness' in terms of port-site wound size is perhaps overrated, the large instrument tips of many standard 5 mm laparoscopic instruments (used in humans and canines) are simply too large to manoeuvre in the limited operating space available. Large instrument tips may be too crude to dissect delicate structures; in contrast, 3 mm paediatric instrumentation has the advantage of having fine tips, and also shorter jaws for working in small spaces. The shorter 20 cm length also offers better ergonomics than standard 30–45 cm-long instrumentation, which again helps with precise surgery in restricted spaces. In the smallest patients, even shorter instrument lengths would be desirable, but are not commonly commercially available. In laboratory rat surgical studies small arthroscopy instruments have been used without ports, due to their short shaft lengths, and this may perhaps be applicable for simple procedures in small mammals when instrument changes are not needed.

These patients have thin body walls, which are poor at retaining smooth shaft cannulae when changing instruments. Some 3 mm cannulae have a thick silicon valve, which has higher friction against the instrument shaft than the cannula shaft has against the port site. This results in frustrating motion at port sites during a procedure, and even in port loss, with subsequent deflation of the abdomen or coelom. Threaded cannulae can be used, but these are more traumatic, and result in a larger wound defect. An alternative is to use cannulae with finely grooved shafts and a low-friction disposable silicon valve. These are available in 3 and 5 mm as well as larger sizes (YelloPort+, Surgical Innovations).

Lightweight, clear plastic drapes are an obvious advantage in small exotic pets. Endosurgery needs wide sterile draping if light, camera and electrosurgery cables are not to drag from non-sterile to sterile draped areas, even if the patient is small and completely covered by the drape. This of course limits the anaesthetist's access to and visualisation of the patient during surgery (Fig. 10.3).

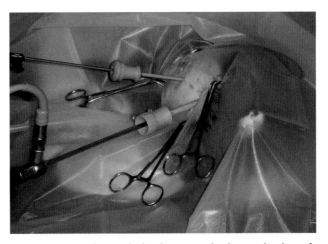

Fig. 10.3 Transparent drapes help the anaesthetic monitoring of small mammals such as this rabbit during laparoscopy. The finely grooved YelloPort+ cannulae are smaller and less traumatic than threaded cannulae, and have better tissue retention in small mammals with their thin body wall, due to low instrument friction with a lubricated silicon valve.

If using an open-access approach to placement of the primary optical trocar in small mammals, a flexible, low-profile ring retractor such as the Lonestar retractor (ARK Surgical UK) can be extremely useful, especially in obese rabbits. It can also aid laparoscopy-assisted procedures, such as laparoscopy-assisted gastrotomy for foreign bodies in ferrets or iguanas, or laparoscopy-assisted cystotomy for urolithiasis in male rabbits, by replacing the need for stay sutures, with the time-saving use of fine blunt-ended elastic stays. This reduces the risk of any abdominal or coelomic contamination from an opened viscus.

Birds

Avian endoscopy and coelioscopy has been performed since the 1970s, originally for sexing in species without obvious sexual dimorphism (Bush et al., 1978; Harrison, 1978). Avian endoscopy is arguably the most well established of all endoscopy techniques in exotic pet animals. This is perhaps not necessarily due to its ease, as these are small patients, with a limited operating space, and until fairly recently there was a limited range of suitable small instruments for multiple puncture techniques. In fact, it is almost certainly due to the fact that the alternative, open coelomic surgery, is a much poorer option, with a notably higher morbidity and mortality, as well as severe limitations in access and visualisation.

Careful handling of the endoscope and support of the camera, light cable and endoscope eyepiece region are needed to prevent inadvertent injury to delicate avian structures during endoscopy (Divers, 2011). It is highly recommended that practitioners practice on avian cadavers of different species, to familiarise themselves with normal avian anatomy, species differences and their appearance during endoscopy.

The so-called universal 2.7 mm-diameter, 30° viewing angle, 18 cm endoscope and associated operating sheath truly justifies its name in pet avian endoscopy, and is well suited to psittacines and raptors that make up a majority of avian pet patients. In larger avian patients such as large raptors, a 4 mm endoscope is advantageous, being less fragile and yielding enhanced visualisation and illumination. A 1.9 mm endoscope is useful for tracheoscopy, and can be used in small patients, but is fragile and easily damaged. A 30° endoscope is extremely useful, if not essential, for maximising visualisation in the small coelomic space of most birds.

Avian patients share the fortunate factor for the endoscopist of having their viscera suspended within the air sacs of the coelom, making insufflation unnecessary. Carbon dioxide insufflation would actually kill the patient through asphyxia. Anaesthesia requirements are the same for any surgical intervention, and while anaesthetic gases escape from any coelomic wounds, this is negligible in coelomic endoscopy and can generally be ignored. While brief procedures (less than 20 min total anaesthesia) are possible under maintenance with a face mask, it is advisable, and certainly necessary in longer procedures, to maintain anaesthesia via an endotracheal tube. Intermittent positive-pressure ventilation (IPPV) should be provided as birds usually hypoventilate under anaesthesia and with increasing anaesthetic duration, so there is an increased likelihood of a fatal hypercapnia developing. Capnography is far more useful in monitoring avian anaesthesia than pulse oximetry.

Tracheoscopy

Tracheoscopy is useful for syringeal *Aspergillus* species fungal granulomas, which usually manifest in parrots as a sudden 'change in voice', and small foreign bodies such as inhaled seeds, that typically lodge at the tracheal bifurcation. It is of course essential to adequately stabilise these patients, which may be in respiratory distress, before undertaking anaesthesia and endoscopic examination. The major hurdle to tracheoscopy in birds is the narrow tracheal lumen which tapers towards the tracheal bifurcation, where pathology often occurs, and the relative length of the trachea. However, while tracheal occlusion and asphyxiation would be a real risk in small mammals, birds have the advantage that a coelomic air-sac tube can be inserted to allow ventilation and anaesthesia, even if the tracheal lumen is completely obstructed by the endoscope. A coelomic air-sac tube can be inserted into the same left lateral coloemic location as coelioscopy is performed (see below). Some practitioners do not insert an air-sac tube, choosing very brief intermittent tracheoscopy periods. However, it should be remembered that – as most patients are being examined via this method because of respiratory distress or disease – there are high risks with anaesthesia, which should be explained to owners. In smaller parrots a 1.9 mm, 18 cm-long endoscope is needed. This has the disadvantages of being fragile, and giving a smaller image; also, due to its thin and hence sharp nature, it can also cause traumatic injury to the trachea. In larger birds the 2.7 mm or even 4 mm endoscope can be used, but in these cases prior placement of a coelomic air-sac tube is strongly advised. These larger-diameter endoscopes also allow the opportunity for a brief initial coelioscopy to evaluate any lower air-sac or pulmonary disease before tracheoscopy. In raptors it should be noted that tracheal nematodes such as *Syngamus* spp. or *Capillaria* spp. may be encountered, and these can be pushed by the inserted endoscope to form an obstructive tracheal plug, with subsequent asphyxiation on recovery.

Cloacoscopy

Cloacoscopy is useful in birds for haematochezia/haematurea, in visualising typical cauliflower-shaped cloacal papillomas, cloacitis (which may manifest as raised or pseudomembranous plaques), salpingitis and enteritis. Biopsy techniques need to be careful, as exuberant taking of biopsies can result in cloacal perforation and resultant coelomitis. A sheathed endoscope may be used for inflation with warmed saline for visualisation, or, alternatively, fluids supplied via a rubber catheter and the cloaca simply pinched closed around the endoscope's inserted shaft. Inside the cloaca the entrances to the rectum, ureters and in female birds the oviduct (uterus) can be visualised. In some cases the caudal oviduct may be entered and examined. The resultant increase in coelomic pressure during cloacoscopy can result in oral regurgitation of fluid during anaesthesia, and it is preferable that birds are intubated. Hernandez-Divers (2006) evaluated the quality of cloacoscopically taken bursa of Fabricius biopsies in pigeons, but found that only 30% of cases yielded a diagnostic-quality histological sample.

Rhinoscopy

The operculum prevents entrance of endoscopes into the nares, although the endoscope can still be used to give a magnified external view. The alternative is to examine the caudal nasal passages entering via the choanal slit in the roof of the upper beak inside the mouth. This may demonstrate discharge, foreign material or parasites, such as leeches in waterfowl.

Otoscopy

Most birds have a shallow, wide external ear canal, with a tympanic membrane that is easily visible to the eye. External ear disease, with the exception of trauma, is also uncommon in birds, making otoscopy of little useful application in birds.

Oral endoscopic examination or 'stomatoscopy'

While the oral cavity and pharynx of raptors and soft-billed birds may be examined in consciously restrained birds, parrots will easily break an endoscope with their powerful beak, and need anaesthesia for safe examination. Oral examination can demonstrate necrotic plaques encountered with *Trichomonas* or *Candida* infections, *Capillaria* nematodes, or injuries and foreign bodies.

Rigid endoscopy of the upper gastrointestinal tract

The 2.7 mm endoscope and sheath is well suited to endoscopy of the upper gastrointestinal tract in birds, allowing one to examine the oral cavity, oesophagus, crop (present in parrots and diurnal raptors, but absent in owls) and proventriculus. It can be used for retrieval of some ingested foreign bodies, such as bitten-off pieces of plastic tubing, from the crop or proventriculus. Distension of the lumen to allow visualisation can be performed by either insufflation with air via a syringe attached to the sheath, or flushing the crop and stomach with saline after the bird has been placed head down and intubated. Fluids used should be warmed to prevent patient hypothermia. Endoscopy is not advisable for crop or proventricular biopsy in the diagnosis of proventricular dilatation syndrome, a gastrointestinal motility disorder, due to the risk of perforation.

Coelioscopy

Coelioscopy is without doubt the mainstay of avian endoscopy, and essential in diagnostic investigation of conditions such as *Aspergillus* fungal air sacculitis, and differentiating causes of avian hepatitis.

Coelioscopy entry sites

The selection of the entry site is dependent on the results of other imaging modalities such as radiography, and the anticipated pathology and its location. The left lateral approach is most common, due to avian endoscopy's original application for sexing. Most avian species in fact only have an ovary on the left side. A right lateral approach may be used to assess the pancreas in some birds, or to investigate a right-sided lesion visualised on radiographs. A ventral midline approach is particularly useful in visualising the liver. The ventral approach can generally be safely used in cases of ascites, as the endoscope enters the hepatoperitoneal cavity without entering the air-sac system. An interclavicular approach can be used to assess the cervical air sacs, external trachea and syrinx, and in some species the thyroid glands. Care needs to be taken not to perforate the crop in species that possess one, and this may require a larger entry incision. While this approach is useful in larger zoo avian species such as penguins, it is rarely used in pet psittacines and diurnal raptors.

Any space-occupying structures, such as eggs, will notably reduce the space available for coelioscopic examination.

Birds should preferably be starved before endoscopy to reduce the risk of perforating the proventriculus, which can result in fatal coelomitis. Feathers should be plucked rather than cut, as these will then rapidly regrow. Minimal plucking is generally required. Surgical skin preparation is as for any sterile surgery.

Left lateral coelioscopy approach

Birds are positioned on their right side and the left wing secured dorsally. Lack of muscle tension in this wing also helps determine whether anaesthetic depth is sufficient to proceed with coelioscopy. The left leg may be either pulled caudally or cranially. When the leg is pulled caudally, the endoscope is inserted in the middle of a triangle formed by the caudal border of the last rib, the spine dorsally and the cranial edge of the iliotibialis muscle (Fig. 10.4). If the leg is pulled cranially, the endoscope is again inserted behind the last rib, and ventral to the flexor cruris medialis muscle, which runs from caudal to the stifle to the ischium. In

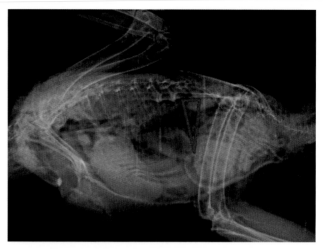

Fig. 10.4   With the leg pulled caudally, the endoscope is inserted in the middle of a triangle formed by the caudal border of the last rib, the spine dorsally and the cranial edge of the iliotibialis muscle.

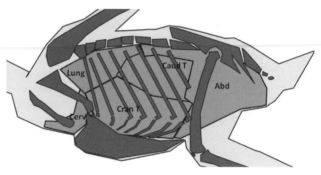

Fig. 10.5   The distribution of the avian air-sac system. Abd, abdominal air sacs; Caud T, caudal thoracic air sacs; Cran T, cranial thoracic air sacs; Cerv, cervical air sacs.

both cases following a small skin incision, careful blunt dissection with mosquito artery forceps, and gentle blunt penetration of the caudal thoracic air sac, need to be performed to prevent injury to the underlying organs. The caudal thoracic air sac is best suited for entry and examination of the organs from a lateral approach. Occasionally endoscope placement may be found to be in the cranial thoracic or abdominal air sacs instead. There is less chance of entering the cranial thoracic air sac if the approach caudal to the leg is used. For the distribution of the air sacs see Fig. 10.5. Lateral coelioscopy is contraindicated in cases of ascites, as resultant connections between the hepatoperitoneal cavity and the respiratory air-sac system will drown the bird.

Normal clear air-sac walls will allow visualisation through them, although they may have to be gently punctured or incised to allow entry.

The cranial kidney, gonad and adrenal gland are visible through the abdominal air sac, with the ureter and uterus or ductus deferens ventral to them. Cranial to this the left lung may be visualised, and in larger birds the endoscope can be advanced into the ostium to examine the bronchi. The heart, edge of the liver and medial aspect of lung can be visualised by directing the endoscope cranially into the cranial air-sac space. The spleen is normally located within the abdominal air sac, ventral to the kidney, in the junction between proventriculus and gizzard, but may be obscured in female birds with an active ovary.

Avian endosurgical organ biopsies are extremely small (1–1.5 mm) when using flexible biopsy forceps via the 2.7 mm endoscope and operating sheath. While this limits tissue trauma, it can also limit the diagnostic value unless care is taken. Any visible lesions should be targeted for sampling, as pathological changes may not be diffusely distributed. When performing a liver or lung biopsy it is advisable to first incise the overlying air sac and serosal membranes. This minimises crush artefact as well as ensuring that hepatic parenchyma is indeed sampled. If possible more than one biopsy should be taken. Prior use of scissors is not generally necessary when biopsing the kidney, spleen, adrenal glands and many obvious visual lesions (Fig. 10.6). Post-biopsy haemorrhage is usually minor in birds, which tend to have good extrinsic clotting ability.

Ventral coelioscopy approach

Birds are positioned in dorsal recumbency, and entry is made on midline just caudal to the end of the keel. A layer of adipose tissue may be present

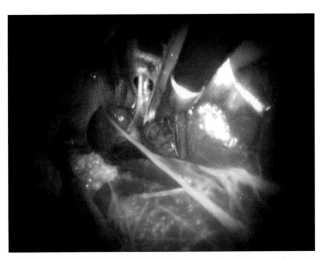

Fig. 10.6 Larger biopsies are possible in birds if using multiple ports. Here a kidney biopsy is being taken. The overlying capsule does not need prior incision.

just beneath the linea alba caudal to the sternum. This is particularly common in obese Amazon parrots. Care is needed not to traumatise the duodenum and pancreas. The ventral approach is indicated in cases of ascites, as fluid remains localised in the hepatoperitoneal cavity, and does not enter the respiratory air-sac system. The hepatoperitoneal cavity is separated into left and right sides, and the central separating membrane can be perforated to allow bilateral access. The surface of most of the liver can be examined from this approach, and pancreas and duodenum are also visualised.

Coelioscopy risks and complications

While minimally invasive, coelioscopy is not without risks. The main complication is haemorrhage. While minor haemorrhage is inconvenient, obscuring endoscopic examination, major haemorrhage can be life-threatening. Haemorrhage most commonly occurs from penetration of the kidney at the start of lateral endoscopy. This may occur if the operator inadvertently directs the endoscope or sheath dorsally when entering the coelomic cavity. If major haemorrhage occurs, and the source cannot be identified or stopped, the cranial portion of the bird's body should be elevated to limit haemorrhage to the caudal air sacs and prevent blood entering the lungs.

Closure of small punctures in the air sacs is generally not required. Occasionally a postoperative subcutaneous emphysema may develop at the entry site if only skin closure is performed. While some authors recommend repeated air drainage until healing occurs (Lierz, 2006), most cases heal on their own without intervention. Divers (2011) recommends either a two-layer closure or use of a single suture incorporating muscle and skin to prevent this occurrence.

As the majority of avian coelioscopy cases are diagnostic in nature, single-puncture techniques using an operating sheath to allow small biopsy or grasping forceps are sufficient. Coelioscopy techniques using multiple instrument ports in birds are possible, but technically demanding in small species due to the limited space available, and require 2 or 3 mm instrumentation and radiosurgery. Endosurgical sterilisation of females is simpler than castration of males, but experience is needed in differentiating the inactive oviduct from the ureter. The ureter may not always contain visible urates, but does tend to demonstrate regular contractions (Lierz, 2006). Other such multiple-port procedures include granuloma and tumour removals.

Other applications

Other more unusual applications of rigid endosurgery in birds include its use for the debridement of bone sequestra (Fig. 10.7). Not all cases are amenable to this method, and whenever possible it is preferable to perform larger access and osteotomy for debridement.

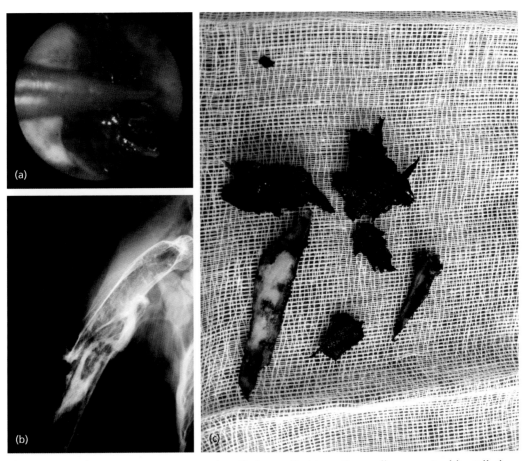

Fig. 10.7 Endosurgery can even occasionally be applied to orthopaedic cases. A white-tailed sea eagle (*Haliaeetus albicilla*) with a large sequestrum that formed after a humerus fracture had this removed minimally invasively under endoscopic visualisation. (a) Removal of pieces of the sequestrum using forceps. (b) X-ray visualisation of the fractured humerus. (c) The removed pieces of bone.

Reptiles

Minimally invasive endosurgical techniques are particularly advantageous in reptiles, as wound healing progresses much more slowly than in birds and mammals.

Rhinoscopy

The small entrance to the nares precludes the use of rhinoscopy in anything but large tortoises and turtles. If performing anterior rhinoscopy, the patient must be intubated, and preferably a swab placed over the tracheal entrance to prevent aspiration of fluid instilled via the nares.

Just as in birds, the choanae themselves in the dorsal roof of the oral cavity can be examined with the endoscope in a retrograde manner.

Tracheoscopy

Tracheoscopy can be performed, as in birds, with a long, slender endoscope. Many chelonia have a trachea that bifurcates cranially, behind the head. This allows retraction of the head into the shell without resultant kinking or compression of the trachea. Combined with tortuous primary bronchi, this makes tracheoscopy difficult in these patients. The trachea of snakes can be particularly long and narrow, and it is often not possible to reach the lung lumen by this method. The outer surface of the lung can be visualised by coelioscopy; surgical endoscopy of the interior of the faveolar lung is also possible (see below, under coelioscopy). Tortoises, like birds, have complete tracheal rings, making the trachea much more susceptible to trauma if endotracheal tubes are cuffed. In contrast, lizards and snakes have C-shaped tracheal cartilage rings, similar to mammals.

Otoscopy

Similar to birds, otoscopy has very limited application in reptiles. Lizards have a shallow, wide external ear canal, if any, with a tympanic membrane that is easily visible to the eye. Tortoises have a tympanic membrane flush with the skin and no external ear canal at all, and snakes have no ears. Skin mites could be visualised in the ear, but are usually easily demonstrated elsewhere on the body by simpler means. Endoscopic examination of the middle ear can be used after a myringotomy has been performed in lizards and tortoises to remove an ear abscess, to help visualise whether all necrotic and purulent material has been removed.

Oral endoscopy or stomatoscopy

While the majority of reptiles have relatively widely opening mouths, and hence are easily visualised in comparison to birds and small exotic mammals, oral endoscopy can be used to enhance visualisation of the back of the mouth in small chelonians, and can help visualise the entrance to the Eustachian tube which may contain caseous material in tortoises with middle-ear infections and abscessation.

Rigid endoscopy of the upper gastrointestinal tract

As in birds, a sheathed endoscope can be used to examine the pharynx, oesophagus and stomach, and insufflation can be provided with a syringe of air attached to the sheath, or a visual space created by instillation of warm fluid. Rigid oesophagoscopy and gastroscopy is particularly useful

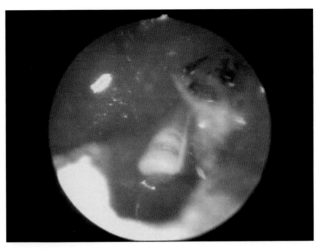

Fig. 10.8 A rigid 2.7 mm endoscope and grasping forceps inserted via the operating sheath being used to retrieve a piece of stomach tube bitten off and swallowed by a bearded dragon (*Pogona vitticeps*).

in retrieving recently swallowed foreign bodies, such as bitten-off fragments of feeding tubes (Fig. 10.8).

Cloacoscopy and cystoscopy

Cloacoscopy with warm saline infusion is performed as in birds, and is well established as a diagnostic technique (Coppoolse and Zwart, 1985). Cystoscopy is particularly useful in chelonia, as the voluminous bladder has a thin wall, and allows a degree of visual examination of the adjacent coelomic organs such as the edge of the liver, ovaries and stomach surface through the bladder wall (Fig. 10.9). Biopsies of the organs visualised in this manner cannot, however, be obtained across the bladder wall, and coelioscopy is necessary. Care needs also to be taken not to puncture the bladder wall and cause a coelomitis. Cystoscopy is also useful in chelonians in determining whether retained shelled eggs visible on radiographs are in the oviduct or are passed into the bladder (Fig. 10.10). These will not respond to calcium and oxytocin administration, and require surgical removal. Cloacoscopy is also useful in cases of cloacal prolapses as an aid in assessing what organ has prolapsed and the possible causes.

Coelioscopy

Coelioscopy is an important adjunctive diagnostic modality in addition to radiography and ultrasonography in reptiles. It allows direct visualisation of organs and targeted biopsy of any pathology seen for histology and microbiological culture. Whereas sterile skin preparation is needed as for other species, particular care needs to be taken to clean the skin

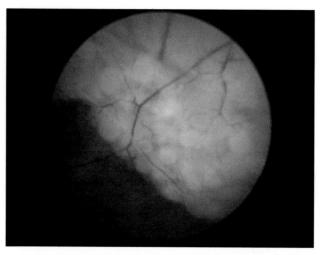

Fig. 10.9   Due to their thin bladder wall, cystoscopy allows a degree of transmural visualisation of some coelomic organs in chelonians. In this case the right ovary, which is inactive, and the edge of the liver are evident.

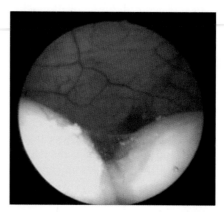

Fig. 10.10   Cystoscopy in a Hermann's tortoise (*Testudo hermanni*) demonstrating a dystocia due to eggs having been passed into the bladder. This can usually not be determined by radiography.

of dirt and debris, as their entry into the coelom can still result in sterile granuloma formation. Scrubbing scales and the tiny spaces between them with an old toothbrush in thick skinned reptiles is ideal. Conversely, some geckos have extremely friable skin, and care must be taken not to tear it during skin preparation.

IPPV, either by hand-bagging or a dedicated ventilator, is needed for reptile coelioscopy. A surgical plane of anaesthesia results in notable respiratory depression or apnoea in these species. Insufflation also causes lung compression, most notably in lizards with a single coelomic cavity.

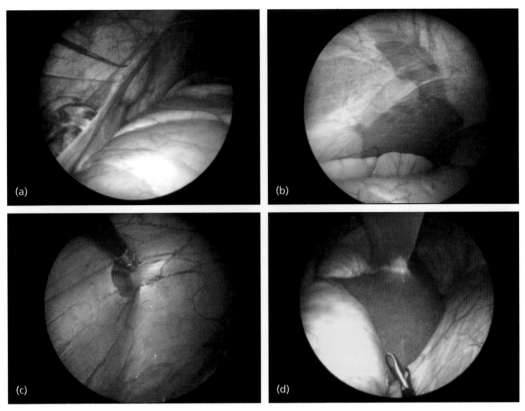

Fig. 10.11 In *Varanus* monitor lizards a well-developed septum divides the coelomic cavity. (a) In this ornate monitor (*Varanus ornatus*) only the kidney, adipose bodies and vas deferens lie in the caudal section. (b) The liver and other organs can be visualised through the septum. (c) An incision needs to be made to access the other coelomic organs, such as the liver (d) for biopsy.

The majority of pet lizard species have a single pleuroperitoneal or coelomic cavity, allowing unimpeded examination from the thoracic inlet to the pelvis, with only the pericardium separated from the rest of the cavity. In monitor lizards, however, the coelomic cavity is separated by a well-developed transverse postpulmonary septum. The lungs, liver, stomach and other organs may also be situated in the cranial portion, dependent on species. The septum needs to be incised to access organs for biopsy (Fig. 10.11).

In dorsoventrally flattened lizards such as bearded dragons, a ventral approach is favoured, while in laterally flattened species such as chameleons and roundbodied lizards such as the green iguana a lateral paralumbar fossa approach is used. The lateral approach is well suited to multiple port procedures such as orchidectomy or ovariectomy. The ventral approach allows more limited exposure due to the presence of the midline abdominal vein (Fig. 10.12). This is formed by the bilateral pelvic veins and runs deep to the abdominal muscles from just cranial

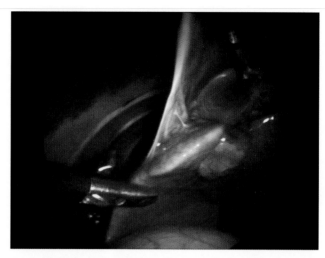

Fig. 10.12   A ventral approach to coelioscopy in lizards, such as for this liver biopsy, yields reduced access and visualisation due to the midline abdominal vein, caudal to the liver.

to the pelvis until just cranial to the umbilicus, where it then joins the hepatic vein. This vein and its suspensory membrane can hinder visualisation and exploration via ventral coelioscopy. Access should either be made caudal to the junction between the bilateral pelvic veins, or just off midline, and is usually accomplished by an open technique. A small skin incision is made and blunt dissection with haemostats performed until the coelom is entered, and the cannula placed.

Tortoises and other chelonians are ideal candidates for coelioscopy, as the alternative, transplastral coeliotomy, requires an osteotomy and bone flap, and has a notably higher morbidity and mortality associated with it. The normal access site is in the middle of the prefemoral fossa. While either can be used, it is more ergonomic for right-handed surgeons to operate in the left prefemoral fossa. As most tortoises can have a voluminous bladder that will interfere with coelioscopy, it is advisable to encourage urination before anaesthesia, by stimulating the cloaca. Access is open, with dissection using a blunt-tipped haemostat as in lizards.

Despite the simple anatomy of snakes, coelioscopy yields poor visualisation in most cases. Insufflation usually fails to result in any meaningful operating space, as the coelom is constrained by the encircling rib cage, and snakes also have more diffuse coelomic adipose tissue. There may also be fibrous connections between organ surfaces. Recently, visualisation and access to organs such as the liver has been described from across the lung surface (see below).

After visualisation of any pathology and target organs, biopsy technique is generally routine. Multiple biopsies are recommended, as samples are typically small, pathology may not be diffusely distributed and some biopsies may suffer from crush artefact. The kidneys are extracoelomic, and in many species may either be difficult to visualise behind the pigmented coelomic membrane, or positioned in the pelvis where they cannot easily be accessed. In those species, such as terrapins, where they are accessible, it is recommended to incise the overlying coelomic membrane for biopsy access; otherwise samples will suffer from notable crush artefact.

The saurian lung is a unicameral balloon-like structure, with spongy faveolar gaseous-exchange tissue, rather than alveoli. The faveolar structure gradually reduces caudally through the lung, leaving the caudal section as a relatively avascular thin-walled air sac.

Jekl and Knotek (2006) and Stahl et al. (2008) described the endoscopic examination of the inner lung surface in snakes, and Divers (1999) described a similar technique in green iguanas. This not only allows visual examination but also sampling for microbiological culture, biopsies for histology and removal of pentastomid parasites in the lungs (Greiner and Mader, 2006). A small surgical incision is made into the lung at maximum inflation, and the endoscope entered to examine the inner structure (Fig. 10.13). In snakes the transition from vascular respiratory lung to the relatively avascular caudal section of non-respiratory lung and air conveniently lies approximately cranial to half the snake's snout-to-cloaca length. A small skin incision between the ventral most two rows of lateral scales is made midway down the snake's body on the right side (Taylor, 2006) as many species only have a right lung. However, Divers (2010) advises using 35–45% of the snout-to-cloaca length as the site for entry. Blunt dissection into the coelomic cavity helps

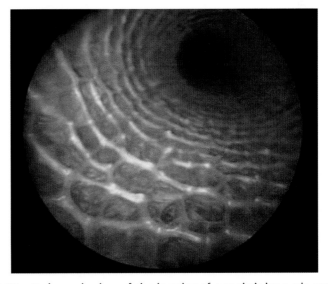

Fig. 10.13 Endoscopic view of the interior of a snake's lung, via surgical access, viewed from caudal to cranial, demonstrating the faveolar structure.

expose the lung when it is held maximally inflated: the lung is grasped, a small incision made for entry of the endoscope and the lung edges sutured to the skin incision. The lung edges can otherwise be held with stay sutures or atraumatic elasticated hook stays used on a flat retractor ring (Lonestar retractor). In iguanas and similar lizards, the lung can be grasped when maximally inflated via a small, mid-lateral intercostal approach. In monitor lizards the lung is adherent to the dorsal body wall, and may be similarly accessed from a dorsal approach. The lung is closed at the end of the procedure with an absorbable suture. Incisions in the lung made during coelioscopy for internal examination are not recommended as these may not heal due to pressure effects and lung wall movements.

A similar technique has also been described in chelonians, where the lung is entered after an access hole is burred or drilled into the carapace at a point selected on radiography. Care should be taken not to introduce debris or contamination from the carapace into the lung, and use of a second sterilised burr to make the final entry into the pleural cavity is advisable. The lung is again grasped, and punctured or incised when maximally inflated.

Divers (2011) has most recently reported using access from within the avascular caudal region of the lung to perform liver biopsies in snakes. The liver is localised and the overlying air sac and liver capsule incised, before a biopsy is taken. This appears preferable to a coelioscopic approach, which in snakes yields poor visualisation.

In larger lizards, such as the green iguana, multiple entry techniques such as orchidectomy and oophorectomy (ovariectomy) (Fig. 10.14) are possible using a paralumbar fossa approach when the ovary is inactive. Radiosurgery is recommended and low settings are necessary to avoid damaging the closely associated adrenal glands and vena cava.

In tortoises and terrapins, a coelioscopy-assisted oophorectomy can be performed. Via a left prefemoral fossa approach the ovary is localised and the fibrous non-follicular tissue is grasped with 3 mm atraumatic grasping forceps. The ovary is then exteriorised before standard removal using radiosurgery or haemostatic vascular clip application. Innis et al. (2007) report that in the majority of pet species both ovaries can be removed through the same left prefemoral incision. Care should be taken not to damage or rupture a follicle during coelomic retrieval, as this will lead to postoperative yolk-induced coelomitis.

Reptile skin has a tendency to invert, and this can impede healing. Normal skin healing is prolonged in reptiles, and sutures should be left in place for a minimum of 4–6 weeks (Mader et al., 2006). An everting suture pattern should be used for closure of port sites, such as simple interrupted horizontal mattress sutures, and monofilament non-absorbable suture material is recommended. The raw everted wound edges can further be sealed with tissue adhesive to reduce the risks of both contamination and subsequent wound infection, as well as wound-edge irritation or pain.

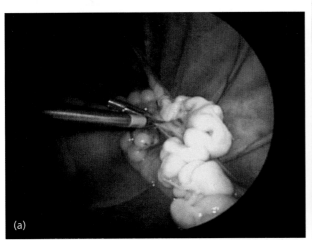
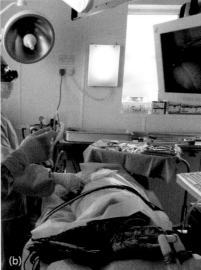

Fig. 10.14 (a) Larger lizards are well suited to multiple puncture endosurgical techniques such as this ovariectomy in a green iguana (*Iguana iguana*) in lateral recumbency. (b) Medium and larger lizards, such as this 24 kg ornate monitor (*V. ornatus*), are best placed in sternal recumbency for anaesthesia and approached coelioscopically via lateral paralumbar fossa access.

Small mammals

Oral endoscopy or stomatoscopy

Dental disease is one of the most common reasons for presentation of rabbits, guinea pigs and chinchillas to veterinary surgeons. In conjunction with skull radiography, oral endoscopy can help provide a thorough assessment of the extent of oral pathology, and allows excellent illumination and magnification of the caudal aspects of the dental arcade. Jekl and Knotek (2007) demonstrated that a rigid endoscope was superior to a laryngoscope for intraoral visualisation of dental disease in 170 rabbits, guinea pigs, chinchillas, degus and prairie dogs. However, they found that while the laryngoscope could be safely used in manually restrained animals, use of the endoscope necessitated anaesthesia. A 30° endoscope is highly recommended to be able to best visualise the lingual, buccal and occlusal surfaces of both upper and lower arcades. If available, a 70° endoscope can enhance visualisation of the occlusal surfaces of the caudal most molars in smaller animals (Jekl and Knotek, 2007). The author's preference is to use 4 mm, 18 cm-long endoscope as this is much sturdier than the commonly used 2.7 mm one, and provides a better image. It is also more likely to survive should a patient attempt to chew the inserted endoscope. In any case, the use of dental gags is recommended even under anaesthesia. A dental probe is needed to properly assess any loose teeth or small inapparent diastemas between teeth that could lead to dental root abscesses. As visualisation is easier with the oral endoscope there is a reduced risk of post-dental examination pain and anorexia due to spreading the oral gag too widely, with resultant masseter muscle tears or temporomandibular joint injuries. The endoscope can be periodically inserted during the hand-filing or motorised burring of overgrown molar spurs.

Endoscopy-assisted intubation

The intubation of rabbits can be difficult (as in guinea pigs and chinchillas) due to their long narrow mouths and long soft palate that normally overlies the epiglottis (as obligate nasal breathers). Recommendations for assisting with intubation include using an otoscope, or intubating blindly by listening to the rabbit's respiratory sounds emanating from the tube. Practice has much to do with ease and success of blind intubation. Texts advise the use of an endoscope inserted down the endotracheal tube to aid intubation (Harcourt-Brown, 2002), and this can certainly be useful in difficult cases. There are disadvantages, however. The endotracheal tube may need to be cut shorter, to allow the endoscope to reach the end for visualisation. In small rabbits and rodents a 1.9 mm endoscope is needed to fit within the narrow endotracheal lumen, and these scopes are very delicate and easily damaged. They can also result in laryngeal injuries. The use of a larger, less fragile 4 mm, 30° endoscope outside the endotracheal tube is easier to use in aiding intubation of rabbits and small mammals (Fig. 10.15). Endoscopes should always be used with a mouth gag. No matter whether intraluminal or extraluminal

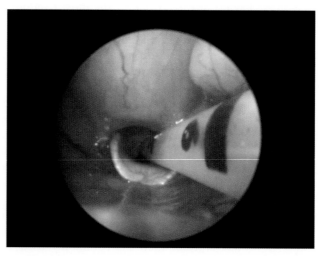

Fig. 10.15   The use of a 4 mm, 30° endoscope outside the endotracheal tube to aid intubation of a rabbit.

endoscopy-aided intubation is performed, positioning is vital to success. The rabbit's neck needs to be held vertically and extended, slightly lifting the front of the rabbit's body from the table, to allow dislocation of the soft palate from above the epiglottis. If this is not performed, intubation, even if aided with an endoscope, is almost impossible. The rabbit also needs to have reached a reasonable plane of anaesthesia after induction, otherwise the strong swallowing reflex makes intubation difficult. Sufficient time is needed after intramuscular induction.

Vaginoscopy

Vaginoscopy as part of the diagnostic work-up for haematurea in rabbits is unfortunately not usually helpful in determining whether the underlying cause is a uterine adenocarcinoma. The double cervix is usually unremarkable in appearance and closed. Vaginoscopy is however useful in determining if a female rabbit has been previously neutered. The technique is performed under anaesthesia. The endoscope and sheath are inserted in the vulva and the vagina inflated with saline while the vulva is pinched closed by the operator's fingers. Most clinicians will perform rabbit ovariohysterectomies including the cervix to prevent the risk of later development of an adenocarcinoma in the remnant uterine tissue. Neutered rabbits will hence only show a vaginal scar (Fig. 10.16) while in intact rabbits the normal double cervix will be apparent (Fig. 10.17). If the ovariohysterectomy has been incorrectly performed in front of the cervix the scar may of course not be evident.

Cystoscopy

Cystoscopy can be useful in investigation of haematurea in female rabbits. However, the most common cause of true haematurea in female

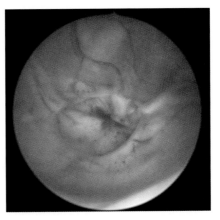

Fig. 10.16 Vaginoscopy demonstrating the cranial vaginal scar in a neutered rabbit.

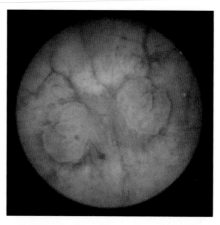

Fig. 10.17 Vaginoscopy demonstrating the normal double cervix in an intact rabbit.

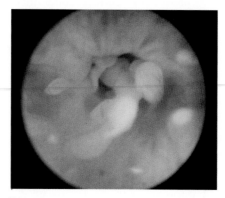

Fig. 10.18 Not all haematurea in intact female rabbits is due to uterine adenocarcinomas. In this case, multiple benign urethral polyps, visualised at cystoscopy, were the cause.

rabbits is uterine adenocarcinoma (see below). Porphyrins in the urine, due to a diet high in dark leafy green vegetables, can be differentiated from true haematurea by means of urine dipstick testing. Occasionally haematurea in female rabbits may result from other bladder neoplasia or benign urethral polyps (Fig. 10.18).

While cystoscopy is not needed for diagnosis of bladder urolithiasis in rabbits, guinea pigs, and chinchillas (uroliths are made of radiodense calcium carbonate and/or calcium oxalate), it can be a useful aid in performing voiding urohydropropulsion. This technique has been well described in canines by Lulich et al. (1993). Despite their small body size, rabbits have a surprisingly wide urethra, making this technique useful in reducing the need for surgical management of uroliths in female rabbits. The urethra of a 2.5 kg female rabbit is actually wider than that of a 35 kg dog, and urohydropropulsion has been used to remove uroliths up to 1.1 cm in diameter without surgery (R. Pizzi, unpublished results). Cystoscopy-assisted voiding hydropropulsion can only be performed in females. The cystoscope is inserted and the urolith visualised. The vulva is pinched/held closed with fingers while fluid is instilled into the bladder to fill it completely. The rabbit is then held vertically, head up, with the cystoscope still in place, to keep the bladder filled, and the cystoscope is gradually withdrawn, still keeping the vulva pinched closed. This results in the urolith falling to the neck of the bladder or entering the wide urethra. While the rabbit is held in this position by an assistant, the bladder is firmly but gently squeezed while the vulvar lips are released. The urolith is thus flushed down the fluid-distended urethra. The procedure may need to be repeated a few times. While it can be performed blindly, the cystoscope is useful in assessing the bladder mucosa and checking for signs of trauma. If the mucosa is markedly thickened from a chronic cystitis, this may grip the uneven surface of the urolith, preventing its hydropropulsion. Just as in other species there is a risk of iatrogenic bladder rupture. This occurrence is not catastrophic, as to remove a symptomatic urolith a cystotomy would otherwise have to be performed. Owners should nevertheless be warned and consent to the procedures. Because of this risk, it is essential to copiously lavage the bladder with sterile physiological saline before attempting urohydropropulsion, in order to remove any other bladder 'sand', which consists of calcium carbonate and calcium oxalate microliths.

Voiding urohydropropulsion is not possible in guinea pigs, as they have separate vagina and urethral openings, the latter of which is relatively narrow. While cystoscopic removal of uroliths has been described using small flexible graspers inserted via the operating channel of the endoscope sheath (Pizzi, 2009), the author no longer performs this technique. The uneven surface of the urolith may be traumatic to the urethra, and this technique is not practical with anything but very small, solitary uroliths.

In male rabbits, guinea pigs and rodents a laparoscopy-assisted cystotomy can be performed, as in canine and feline patients (see Chapter 5 in this volume). It must be remembered that the urethra is still very wide in male rabbits, and uroliths can slip into it. These can be missed during surgery, or prove difficult to retrieve. Male rabbits should always be catheterised to allow retropulsion of any uroliths into the bladder during the procedure for retrieval. Uroliths may slip into the urethra alongside narrow urinary catheters and the surgeon should be careful to correlate retrieved uroliths with those seen preoperatively on radiography.

Mechanical cystoscopic lithotripsy using cystoscope stone-crushing forceps is generally not an option in rabbits and pet rodents, as the calcium carbonate/oxalate uroliths normally encountered are extremely dense and hard, and not effectively broken by the small optical forceps that can be used in these species.

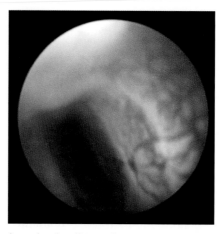

Fig. 10.19   Lateral tracheal collapse due to suspected chondromalacia in a pet rabbit.

Tracheoscopy

Most small pet mammals have a very narrow-diameter tracheal lumen. This makes bronchoscopy (either with a flexible or rigid endoscope) far more risky in these species, as it results in significant luminal reduction. It should also be considered that many rabbits have a degree of lung pathology that may not be clinically apparent, as they are a prey species and will hide signs of illness. Brief intermittent tracheoscopy with a 2.7 or 1.9 mm endoscope is possible. Oxygen should always be immediately available in case of a respiratory crisis. The author has used tracheoscopy to diagnose symptomatic lateral tracheal collapse due to suspected chondromalacia in pet rabbits (Fig. 10.19). This condition manifested as recurrent tracheitis and a stridorous noise.

Otoscopy

A 1.9 or 2.7 mm endoscope can be used for otoscopic examination in ferrets and rodents. However, the author has found otoscopy to be impractical in many rabbits with otitis externa or otitis media. Both the horizontal and vertical cartilages of the external ear canal are vertical in rabbits, and extremely narrow. The ear canal is highly sensitive, particularly to any stretching, which is painful in rabbits. Chronic inflammation only exacerbates this. Rabbits have thick, tenacious pus, and also often appear to have thick cerumen. Not only are pus and these thick ceruminous/waxy deposits difficult to differentiate visually, both being white, but attempts to flush this thick debris from the ear canal very easily result in tympanic-membrane rupture, as the inserted cannula seals the narrow ear canal. Rough otoscopy can also result in tearing of the ear canal at the small junction of the cartilage rings and this may lead to leakage of wax into the peri-auricular and subcutaneous tissues and formation of a sterile granuloma. These can be later mistaken for sub-cutaneous abscesses. Attempted removal does not result in resolution, and these cases require a lateral wall resection for the resolution of recurrent clinical signs.

Rhinoscopy

Rhinoscopy is not only technically difficult in small pet mammals due to the small size of the nasal passages, but in rabbits, guinea pigs and chinchillas it also carries a high risk of inhalation pneumonia, due to the fact that they are obligate nasal breathers. Divers (2011) has, however, described rhinoscopy in pet rabbits using fluid flushing similar to that performed in dogs and cats for examination, and even debridement of nasal abscessation, without problems. As retrograde rhinoscopy using a small flexible endoscope is not generally possible in rabbits with their long soft palate, the author has performed surgical retrorhinoscopy through an oesophageal approach. Rabbits need to have an endotracheal tube placed for this technique, which is performed in the same manner as the placement of an oesophageal feeding tube. Long, curved haemostats are inserted through the mouth, past the pharynx and into the proximal oesophagus. The jaw tips are raised against the skin, and, after a small skin incision, pushed through the oesophageal wall. The sheathed endoscope is then inserted between the jaws, before the haemostat is removed. This allows access to the caudal aspect of the nasal cavity. Forceful flushing of the nasal passages in a cranial direction to help remove a foreign body or clear the nasal passages of caseous purulent material is also possible. The technique does, however, carry a small risk of post-surgical cellulitis if copious flushing of purulent debris is performed.

Laparoscopy

A number of laparoscopic procedures are possible in small exotic mammals, just as in dogs and cats, but only general principles and some of the most common procedures can be mentioned here. Intubation is mandatory for safe anaesthesia during laparoscopy in small exotic mammals, and IPPV should also be performed. Many species have small pulmonary capacities and ventilate poorly under anaesthesia. Subclinical respiratory disease is not uncommon in rabbits.

In almost all mammal species laparoscopic access is possibly the most difficult part of a procedure, with the most risk associated with it. Small mammals such as rabbits have a very thin abdominal wall, and are well suited to an open-access approach to placement of the primary optical cannula for subsequent insufflations. The voluminous, thin-walled and easily injured caecum in rabbits, guinea pigs and chinchillas carries a risk of bowel perforation with either the Veress needle or sharp primary cannula. These species are also highly prone to abdominal adhesion formation, and this further increases the risks associated with a blind-access approach. Elhage et al. (1996) demonstrated that open access was statistically significantly safer than blind-access techniques such as the use of a Veress needle in rabbits with abdominal adhesions, and this resulted in fewer bowel injuries. The Ternamian EndoTIP cannula also appears poorly suited to these species, particularly if there are abdominal adhesions present, as the spiral end can catch and penetrate a section of gas-distended caecum.

The author's preference is to use a 4 mm, 30°, 18 cm-long laparoscope for most small mammals, and a 5 mm, 30°, 30 cm laparoscope for larger rabbits, as these give markedly more illumination and better visualisation than a 2.7 mm endoscope. If using an open-access technique it can be difficult to achieve a 3 mm-sized skin wound for safe insertion of the primary optical cannula for initial insufflation anyway. One disadvantage of a standard 5 mm endoscope used in canine surgery is that its length can interfere with the surgeon's position standing behind the scope. The laparoscope can alternatively be held by the camera operator beneath one of the surgeon's arms.

Diagnostic applications of laparoscopy in small pet mammals are particularly useful. The large gas-filled caecum in rabbits and hystrico-morph rodents limits the use of abdominal ultrasound. Useful applications include exploration of abdominal masses and staging of suspected uterine adenocarcinomas and other neoplasia and metastasis in rabbit does. Not all abdominal masses are neoplastic, and well-encapsulated abdominal abscesses due to a bite from a cage mate are also common in rabbits and hold an excellent prognosis.

While the main application for small pet mammal laparoscopy in first-opinion practice is diagnostic in nature, more complex procedures are also possible (Fig. 10.20). Laparoscopy-assisted procedures can be especially useful, as the operating space is very small in these patients, making intracorporeal suturing difficult, even with dedicated 3 mm needle holders. Some instrumentation used in larger animals is also unsuitable. Endoscopic staplers are simply too large to insert into even giant-breed rabbit intestines for anastomosis, or chests for lung biopsy. The relatively thin body wall in these small mammals also facilitates laparoscopy-assisted procedures. Techniques such as laparoscopy-assisted cryptorchidectomy (Fig. 10.21), cystotomy and enterotomy use the same fundamental techniques as in dogs and cats.

Laparoscopic neutering of female rabbits is possible. Rabbits are primarily neutered to prevent the development of malignant uterine adeno-carcinomas. These have an extremely high incidence in rabbits, with a frequency as high as 80% in 5–6-year-old rabbits in one study (Percy and Barthold, 2001). Unfortunately there is no evidence to demonstrate that ovariectomy is sufficient to prevent their development, and therefore ovariohysterectomy distal to the cervix is recommended in rabbits. Rabbits deposit fat in the uterine suspensory ligaments, making a lapar-oscopic or laparoscopy-assisted ovariohysterectomy difficult, unless

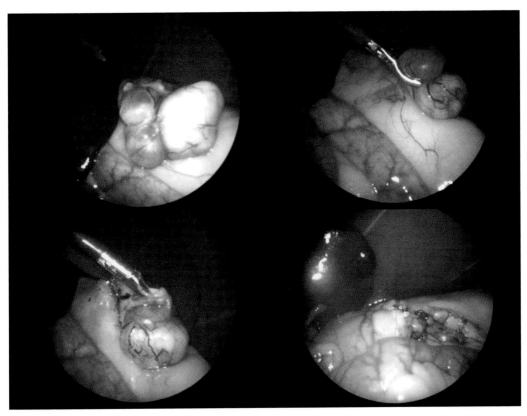

Fig. 10.20 Removal of an ovarian remnant in a 650 g ferret. Despite the patient's small body size, insufflation provides a good operating space and visualisation for use of 3 mm instruments.

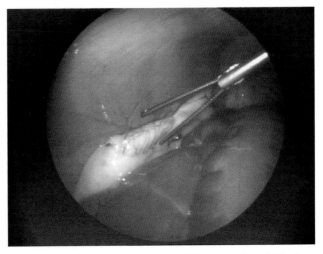

Fig. 10.21 Laparoscopy-assisted cryptorchidectomy in rabbits is essentially identical to that performed in dogs and cats.

performed in young prepuberal rabbits (less than 6 months of age). The author has safely performed laparoscopic ovariohysterectomies in giant-breed rabbits as young as 12 weeks old.

Laparoscopy has been clearly demonstrated to result in lower post-operative abdominal adhesion formation than open surgery in rabbits (Luciano et al., 1989; Jorgenson et al., 1995; Tittel et al., 2008), and also in lower postoperative mortality rates than laparotomy in rabbits with peritonitis (Chatzimavroudis et al., 2009).

A disadvantage of laparoscopy is that unrecognised bowel injuries in rabbits, typically incurred during access, result in delayed clinical manifestations compared to open abdominal surgery. This appears due to the fact that less of an inflammatory response occurs with the minimally invasive nature of laparoscopy (Aldana et al., 2003; El-Hakim et al., 2004, 2005). In contrast to rabbits with intestinal leakage deteriorating within 12–24h of open surgery, clinical impairment may be delayed for 2–3 days in rabbits undergoing laparoscopy. Laparoscopic lavage also appears to be less effective in removing abdominal contamination, and has a higher associated risk of postoperative adhesion formation than in humans (Roberts et al., 2002). This is likely due to the fact that the small operative space makes truly effective lavage difficult. It is hence essential that the abdomen is always carefully examined immediately after entry of the laparoscope for any signs of bowel trauma or intestinal leakage before proceeding further.

Care must be taken with electrosurgery in rabbits, as inadvertent peritoneal cautery or excessive charring will result in adhesion formation (Balbinotto et al., 2010). The thick fur of rabbits, combined with their low body weight, may also result in poor ground-plate contact when using monopolar electrosurgery and result in burns. Radiosurgical frequencies carry a lower risk. Alternatively the area to lie against the contact plate may be clipped and wet swabs used to improve contact.

Thoracoscopy

While thoracoscopy is certainly possible in small pet mammals, size constraints limit its applications, as well as making inadvertent pulmonary trauma a much higher risk than in larger mammals. It can in fact be very difficult to always enter instruments through ports under safe visual control (Fig. 10.22). Small rib spaces preclude the use of endoscopic staplers, which are 12mm in diameter, in even the largest rabbits. Lung biopsies require the use of commercially available pre-tied loop ligatures, or the surgeon employing a self-tied extracorporeal knot, such as the Meltzer knot (see Chapter 6). An advantage of self-tied knots is that they may be applied through 3mm ports, unlike commercially available knots which require 5mm ports. In some patients even 3mm instruments are too large. The extremely limited operating space remains the main constraint, although more technically difficult procedures have been performed, such as thymic cyst removal (Fig. 10.23).

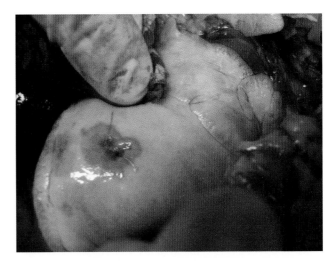

Fig. 10.22 Although thoracoscopy is possible in small mammals, the limited operating space carries an increase risk of injury. Inadvertent lung puncture from instrument entry is evident in this rabbit at post-mortem examination.

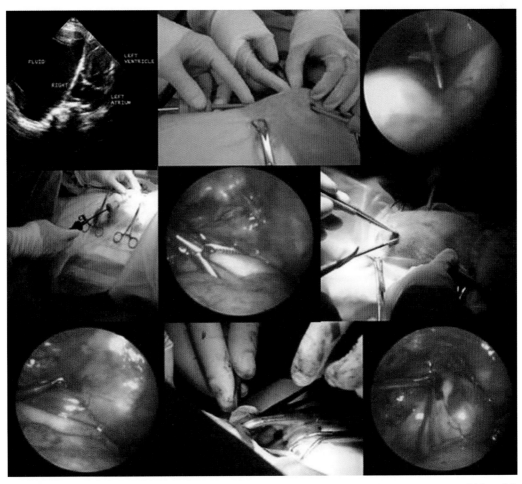

Fig. 10.23 A thoracoscopic assisted resection of a large benign thymic cyst in a pet rabbit, with the aid of a 3 mm monopolar hook and radiosurgery, demonstrates that complex procedures are possible using thoracoscopic techniques with 3 mm instrumentation in small mammals.

Online resources

Videos of many of the exotic pet animal endosurgical procedures are available to view online at the internet portal www.veterinarylaparoscopy.com.

Further reading

Bush, M. (1980) Laparoscopy in birds and reptiles. In *Animal Laparoscopy*, Harrison, R.M., and Wildt, D.E. (eds), pp. 183–197. Williams and Wilkins, Baltimore, MD.

Dukelow, W.R. (1980) Laparoscopy in small animals and ancillary techniques. In *Animal Laparoscopy*, Harrison, R.M., and Wildt, D.E. (eds), pp. 95–105. Williams and Wilkins, Baltimore, MD.

Hernandez-Divers, S.J. (2009) Small mammal endoscopy. In *Ferrets, Rabbits, and Rodents, Clinical Medicine and Surgery*, Quesenberry, K.E. and Carpenter, J.W. (eds), pp. 392–394. Elsevier, St Louis, MO.

References

Aldana, J.P., Marcovich, R., Singhal, P., Reddy, K., Morgenstern, N., El-Hakim, A., Smith, A.D. and Lee, B.R. (2003) Immune response to laparoscopic bowel injury. *Journal of Endourology* 17, 317–322.

Balbinotto, R.P., Trindade, M.R., Muller, A.L., Nunes, A.G., Da Silva, R., Meyer, F.S. and Cerski, C.T. (2010) Experimental model of the formation of pelvic adhesions by videolaparoscopic in female rabbits. *Acta Cirurgica Brasileira* 25, 34–36.

Bush, M., Kennedy, S., Wildt., D.E. and Seager, S.W.J. (1978) Sexing birds by laparoscopy. *International Zoo Yearbook* 18, 197–199.

Chatzimavroudis, G., Pavlidis, T.E., Koutelidakis, I., Giamarrelos-Bourboulis, E.J., Atmatzidis, S., Kontopoulou, K., Marakis, G. and Atmatzidis, K. (2009) CO(2) pneumoperitoneum prolongs survival in an animal model of peritonitis compared to laparotomy. *Journal of Surgical Research* 152, 69–75.

Cook, R.A. (1998) Minimally invasive surgery in nondomestic animals. In *Veterinary Endosurgery*, Freeman, L.J. (ed.), pp. 251–266. Mosby, St Louis, MO.

Coppoolse, K.J. and Zwart, P. (1985) Cloacoscopy in reptiles. *Veterinary Quarterly* 7, 243–245.

Divers, S.J. (1999) Lizard endoscopic techniques with particular reference to the Green iguana (*Iguana iguana*). *Seminars in Avian and Exotic Pet Medicine* 8, 122–129.

Divers, S.J. (2010) *Minimally-invasive endoscopy & endosurgery of birds, reptiles, and fish*. Thesis, Royal College of Veterinary Surgeons.

Divers, S.J. (2011) Exotic pets. In *Small Animal Endoscopy*, Tams, T.R. and Rawlings, C.A. (eds), pp. 623–654. Elsevier, St Louis, MO.

Elhage, A., Lanvin, D., Qafli, M. and Querleu, D. (1996) The advantage of an umbilical micro-laparotomy, 'open laparoscopy', for laparoscopic surgery, experimental study. *Journal of Obstetrics & Gynecology and Reproductive Biology (Paris)* 25(4), 373–377.

El-Hakim, A., Chiu, K.Y., Sherry, B., Bhuiya, T., Smith, A.D. and Lee, B.R. (2004) Peritoneal and systemic inflammatory mediators of laparoscopic bowel injury in a rabbit model. *Journal of Urology* 172, 1515–1519.

El-Hakim, A., Aldana, J.P., Reddy, K., Singhal, P. and Lee, B.R. (2005) Laparoscopic bowel injury in an animal model: monocyte migration and apoptosis. *Surgical Endoscopy* 19, 484–487.

Greiner, E.C. and Mader, D.R. (2006) Parasitology. In *Reptile Medicine and Surgery*, 2nd edn, Mader, D.R. (ed.), pp. 343–364. Saunders Elsevier, St Louis, MO.

Harcourt-Brown, F. (2002) *Textbook of Rabbit Medicine*. P. 132. Butterworth Heinemann, Edinburgh.

Harrison, G.J. (1978) Endoscopic examination of avian gonadal tissue. *Veterinary Medicine & Small Animal Clinician* 73, 479–484.

Hernandez-Divers, S.J. (2006) Evaluation of coelioscopic splenic biopsy and cloacoscopic bursa of Fabricious biopsy in pigeons (*Columba livia*). *Journal of Avian Medicine and Surgery* 20, 234–241.

Innis, C., Hernandez-Divers, S.J. and Martinez-Jiminez, D. (2007) Coelioscopic-assisted prefemoral oophorectomy in chelonians. *Journal of the American Veterinary Medical Association* 230, 1049–1052.

Jekl, V. and Knotek, Z. (2006) Endoscopic examination of snakes by access through an air sac. *Veterinary Record* 158, 407.

Jekl, V. and Knotek, Z. (2007) Evaluation of a laryngoscope and a rigid endoscope for the examination of the oral cavity of small mammals. *Veterinary Record* 160(1), 9–13.

Jorgensen, J.O., Lalak, N.J. and Hunt, D.R. (1995) Is laparoscopy associated with a lower rate of postoperative adhesions than laparotomy? A comparative study in the rabbit. *ANZ Journal of Surgery* 65, 342–344.

Lierz, M. (2006) Diagnostic value of endoscopy and biopsy. In *Clinical Avian Medicine*, Harrison, G.J. and Lightfoot, T.L. (eds), pp. 631–652. Spix Publishing, FL.

Luciano, A.A., Maier, D.B., Koch, E.I., Nulsen, J.C. and Whitman, G.F. (1989) A comparative study of postoperative adhesions following laser surgery by laparoscopy versus laparotomy in the rabbit model. *Obstetrics & Gynecology* 74, 220–224.

Lulich, J.P., Osborne, C.A., Carlson, M., Unger, L.K., Samelson, L.L., Koehler, L.A. and Bird, K.A. (1993) Nonsurgical removal of urocystoliths in dogs and cats by voiding urohydropropulsion. *Journal of the American Veterinary Medical Association* 203, 660–663.

Mader, D.R., Bennet, R.A., Funk, R.S., Fitzgerald, K.T., Vera, R. and Hernandez-Divers, S.J. (2006) Surgery. In *Reptile Medicine and Surgery*, 2nd edn, Mader, D.R. (ed.), pp. 581–630. Saunders Elsevier, St Louis, MO.

Percy, D.H. and Barthold, S.W. (2001) *Pathology of Laboratory Rodents and Rabbits*, pp. 303–304. Blackwell Publishing, Ames, IA.

Pizzi, R. (2009) Cystoscopic urolith removal in a pet guinea pig (*Cavia porcellus*). *Veterinary Record* 165, 148–149.

Pizzi, R. (2010) Invertebrates. In *BSAVA Manual of Exotic Pets*, 5th edn, Meredith, A., Johnson Delaney, C. (eds), pp. 373–385. British Small Animal Veterinary Association, Gloucester.

Roberts, L.M., Sanfilippo, J.S. and Raab, S. (2002) Effects of laparoscopic lavage on adhesion formation and peritoneum in an animal model of pelvic inflammatory disease. *Journal of the American Association of Gynecology and Laparoscopy* 9, 503–507.

Stahl, S.J., Hernandez-Divers, S.J., Cooper, T.L. and Blas-Machado, U. (2008) Evaluation of transcutaneous pulmonoscopy for examination and biopsy of the lungs of ball pythons and determination of preferred biopsy specimen handling and fixation procedures. *Journal of the American Veterinary Medical Association* 233, 440–445.

Taylor, W.M. (2006) Endoscopy. In *Reptile Medicine and Surgery*, 2nd edn, Mader, D.R. (ed.), pp. 549–563. Saunders Elsevier, St Louis, MO.

Tittel, A., Treutner, K.H., Titkova, S., Ottinger, A. and Schumpelick, V. (2008) Comparison of adhesion reformation after laparoscopic and conventional adhesiolysis in an animal model. *Langenbecks Archives of Surgery* 386, 141–145.

Index

Note: page numbers in *italic* refer to figures and tables.

Clinical Manual of Small Animal Endosurgery, First Edition. Edited by Alasdair Hotston Moore and Rosa Angela Ragni.
© 2012 Blackwell Publishing Ltd. Published 2012 by Blackwell Publishing Ltd.